Clinical Teaching in Nursing Education
Second Edition

Clinical Teaching in Nursing Education

Second Edition

Dorothy E. Reilly, EdD, RN, FAAN
*Professor Emeritus of Nursing
College of Nursing
Wayne State University
Detroit, Michigan*

Marilyn H. Oermann, PhD, RN
*Associate Professor of Nursing
College of Nursing
Wayne State University
Detroit, Michigan*

National League for Nursing • New York
Pub. No. 15-2471

To our students

Copyright © 1992
National League for Nursing
350 Hudson Street, New York, NY 10014

All rights reserved. No part of this book may be reproduced in print, or by photostatic means, or in any other manner, without the express written permission of the publisher.

ISBN 0-88737-549-9

> The views expressed in this publication represent the views of the authors and do not necessarily reflect the official views of the National League for Nursing.

This book was set in Goudy by Publications Development Company. The editor was Nancy Jeffries. Port City Press, Inc. was the printer and binder. The cover was designed by Lillian Welsh.

Printed in the United States of America

Contents

Preface to the Second Edition ... ix

Foreword ... xiii

1. A Theoretical Perspective of Clinical Practice ... 1

   Meaning of Professional Practice/Theories of Practice/
   Purposes of Clinical Practice in an Educational Program/
   Nursing as a Practice Discipline/Theory of Practice in
   Nursing/Historical Perspective of Clinical Practice in
   Nursing Education

2. Conceptual Framework of the Teaching–Learning Process ... 23

   Rationale for a Conceptual Framework of the Teaching-Learning
   Process/Learning Concept Rooted in Human Science Theory/
   Concept of Learning/Concept of Teaching/The Dynamic: Teaching
   and Learning/Relevance of Conceptual Framework of the
   Teaching-Learning Process to Teaching in the Clinical Setting

3. Nursing Process: A Practice Modality ... 55

   A Concept of Nursing Process/Derivation of the Nursing
   Process/Nature of Nursing Process/Nursing Process—Nursing
   Frameworks/Teaching the Nursing Process in the Clinical
   Setting/Concerns Regarding the Teaching of Nursing Process

CONTENTS

4. Clinical Practice Setting: A Learning Environment — 109

   Clinical Settings for Nursing Education/Development of Learning Environment/Selection of Clinical Settings

5. Student-Teacher Interactions Within the Clinical Practice Setting — 139

   Qualities of Teacher in Clinical Setting/Teacher-Student Relationship/Selection of Learning Experiences/Instructional Process

6. Teaching Methods — 161

   Criteria for Selection of Teaching Methods/Clinical Teaching Methods

7. Cognitive Learning in the Clinical Setting — 207

   Concept Learning/Problem Solving/Decision Making/Critical Thinking/Clinical Judgment/Teaching/Teaching Methods

8. Psychomotor Learning in the Clinical Setting — 247

   Concepts Relevant to Psychomotor Skill Development/Learning Process Framework for Psychomotor Skill Development/Practice/Teaching/Taxonomy of Psychomotor Skill Performance/Use of a Performance Taxonomy/Teaching Methods

9. Affective Learning in the Clinical Setting — 291

   Concepts Relevant to Affective Skill Development/Affective Component in Nursing/Approaches to Teaching/Clinical Setting for Experiential Affective Learning/Preparation of Objectives/Teaching Strategies

10. Place of Clinical Practice Within a Nursing Curriculum — 341

    Concept of Curriculum/Components of the Curriculum/Planning the Clinical Component/Model for a Unit of a Clinical Course

11. Clinical Evaluation — 379

Concept of Evaluation/Nature of Clinical Evaluation Process/Relationship of Clinical Evaluation to Objectives/Methods of Evaluating Clinical Practice/Use of Multiple Strategies for Clinical Evaluation/Evaluation Protocol for Unit on Chronic Pain

12. Grading of Clinical Experience — 421

Meaning of Grades/Uses for Grades/Types of Grading Systems/Issues on Grading Clinical Performance/Grading Systems for Clinical Practice Experience

13. A Future Perspective: The Clinical Setting — 451

The Information Society/Health Care Delivery Costs/The Use of the Clinical Setting in the Future/Effect of Change on Use of Clinical Setting for Preparation of Practitioners

Index — 497

Preface to the Second Edition

Nursing, our profession and our practice, is evolving at a rapid pace not only in its practice domain, but also in its role within the health care delivery system, locally, nationally, and internationally. Changes occurring within nursing as knowledge expands its meaning, opportunities, and mandates as well as societal changes which affect the health of individuals and the health care services they receive, have altered considerably the traditional notion of nursing.

These dynamic changes have posed a challenge to the two authors of this textbook to critique their text in terms of its relevancy to the preparation of the kind of nurse society needs now and will need in the future. The second edition is the response by the authors to the critique and provides a text for educators in the clinical practice setting, faculty in schools of nursing, graduate students preparing for a teaching career in nursing, and staff educators and clinical specialists within a wide variety of health care agencies.

The title of the text has been altered to reflect more clearly the intent of the book, a philosophical, theoretical, and practical resource on clinical teaching for teachers in the clinical setting, so as to maximize the potentials of such an environment for providing dynamic teaching and learning experiences. It is felt that perhaps the previous title suggested the clinical environment rather than the critical process of teaching.

The general format of the first edition, its organization and presentation, has been maintained. The content within each chapter has been substantively changed in accord with new knowledges of nursing and the educational process and the new directions for which nursing is accountable. The basic premise of this text is that educational programming for nursing is neither content-driven nor process-driven, but rather it is driven by the nature of nursing practice and the educational experience which encumber both content and process. In addition to the new substance in each chapter, an extensive new reference and bibliography are presented for each chapter which reflect, for the most part, the latest thinking of authorities in the relevant domains of knowledge, inclusive of reports of research findings.

Several significant changes have been instituted. The content of the original fourth chapter, *The Clinical Milieu: A Learning Environment*, has been divided into two chapters. The first new chapter (Chapter Four) is *Clinical Practice Setting: A Learning Environment*, which presents many of the structural factors that are essential if the clinical setting is to be appropriate for learning experiences involving students and faculty.

The second new chapter (Chapter Five) is *Student-Teacher Interactions Within the Clinical Practice Setting*. This chapter facilitates the exploration of the many dimensions of student-teacher interactions within a multipurpose environment. The research which has been undertaken and reported in this critical component of the teaching-learning process is presented in a succinct, yet scholarly way, to enable teachers to examine their own interactional patterns as they affect the dynamics of their teaching and learning experiences.

The last chapter proposes future directions in nursing that will influence the kinds and purposes of clinical settings in the future. Much emphasis is placed on the future directions of nursing as a professional participant in health care policies and decisions, for the educational process that will be needed mandates new strategies, new use of knowledge from nursing and related fields, and new competencies in addition to the fundamental humanistic care for which nursing is known.

The authors wish to acknowledge the contributions of colleagues and users of the previous edition of this book for their encouragement to write a new edition of this text. We have been most appreciative of the favorable comments that we have received from teaching colleagues who used the first edition and it is our sincere wish that this new edition will be a valuable resource to all teachers.

We are most grateful to our skillful and knowledgeable typist, Julia Ploshehanski, who prepared the final transcript. We also acknowledge the sustaining support of our friends and family, especially David, Eric, and Ross Oermann.

We are pleased to have had the opportunity to prepare this second edition for our colleagues in nursing education.

DOROTHY E. REILLY
MARILYN H. OERMANN

Foreword

Because more than 60 percent of professional nurses work in acute care settings, changes in the health delivery system affect nursing practice immediately. New demands in the practice environment also influence curriculum development and the teaching of the discipline. The decade of the eighties was a period of radical change in healthcare delivery as the prospective payment initiatives changed the configuration of acute care delivery. Prospective payment also stimulated a growth in ambulatory and home care programs because the new payment formulas of Medicare discouraged the use of acute care and skilled nursing home beds for persons able to be treated in less costly and intensive settings. Day surgery in surgi- and emergi-care centers conveniently located in shopping malls, home-based chemotherapy and ventilator-care programs, out-patient diagnosis and therapy, and hospice programs illustrate new treatment modalities which have caused faculties of nursing to reexamine traditional clinical education and evaluation and the design of the curriculum itself.

For generations, nursing students have learned patient care at the bedside of sick persons and from observing and listening to experienced nurses assess patients and make decisions about their care. Today the experience of illness is not contained within hospital walls. Many people find ambulatory centers and their own homes have replaced hospitals in their treatment plans. The challenge of creating clinical experiences in multiple settings, coupled with the intensity of high technology treatment and the aging of the patient population, enlivens discussions of clinical instruction. Perhaps the dialogue will bring about a much desired reform in nursing education and help young nurses see patients' needs more clearly than institutional routines and procedures.

Dorothy Reilly and Marilyn Oermann's latest text, *Clinical Teaching in Nursing Education*, provides a fresh look at an old problem—how to organize and present clinical nursing to students of the discipline. The authors have been on this road before. Their latest text reveals their own struggles to integrate a scientific and theoretical basis for practice into the curriculum and its clinical implementation. This book should be on the reading list of novice and expert teachers. The rapid change in the health care delivery system has made each of us somewhat of a beginner.

SISTER ROSEMARY DONLEY, PhD, RN, FAAN
Executive Vice President
The Catholic University of America
Washington, DC

1

A Theoretical Perspective of Clinical Practice

Professionals practice. This statement determines the entire spectrum of professional education: substance, methodology, setting, and future directions. It is therefore clear that professional education must provide for a practice component where the student learns to think and act like the professional in the specific discipline. The practice component differentiates a professional discipline from an academic discipline. Donaldson and Crowley (1978) note the distinction between the two disciplines. "Academic disciplines emphasize knowing and the theories are descriptive. Professional disciplines are directed toward practical aims and thus generate prescriptive as well as descriptive theories" (p. 115).

MEANING OF PROFESSIONAL PRACTICE

Professionals in a society serve in an area important to that society and through possession of expertise in a specific domain of knowledge serve in behalf of particular needs of designated clients. The practice of professionals in service fields comprises clinical judgments derived from theories, laws, knowledge, principles, and some intuition; use of specialized skills; and acceptance of the client as an autonomous being with inherent rights. Practice is defined as a deliberately planned sequence of actions carried out by highly skilled individuals in response to particularized needs of clients.

Practice, so described, suggests that a professional makes a commitment of service to a particular clientele and that this commitment requires a lifetime career. An additional component of the service element is its legitimization granted by society to members of the profession as long as those members perform their tasks for the good of society. Society in some ways declares ownership of the professional; for the right to practice can be withdrawn whenever society deems that its needs are not being served in accord with accepted standards.

Two notions are significant. One is that the professional possesses a unique body of knowledge and skills used in service to clients in a community; the other is that this service represents a lifelong career commitment. A professional's practice occurs in juxtaposition with the practice of other professionals within a larger society, which itself is in a constant state of flux as it responds to multiple currents in the world of ideas and actions. The body of knowledge and skills that the professional brings to practice in that society can be no more static than the events occurring in society at large at any given time. Client systems may change, client problems may change, the expectations of service may change, indeed, the nature of the professional's knowledge and skills may be markedly altered over a career span. The role of the professional is subject to change as society becomes more knowledgeable and more differentiated relative to the services it demands.

The education of the professional requires more than the use of current knowledge and skills within a delineated practice mode. Preparation for practice addresses skills in learning to learn, initiating or responding to change, and maintaining a realistic perspective of one's practice within the framework of ideas and events of society at any point in time. Society's tendency toward differentiation of services means that no one professional's area of practice is "turf bound"; thus skills of interdisciplinary collaboration in addressing client needs are required. Practice must be viewed continuously within spatial and temporal dimensions.

Schön (1987) raises questions about the relevancy of professional education to the problems and demands of practice today when he says,

"Can the prevailing concepts of professional education ever yield a curriculum adequate to the complex, unstable, uncertain and conflictual world of practice?" (p. 12). The present model of professional education characterized by technical rationality—problem solution based only on scientific research and knowledge—leads Schön (1983) to the conclusion that there is a mismatch between education and the situations of practice where students will eventually practice.

Nursing educators are raising similar questions relative to nursing curricula which still reflect to a large degree the technical rational approach. Tanner (1990) identifies four themes underlying current curriculum revolutions: social responsibility, centrality of caring, interpretive stance and theoretical pluralism. Moccia (1990) recommends returning nursing education to the clinical setting and redefining that setting so that students, faculty, and patients can develop a sense of agency (the individual power to affect nursing's movement), a sense of responsibility, and a sense of connectedness to community and self. Reilly and Oermann (1990) support Schön's (1987) warning on present day nursing curriculum and suggest that curriculum expand from its present tendency to hold a parochial view of nursing and prepare students to meet the problems of an ambiguous world which can not rely on previous solutions. Other nurse educators and scientists, such as, Watson (1985), Benner and Wrubel (1989), Stevenson (1990), Leininger (1990), and Fry (1989), are addressing the danger of loss of humanity in meeting needs of patients in a time of high-technological therapy and decreased resources, financial, personnel and facilities, by developing the caring component of nursing through research and experience in practice.

Present day curricula in nursing no longer can adhere to the content driven, repetitive mode of the past. The role of nursing practice as an initiator as well as follower of change in the health care of society demands a broader perspective of clinical practice than a setting to "practice what is learned in class."

THEORIES OF PRACTICE

The charge to educators of professionals is to prepare practitioners who not only possess the requisite knowledge and skills inherent in their practice, but who also have the ability to evolve their own theory of practice, which is congruent with the expectations of the discipline as it interfaces with society. Such a practitioner does not limit the perception of his or her own actions to the ability to meet client needs, but also sees the opportunity these actions provide for reflection on their meaning, significance, and potential for generating new knowledge for future practice.

Argyris and Schön (1974) define a theory of action as it pertains to the activities of an individual in practice: "A theory of action is a theory of deliberative human behavior which is for the agent a theory of control, but which, when attributed to that agent serves to explain or predict behavior" (p. 6). Within the scope of practice, the activity selected by the practitioner to meet a particular client need is defined by the practitioner in terms of a specific knowledge referent. The consistency with which the individual uses an action in practice for a specifically determined purpose results in that person's identification with the act and the nature of the practice in use. The scope of theories of action with any one profession's practice is extensive because of the complexity of client needs and the environment in which the practice occurs.

Does a theory of practice exist? What are the dimensions? Argyris and Schön (1974) support the notion of a theory of practice with the following definition:

> *A theory of practice, then, consists of a set of interrelated theories of action that specify for the situations of practice, the actions that will under relevant assumptions yield intended consequences. Theories of practice usually contain theories of intervention, that is theories of action aimed at enhancing effectiveness; these may be differentiated according to roles in which intervention is attempted.* (p. 6)

A discipline's theory of practice incorporates theories relevant to the nature of the services it renders, theories of communication and interaction relating to the mode of interaction of the participants, and social and political theories which provide knowledge of the dynamics of structures within which the practice occurs. The profession identifies the theories of action pertinent to its practice and then assumes responsibility for assuring that its practitioners are competent in their use.

The inclusion of practice in a profession implies activity: a "doing," an experiencing. It is more than engaging in an intellectual process relative to theories of action. It means participation in activities which lead to competent use of these theories of action. Practice entails thoughtful consideration of a setting where students have the opportunity to develop skill in use of the theories. Schein (1972) refers to practice as putting the students in a position where they deal with *real problems*. Thus, the nature of the practice setting is determined by the opportunities it provides for students to apply the theories of action with real clinical problems. The emphasis of the reality dimension on the *clinical problem* rather than the setting is significant. Too often the practice setting is described as the real world when in reality it may be the opposite in terms of career practice goals of many students. Furthermore, because of specialization in health care, many settings are a distortion of the real world; for example, an acute children's hospital in a medical center is not the real world to learn about the health care needs of children, for most children's health care is delivered in ambulatory settings.

PURPOSES OF CLINICAL PRACTICE IN AN EDUCATIONAL PROGRAM

Clinical practice provides the opportunity for students to become skillful in the use of theories of action. This statement is a technical perspective whereby one learns the skills necessary to address client problems. A traditionalist might support this perspective as the sole purpose, but teachers of professional students need to recognize that clinical practice experience provides many other learnings essential for competent professional practice. Clinical practice is envisioned as more than the opportunity to put theory learned in the classroom into practice. Benner (1983) notes that "theory offers what can be made explicit and formalized, but clinical practice is always more complex and presents many more realities than can be captured by theory alone" (p. 36). Faculty who conceptualize clinical practice from a narrow perspective limit the opportunities for growth in other dimensions which the individual needs to function with confidence in an evolving society and profession.

Learning How to Learn

A "society of knowledge" now characterizes the world in which professional practice occurs as the twenty-first century approaches. In a period marked by crumbling boundaries of discipline, knowledge, and practice, and development of new patterns of connectedness, learning is a constant, long-term process essential for enabling individuals to meet demands of growing complexity as the society of knowledge unfolds. Mahdi (1987) decries the present stress on maintenance learning which emphasizes pattern reproduction rather than the dynamic process of innovative learning. Professional educators are accountable to assure that the students in their field are prepared for the society of knowledge.

The professional in the knowledge society is an eternal learner throughout the duration of the professional career. Expansions in the frontier of knowledge and the changing expectations of society continuously influence the nature of practice. The student in the profession needs to develop learning skills which facilitate inquiry, pursuit of ideas, concentration, integration, and evaluation. Security in the known as the basis for making clinical decisions is self-serving. Since this knowledge serves others, responsibility for maintenance of current knowledge is a high priority for a professional practitioner.

Clinical practice provides a fertile experience in learning how to learn. The reality of problems guarantees students will encounter variations in "normal" responses that challenge them to seek alternative knowledge and skills for resolution. The multidisciplinary encounters in most clinical practice sites expose the learner to differing approaches to similar problems. The student is challenged to examine and to try new modalities of care. The faculty is challenged to accept risk-taking behavior. This behavior is not chance behavior, but a carefully thought out plan of action in which possible consequences have been noted but the actual outcome remains uncertain. Calculated risk means consideration of risks ranging from reasonable anticipated best outcomes of the action to the potentially worse outcomes of the action for all participants. This process of risk analysis is problem-solving behavior using divergent thinking, a critical element in learning how to learn.

The encouragement of the student for calculated risk-taking in meeting client needs fosters a lifelong learner open to new ideas and experiences. The demand from society for "tried and true" practice stifles learning potential and fosters the development of a practitioner restricted to "what is" and reticent to deal with new ideas.

Handling Ambiguity

Inherent in professional practice are complexity, uncertainty, conflict, and instability. Professional curricula, however, are often limited in helping students to develop a practice modality which provides for competencies in addressing these uncertainties. Schön (1983) attributes much of the difficulty to the model of technical rationality which is used in many professional educational programs emphasizing rigor, status, and knowledge hierarchy. He defines professional activity within this model as "consisting of instrumental problem solving made rigorous by the application of scientific theory and technique" (p. 21).

Many problems encountered in professional practice, however, do not lend themselves to the usual scientific rigor. Schön (1983) identifies a topography of professional practice which incorporates two levels of problems. Problems in the high, hard ground lend themselves to research-based theory and techniques and are most frequently the focus in professional programs. Problems in the swampy low-lands are incapable of technical solutions, but are often the most interesting and challenging. Indeed they may well influence the degree of effectiveness in the use of the scientific solutions. It is in this latter level that one finds such problems as human rights, use of health care resources, cultural variables, conflicts, quality, and types of health care interventions. Professional practice encompasses client needs within a social, cultural, economic, political, and technical milieu. Education preparing practitioners for serving these clients can not rely solely on the scientific competencies in the technical rationality model, but must foster skill development essential for dealing with the reality of the practice world.

Professional practice is concerned with the known and the unknown. Some aspects of practice are convergent (one action is possible) since their rationale is supported by theory. Other components of practice are divergent (multiple actions are possible), since no one theory provides the support for a response. Schein (1972) speaks of the important component of a professional program as "training for uncertainty." He describes the characteristic skills as "maintenance of one's self-confidence even when one does not have a clear answer to the problem; willingness to take responsibility for key decisions that may rest on only partial information, and willingness to make decisions under conditions of high risk" (p. 45). Clinical practice must provide the student with both convergent and divergent components of professional practice. Too often the convergent component receives priority while divergent thinking, which demands dealing with ambiguities and risk taking, is often avoided. The critical question: "What else is possible?" when students suggest an action will help them move from a dualistic approach to a relativistic one.

Skill in handling ambiguity is also a function of the student's ability to deal with role conflict encountered when in the clinical field. Hursh and Borzak (1982) report on this matter in the report of the study of the role of field work in cognitive development. They state, ". . . the student fluctuated between pleasures of giving, relating, helping, doing on the one hand and taking, learning, objectifying, analyzing on the other" (p. 69). Students faced with such a dilemma need to come to a resolution by identifying the common denominators of both the student and caregiver roles. Viewing the situation from both perspectives calls upon problem-solving skill. A reconciliation of these roles is posed by Hursh and Borzak (1982):

> (a) modifying role of the student toward that of scholar, i.e., one who as an adult is interested in learning things in systematic ways, and (b) emphasizing in the role such capacities as a systematic (rather than hunch based) problem solving, informed (rather than speculative) decision making, effective communication and periodic distancing in order to maintain objectivity and allow for careful observation of events (rather than subjective identification with them). (p. 75)

Think Like Professionals

Practice enables the student to develop the process of thinking most appropriate to the profession. Professional knowledge includes the abstract and the concrete. Professionals approach their practice from a problem-solving perspective rather than a task-oriented perspective. The problem-solving approach which incorporates skill in divergent thinking enables the learner to pose questions whose resolution will contribute to the development of a theory of practice for the individual.

Although the posing of practice questions to be resolved comprises a significant pattern of thinking by the professional, more is required. Problem setting, the process by which the elements to be treated in the situation are identified, boundaries established, and context within which elements to be studied are described, is a critical component of professional thinking. (Schön, 1983). Professional practitioners are reflective of their actions and examine them within the context of their relevancy to the need at hand and their significance to patterns of practice.

Professionals are expected to think about their practice within the broader context of the society in which it occurs. Although some professionals have developed tunnel vision about their practice, whereupon the focus is confined to the sphere of their own individual activities, an informed public is demanding that all professionals address their practice within social demands and expectations.

Rigidity of professional thinking is not acceptable practice behavior, for too many problems to be addressed lack convergent solutions. The increase in specialization within professions does increase the potential for parochial thinking as these practitioners tend to confine their thinking within the domain of their clinical focus to the exclusion of the larger world of practice of which they are a part. The practice component of a professional program contributes significantly to the socialization of the student into the professional role and its concomitant values of social consciousness, ethical and moral accountability, and responsibility to society.

Develop Personal Causation

Argyris and Schön (1974) suggest another important outcome of clinical practice learning: the acceptance of the notion of personal causation, the commitment to be responsible for one's own actions. Societal permission for professionals to practice implies that it will hold each professional accountable for all actions relative to practice. The clinical practice experience enables the student to minister to real clients in the management of real problems inherent in their practice. As students, clinical assignments are relegated on the basis of the knowledge and skills possessed at any particular time. Practice enables the student to develop competency to a designated level under the supervision of a faculty or preceptor. Even within this early structured process, the student learns to be accountable for preparation for the learning experience and recording the results according to established protocol. The notion of personal causation learning requires a deliberative process, which is developmental in nature. It must be a positive learning experience, not one of threat, which adds the element of fear to the learning experience.

In summary, clinical practice experience serves a multipurpose role in the education of professionals. It provides experience necessary for the learner to develop knowledge, skills, and values inherent in the theories of action accepted by the profession and necessary for the individual to be self-confident, responsive to society's expectations, and a continuous learner in pursuit of new knowledge that will have an impact on practice. The nature of the contributions of clinical practice experience calls for it to be an integral part of the total curriculum, not an added experience in the final term of studies. The competencies to be achieved are developmental and, thus, must be provided for in increasing complexity in a sequential pattern of experience throughout the total program.

NURSING AS A PRACTICE DISCIPLINE

Nursing is a science and a practice discipline. Nursing research is posing questions as to the nature of a nursing science and its practice element. It is acknowledged that nursing professionals possess expertise in specific areas of knowledge which is used in behalf of particular needs of designated clients. Its practice represents clinical judgments derived from theories, laws, knowledge, principles, and some intuition; the use of specialized skills; and the acceptance of the client as an autonomous being with inherent rights. This description reflects nursing's compatibility with the description of practice noted earlier in the chapter.

Clinical practice may be conceptualized as the medium through which the nurse uses a particular constellation of abilities based on selected theories of action to meet health needs of clients. It is a dynamic comprised of cognitive, psychomotor, and affective behaviors. It is a synthesis of all of these behaviors into a holistic framework called nursing process, the methodology of the practice. It is problem oriented; it involves decision-making; it calls for the best fit when possible between scientifically determined assessed data and intervention strategies reflecting the appropriate theories of action.

Nursing is also responsive to issues and concerns inherent in a practice involving complex human experiences which defy empirical answers, but rather require different types of problem setting in search for appropriate response. Although many current studies of nursing are in accord with logical positivism underlying science, nursing practice has not been unduly influenced by this philosophy throughout its history (Whall, 1989). Its history evidences the moral nature of nursing practice where values of personhood, human rights, caring, feeling, equity, promotion of human welfare through disease prevention, health promotion, and family are inherent. Fry (1981), following her analysis of professional codes of practice and research, concludes that "the concept of nursing embodies scientific (competence), values of technological skills, scientific inquiry and knowledge gained by scientific study, as well as humanistic (moral) values of caring and promotion of human welfare and rights" (p. 5).

Fawcett (1989) describes a metaparadigm on nursing which incorporates the four major concepts generally accepted by nursing theorists: *recipient* of care (individual, family, group, community, society); the *environment*, encompassing relevant inanimate and animate surroundings; *health*, referring to wellness or illness; and *nursing actions*, which include all activities of members of the profession.

Two definitions proposed by nursing authorities are most appropriate to the discussion of the clinical practice component of nursing. The Social Policy Statement of the American Nurses Association (1980) supporting the language in the New York State Practice Act states: "Nursing is the diagnosis and treatment of human responses to actual or potential health problems" (p. 9). Schlotfeldt (1981) provides the following definition: "Nursing is assessing and enhancing the general health status, health assets, and potential of human beings"

(p. 298). These definitions convey the notion of goal-directed services within a defined scope of practice.

Nursing, like other professions, has various categories of practitioners whose level of mastery of knowledge and skill is delineated by the nature of their preparation for entry into the field. Many approaches to differentiating the practice of each of these categories have been proposed with little success in outcome. Delineation is important if the use of the clinical practice experience is to be maximized. Since all groups are involved in making clinical decisions, the nature of the decisions each group makes could serve as the critical criterion for defining boundaries of practice. Relevant to these decisions are the types and depths of interventions for which the nurse will be held accountable and for which learning experiences in the clinical field must be designed.

Practical nursing programs address those clinical decisions that relate to the overt needs of clients' daily living activities. Since these activities are incorporated in the nursing process, practical nurses would be expected to use the process under the direction of the registered nurse. In addition to developing competencies in their own areas of practice, practical nurses would learn those skills essential for a supportive role to the registered nurse.

Programs for associate and diploma students address clinical decisions relating to the overt and covert needs of the client in those areas of care where prescriptive nursing measures are already described for nursing management. Nursing process is developed to a level of mastery with decision making directed toward a differential selection of the appropriate prescriptive management protocol for any given situation.

Programs in baccalaureate nursing address clinical decisions involving overt and covert needs of clients, not only where prescriptive nursing exists, but also where nursing decisions entail developing new modes of nursing management based on analysis of nursing and supportive theories. Nursing process relates to the known and unknown with the nurse having the ability to develop hypotheses that can be tested on the basis of suitable theories of action.

Graduate programs address clinical decision-making involving multivariate or highly specialized client problems which entail the known and unknown. A research posture is in order as the graduate practitioner uses the nursing process to meet specialized client needs. Theories of action are tested and synthesized into a theory of use for each practitioner.

Whatever the level of practice, all categories of nurses providing nursing care to clients have specific skills to perform and a body of knowledge which must be translated into action. The depth and breadth of the practice and the dimensions of accountability are described by the expectations of practice.

THEORY OF PRACTICE IN NURSING

Nursing theory development proceeds on multiple fronts at this time in nursing history, and the processes involved are duly recorded in the nursing literature (Fawcett, 1989; Kim, 1983; Meleis, 1991; Neuman, 1989). A framework particularly useful for the discussion of the clinical practice component of nursing education programs is the theory of practice defined by Argyris and Schön (1974). Elements of the theory include:

1. A set of interrelated theories of action that specify for the situations of practice actions that will, under relevant assumptions, yield intended consequences.
2. Theories of intervention are composed of theories of action aimed at enhancing effectiveness. These may be differentiated according to roles in which intervention is attempted. (p. 6)

Theories of Action

Nursing is an intervention activity for the health of individuals in interaction with their environment during all stages of life in any state of health or illness. Nursing represents multiple theories of action as it seeks to answer to the health-related responses of the clients. The nature of nursing lends itself to three classifications of theories of action, namely, people-centered, health, and nature of practice milieu.

People-Centered Theories of Action
- Caring
- Communication
- Counseling
- Group Process
- Interprofessional interaction
- Interviewing
- Intraprofessional interaction
- Problem solving
- Systems

Health Theories of Action
- Disease/illness intervention
- Disease/illness prevention
- Environmental management
- Health maintenance
- Health promotion
- Human systems functioning
- Mobility
- Observation
- Therapeutic intervention

Nature of Practice Milieu Theories of Action
- Change
- Collaboration
- Conflict resolution
- Decision making
- Leadership
- Management
- Organizational behavior
    - Agency
    - Community
    - Profession
- Power and influence
- Teaching

The relationship of these theories to the practice of nursing in terms of their expression in practice requires much research. Argyris and Schön (1974) differentiate between *espoused theory*, that which is at least tacitly acknowledged and to which the individual gives allegiance when asked, and *theory in use*, that which the individual actually uses as a guide for action. The latter is based upon assumptions about self, others, the situation and connections among action, consequence, and situation. The position of Benner (1983) that there is a lack of knowledge of what occurs over time in actual nursing practice is consistent with Argyris and Schön's position that professions lack knowledge about theory in use. Benner states:

Knowledge development in an applied discipline consists of extending practical knowledge (know-how) through theory-based scientific investigations and through the charting of existing "know-how" developed through clinical experience in the practice of the discipline. (p. 3)

The nurse uses and examines these theories of action on a selective basis as they pertain to a role or function at any particular time. The unique constellation of theories of action developed into theories of intervention and used in a consistent manner becomes the individual's theory of practice.

HISTORICAL PERSPECTIVE OF CLINICAL PRACTICE IN NURSING EDUCATION

Christy (1980) reminds us that clinical practice has always been a function of nursing education, although the role has experienced varied interpretations. Florence Nightingale posited an educational value to clinical practice in the program she established at St. Thomas Hospital. Her emphasis on autonomy for the school from the hospital demanded three requisites, namely:

- It must be an independent educational institution.
- It must have its own independent funds.
- It must have its own board of trustees.

Such a position enabled the school to pursue its educational mission and develop a systematic approach to the theoretical and practice components of the program. The Nightingale system saw the beginning of the unification model in the appointment of a matron responsible to the hospital for care of the patients and to the school for the education of the students. This position reflected Nightingale's belief in the interrelationship of nursing education and service.

Practice in the wards was conducted in an apprenticeship mode under the tutelage of ward sisters, paid by the hospital with an increment for teaching. Teaching emphasis was placed on helping pupils develop skills in *how* to observe, *what* to observe, *how* to think, and *what* to think. Methods included ward teaching, case study, and use of procedure sheets in medical-surgical settings and later in the community. Clinical practice sites in the hospital were selected on the basis of their relevance to the educational program, not in terms of patient care needs.

Although the Nightingale system of nursing education was adopted by three hospitals in the United States in 1873 (The Connecticut Training School, The Boston Training School, and The Bellevue School), the educational value inherent in the system was soon diminished as hospitals realized the potential for nursing schools to provide pupils to meet the need for care of the sick. Roberts (1954) reports that by the end of the first decade in the twentieth century, nursing schools increased from 437 to 1129. Most of these schools were started for economic, not educational reasons, and the primary mode of education was trial-and-error in the ward setting.

This period is often noted as the time of apprenticeship learning in nursing education, but it was not, for there was no one under whom students could serve as apprentices. Instruction in the hospital was by fellow students, seniors, or ward aides, although in a random fashion, doctors did some lecturing and bedside instruction. The first position of instructor to nurses, as noted by Roberts (1954), was the appointment of Jane Delano in the University of Pennsylvania School of Nursing in 1890. In 1885, Isabel McIsaac, principal of the Illinois Training School for Nurses, and a superlative teacher, is believed to be first to institute instruction in nursing procedures. However, by 1910, only one-half of the schools of nursing employed instructors.

In the earlier years of nursing, both nurses and physicians shared in palliative care of patients, for science had not developed sufficiently at the time to effect markedly the course of disease. As science evolved, medical education became established in universities within the milieu of scientific discovery and teaching. As a result of nursing education remaining in hospital setting where service goals superceded educational goals, a significant gap existed between these two types of health care providers. The nurse viewed the patient through the physician's eyes for he/she possessed the scientific knowledge. Nursing then became medically delegated with many of its practice activities defined by another professional (Reilly, 1990).

The change in emphasis of the nursing school from one of education to one of care of the sick had a profound impact on the development of the clinical field as a learning environment. Services to patients superseded the learning needs of the students, and the notion of time in the clinical setting as constituting "work" persisted long after nursing education became more goal directed and structured into a regular educational pattern. The Goldmark Report in 1928 and the Grading School Committee Report in 1934 noted the inequities in nursing programs, particularly in relation to the overuse of clinical practice to the detriment of any theoretical learning. Assignments to clinical areas were based on patient care needs, not learner needs, and instruction occurred after patient demands were met. This practice continued even though collegiate education programs were developing.

The entrance of federal funding into nursing education through the Cadet Corps was a major impetus in changing the role of the clinical setting. Criteria for a school of nursing receiving funds required upgrading of many schools and moneys were made available for the employment of faculty. The directions charted by this government program were compatible with such efforts by nursing leaders to develop truly educational programs in nursing. This movement was further supported by the G.I. Bill after World War II, which enabled many nurses to attend institutions of higher learning for advanced study and degrees.

It was with this movement into higher education by nurses who had experienced considerable autonomy of their practice in the battlefield that questions arose relative to nursing's own identity and the nurses' ability to see the patient through *their own eyes*. Exposure to the world of ideas and research enabled nurses to see their own discipline in a *new* light, and with increase in knowledge, they began the process of developing nursing practice with its own theoretical base controlled and directed by the nursing profession. This movement enabled nursing to become an autonomous profession within the total spectrum of health care providers.

The return of many of these prepared nurses as faculty, knowledgeable about many of the science disciplines supporting nursing, enabled nursing education to find its theoretical base and seek a complimentary relationship between learning in the classroom and the clinical setting. The advent of the control of nursing programs by universities, colleges, and community colleges and the development of accreditation standards and processes moved clinical practice in nursing programs toward the Nightingale model where practice sites are chosen in accord with learner needs and instruction is provided by prepared nurses designated as faculty.

As often happens when a control system is changed, the new order takes over in totality without a careful analysis of the resources developed under the previous control mechanism. The movement from nursing service responsibility for teaching in the clinical setting to the school's responsibility through its own faculty ignored the rich potential that skilled nurses in practice have to contribute to students' learning. The current trend is toward the use of these skilled nurses in a preceptor role in the clinical setting, reflecting the possibility for a true apprenticeship experience for students and new graduates entering the field.

The clinical setting continues to be a significant environment for learning nursing practice, although its potential is still not realized. Its contribution beyond applying classroom learned theory to practice in the care of the patient needs to be identified, planned for, and institutionalized in the educational program.

SUMMARY

Clinical practice is a function of all educational programs preparing professional practitioners, especially in the service fields. To meet the particular type of clinical judgments and specialized skills demanded of such practitioners in a dynamic society, clinical practice provides more than the opportunity to develop the ability to use professional knowledge and skills within a circumscribed practice mode. It facilitates the ability of the student to learn how to learn, handle ambiguity, think like professionals, develop a notion of personal causation, and evolve one's own theory of practice.

Nursing, a practice discipline, encompasses theories of action related to its people-centered mission, concern with matters of health/illness, and the nature of its process within the practice milieu. The theories to be developed and their degree of development are a function of the category of nursing practitioner. The setting in which the learning occurs is a dynamic milieu presenting experiences with real client situations and has the potential to address the multipurpose expectations of clinical practice within an educational program.

Clinical practice has always been a function of nursing. Its historical development evidenced a deviation from its educational commitment to meet the economic expectations of hospitals for nursing care of patients. Through the efforts of nursing leaders, the input of federal funding for nursing programs, the advanced preparation of faculty, and the development of nursing schools within institutions of higher learning, clinical practice is once more viewed as an educational experience in concert with theory and as an integral part of a systematically developed curriculum.

REFERENCES

Argyris, C., Schön, D. (1974). *Theory in practice: Increasing professional effectiveness.* San Francisco: Jossey-Bass.

Benner, P. (1983). *From novice to expert.* Menlo Park, CA: Addison-Wesley.

Benner, P., & Wrubel, J. (1989). *The primacy of caring: Stress and coping in health and illness.* Menlo Park, CA: Addison-Wesley.

Christy, T. (1980). Clinical practice as a function of nursing education. *Nursing Outlook, 28,* 493-497.

Donaldson, S., & Crowley, D. (1978). The discipline of nursing. *Nursing Outlook, 26,* 113-120.

Fawcett, J. (1989). *Analysis and evaluation of conceptual models of nursing.* Philadelphia: F. A. Davis.

Fry, S. (1981). Accountability in research: The relationship of scientific and humanistic values. *Advances in Nursing Science, 4,* 1-13.

Fry, S. (1989). Toward a theory of nursing ethics. *Advances in Nursing Science, 11,* 9-22.
Hursh, B., & Borzak, L. (1982). Toward cognitive development through field studies. *Journal of Higher Education, 50,* 63-77.
Kim, H. (1983). *The nature of theoretical thinking in nursing.* Norwalk, CT: Appleton-Century-Crofts.
Leininger, M. (1990). Historic and epistemologic dimensions of care and caring with future directions. In J. Stevenson, & T. Tripp-Reimer (Eds.), *Knowledge about care and caring: State of the art and future developments* (pp. 19-31). Kansas City, MO: American Academy of Nursing.
Mahdi, E. (1987). Learning needs in a changing world. *The Futurist, 21,* 60.
Meleis, A. I. (1991). *Theoretical nursing: Development and progress* (2nd ed.). Philadelphia: J. B. Lippincott.
Moccia, P. (1990). No sire, It's a revolution. *Journal of Nursing Education, 29,* 307-311.
Neuman, M. (1989). *Theory development in nursing* (2nd Ed.). Philadelphia: F. A. Davis.
Nursing: A social policy statement. (1980). Kansas City, MO: *American Nurses Association.*
Reilly, D. (1990). Research in nursing education: Yesterday-today-tomorrow. *Nursing & Health Care, 11,* 139-143.
Reilly, D., & Oermann, M. (1990). *Behavioral objectives: Evaluation in nursing* (3rd ed.). New York: National League for Nursing.
Roberts, M. (1954). *American nursing history and interpretation.* New York: MacMillan.
Schein, E. H. (1972). *Professional education: Some new directions.* New York: McGraw-Hill.
Schlotfeldt, R. (1981). Nursing in the future. *Nursing Outlook, 29,* 295-301.
Schön, D. (1983). *The reflective practitioner: How professionals think in practice.* San Francisco: Jossey-Bass.
Schön, D. (1987). *Educating the reflective practitioner.* San Francisco: Jossey-Bass.
Stevenson, J. (1990). Quantitative care research: Review of content, process, and product. In J. Stevenson & T. Tripp-Reimer (Eds.). *Knowledge about care and caring: State of the art and future developments* (pp. 97-118). Kansas City, MO: American Academy of Nursing.
Tanner, C. (1990). Reflections in the curriculum revolution. *Journal of Nursing Education, 30,* 295-299.
Watson, J. (1985). *Human science and human caring.* Norwalk, CT: Appleton-Century-Crofts.

Whall, A. (1989). The influence of logical positivism in nursing practice. *Image: Journal of Nursing Scholarship, 21,* 243-245.

BIBLIOGRAPHY

American Nurses Association. (1979). *Entry into professional practice: Proceedings of National Conference.* Kansas City, MO: Author.

Baron, R. J. (1981). Bridging clinical distance: An emphathetic rediscovery of the known. *Journal of Medical Philosophy, 6,* 5-23.

Brown, J. S., Tanner, C. A., & Padrick, K. (1984). Nursing search for scientific knowledge. *Nursing Research, 33,* 26-32.

Carnegie Commission on Higher Education. (1971). *Higher education and the nation's health.* New York: McGraw-Hill.

Chin, P. (1989). Nursing patterns of knowing and feminist thought. *Nursing & Health Care, 10*(2), 71-78.

Donahue, M. (1983). Isabel Maitland Stewart's philosophy of education. *Nursing Research, 32,* 140-146.

Ellis, R. (1982). Conceptual issues in nursing. *Nursing Outlook, 30,* 406-410.

Gordon, D. (1986). Models of clinical expertise in American nursing practice. *Social Science Medicine, 22,* 953-961.

Greene, J. A. (1979). Science, nursing and nursing science: A conceptual analysis. *Advances in Nursing Science, 2,* 57-64.

Johnson, D. E. (1983). *Physicians in the making: Personal, academic and socioeconomic characteristics of medical students from 1950-2000.* San Francisco: Jossey-Bass.

Johnson, J. (1987). Essentials of collegiate and university education for professional nursing. *Journal of Professional Nursing, 3,* 207-213.

Kaler, S., Levy, D., Schall, M. (1989). Stereotypes of professional roles. *Image: Journal of Nursing Scholarship, 21*(2), 85-89.

Kidd, P., & Morrison, E. (1988). The progression of knowledge in nursing. *Image: Journal of Nursing Scholarship, 20*(4), 222-224.

Miller, M., & Malcolm, N. (1990). Critical thinking in the nursing curriculum. *Nursing & Health Care, 11*(2), 67-73.

National League for Nursing. (1989). *Curriculum revolution: Reconceptualizing nursing education.* New York: National League for Nursing.

Nightingale, F. (1859). *Notes on nursing: What it is and what it is not.* London: Harrison & Sons.

Oermann, M. (1991). *Professional nursing practice: A conceptual approach.* Philadelphia: J. P. Lippincott.

Olsen, E. M. (1983). Baccalaureate student's perception of factors assisting knowledge application in the clinical laboratory. *Journal of Nursing Education, 22,* 18-21.

Peplau, H. (1988). The art and science of nursing: Similarities, differences, and relations. *Nursing Science Quarterly, 1*(1), 8-15.

Rodgers, B. (1991). Deconstructing the dogma in nursing knowledge and practice. *Image: Journal of Nursing Scholarship, 23*(3), 177-181.

Saylor, C. R. (1990). Reflection and professional education: Art, science, & competency. *Nurse Educator, 15*(2), 8-11.

Stewart, I. M. (1943). *The education of nurses.* New York: MacMillan.

Styles, M. (1982). *Nursing toward a new endowment.* St. Louis: C. V. Mosby.

Thompson, J. (1987). Critical scholarship: The critique of domination in nursing. *Advances in Nursing Science, 10*(1), 27-38.

Visintainer, M. (1986). The nature of knowledge and theory in nursing. *Image, Journal of Professional Nursing, 18*(2), 32-38.

Warner, S., Ross, M., & Clark, L. (1988). An analysis of entry into practice arguments. *Image: Journal of Nursing Scholarship, 20*(4), 212-216.

2

Conceptual Framework of the Teaching-Learning Process

The clinical setting is a dynamic multipurpose environment in which the various goals of clinical practice in a professional curriculum can be attained. The teacher enters the setting to teach. How does the teacher perceive this action? How does the teacher perceive the learning action in which students are engaged? Each teacher must ponder these questions and arrive at his or her own answers, for the answers will influence significantly the direction of the educational process.

RATIONALE FOR A CONCEPTUAL FRAMEWORK OF THE TEACHING-LEARNING PROCESS

A conceptual framework of the teaching-learning process, representative of a synthesis of compatible beliefs about the nature of both the teaching and learning processes, serves as the basis for all decisions relative to the learning of clinical practice competencies. The framework is descriptive rather than prescriptive. It provides the source for decisions relative to the selection of learning objectives for practice sessions in relation to the total program, the choice of learning experience and teaching strategies, and the determination of expectations in the performance of students and teachers. It is particularly important in assisting both students and teachers to maintain a reality perspective of the learning process so that the learner model, not the practitioner model, provides a referent for performance evaluation.

Instructional decisions must have a rationale supported by theory and fundamental values that reflect the integrity and worth of each student. Teachers need an explicit philosophy of the educational process and must function from a firmly established and supported concept of teaching and learning.

LEARNING CONCEPT ROOTED IN HUMAN SCIENCE THEORY

A conceptual framework of the teaching-learning process is rooted in theory. The teacher has numerous theories of learning, some descriptive and some prescriptive, from which to select and develop an operational concept of learning. The notion of the learning process may be based on one theory or it may be eclectic, derived from compatible elements from several theories. No predictive theory of instruction has been developed, but various descriptions of the process are found in the literature. The teacher must be certain that there is congruence between the concepts of the learning process and the teaching process if the total dynamic is to be developed for use in the clinical setting.

The purpose of clinical practice in a nursing program as described suggests a learning theory that addresses cognitive, developmental, and humanistic processes. Nursing is a cognitive activity. Although its practice entails numerous psychomotor and affective skills, the underlying activities are problem-solving and decision-making skills and clinical judgments. Its charge to act within an ambiguous, ever-changing society demands that its practitioners be skillful in learning to learn and continually relate nursing practice to developing events at any point in time.

The nature of the learning process appropriate for a teacher in a clinical setting is derived from theorists who perceive learning from a human science perspective rather than one of natural science. Two theories characteristic of each of the two perspectives are: natural science (behaviorism) and human science (phenomenology). Milhollan and Forisha (1972) describe the scientific base of each of these theories:

> *Behaviorism.* The laws that govern man are primarily the same universal laws that govern all natural phenomena. Therefore, the scientific method, as evolved by the physical sciences, is appropriate as well for the study of the human organism.
>
> *Phenomenology.* Only a science of man which begins with experience, as it is immediately given in this world of being, can ever be adequate for the study of the human organism. (p. 13)

Theorists subscribing to a human science view of learning are those associated with gestalt/cognitive field theory, development theory, and humanism theory. These theorists are often referred to as phenomenologists because of their approach to the study of mental activities from a meaningful holistic framework rather than the analysis of each part of the activity. The fundamental difference between those who approach learning from a natural science perspective and those who approach learning from a human science perspective is rooted in their basic beliefs about the nature of man. The human science view of man is the most compatible with the nature of nursing and the processes by which learners achieve practice competencies.

Milhollan and Forisha (1972) differentiate man as perceived by these two groups of theorists.

> *The behaviorist orientation considers man to be a passive organism governed by stimuli supplied by the external environment. Man can be manipulated, that is, his behavior controlled through proper control of environmental stimuli. Furthermore the laws that govern man are primarily the same as the universal laws that govern all natural phenomena. Therefore, the scientific method, as evolved by the physical sciences, is appropriate as well for the study of the human organism.*
>
> *The phenomenological orientation considers man to be the source of all acts. Man is essentially free to make choices in each situation. The focal point of this freedom is human consciousness. Behavior is,*

thus, only the observable expression and consequences of an essentially private internal world of being. Therefore, only a science of man which begins with experiences . . . as it is immediately given in this world of being can ever be adequate for a study of the human organism. (p. 13)

Dubos (1981) differentiates between the capacity of man from that of animals. He states, "whereas animal life is a prisoner of biological evolution which is essentially *irreversible*, human life has the wonderful freedom of social evolution which is rapidly reversible and creative" (p. 6).

The phenomenologic perspective sees man as a purposive, goal-directed individual in constant interaction with the environment. Cognitive abilities enable the individual to seek meaning in and order to all experiences. Mental capacities enable the person to be curious, creative, imaginative, and free to make choices. These abilities reflect characteristics of individual uniqueness, human consciousness, complexity, and unpredictability. The possession of mental processes of thinking and discrimination enable one to be both a generator and a transmitter of knowledge.

Each individual, although involved in the events occurring in the environment, lives in a very private, subjective world of feelings, emotions, and perceptions. Thoughts and behavior arise from this inner world and the individual seeks to maintain balance between both the inner and outer worlds. Therefore, any study of man must occur within the context of a human world of meaning and values where the individual demonstrates an active mind and free will.

A concept of learning based on the phenomenologic view of man recognizes the uniqueness of the individual and the mental capacities that enable a person to (1) grasp meaning from experiences in a creative way; (2) make choices and decisions based upon thoughtful deliberations; and (3) be the source of one's own responses to events in both the internal and external environment. This concept accepts the notion that learning behavior is often an internal process which may be inferred from behavior change rather than be primarily dependent upon observation as professed by supporters of learning as studied by a natural science.

The acknowledgment of the individual as an open system in simultaneous mutual interaction with the environment is more compatible with a learning concept fundamental to the instructional process directed toward cognitive, feeling, and action inherent practice, than the more mechanistic, environmentally controlled notion of the individual as a closed system espoused in the behaviorist theory of learning.

The emphasis on the notion of learning from a holistic perspective is congruent with the involvement of the whole person in learning the phenomenon of practice within the field setting. The selection of cognitive theory as the nucleus of the framework differentiates the preparation for nursing practice as an educational experience rather than a training one. Chickering (1976) makes a distinction between the two processes: "Training starts with the task and conforms a person to it; education starts with the learner and uses tasks in service of increased differentiation and integration" (p. 82).

CONCEPT OF LEARNING

Learning and Experience

Learning is a process by which behavior is changed as a result of experience. Hergenhahn (1982, p. 4) sees learning as a process that mediates behavior and acts as the intervening variable between certain experience and behavior change. He diagrams the process as follows:

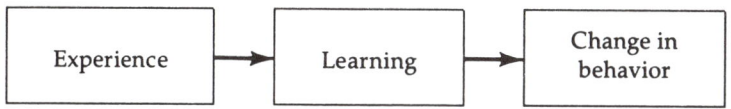

Some individuals conceptualize learning as outcome and state that learning *is* a change in behavior as a result of experience. It is the process of learning that is critical to this presentation and the outcome is perceived as "what is learned."

The notion of experience in any concept of learning is critical, for it differentiates change in behavior which may be the result of maturation or alteration in structure or function in any component of the individual's being. Dewey, the master theorist in the domain of experience as it relates to learning, recognizes the need for experience to be sufficiently challenging to promote cognitive learning, but cautions us that all experience is not equally educational. Stressing the need for quality experience, Dewey (1963) states:

> The central problem in education based in experience is to select the kind of present experiences that live fruitfully and creatively in subsequent experiences. The essence of experience for learning is its meaningfulness to the educational goals of the learner and its ability to prepare the individual for deeper and more complex experiences in the future. (pp. 26–27)

Dewey (1963) provides two criteria to discriminate between educative and miseducative experiences:

1. *Continuity of experience:* every experience both takes something from those which have gone before and modifies in some way the qualities of those that come after. Continuity means continued growth.
2. *Interaction:* consigns equal rights to both factors in experience—objective and internal conditions. An experience is always what it is because of a transaction taking place between an individual and what, at the time, constitutes own environment. (pp. 33–34)

Thus, a meaningful educational experience is one through which the knowledge and skills gained are able to be effective in managing comparable situations which follow. It is the connectiveness of experience that is the essential criterion in any planning for learning.

Steinaker and Bell (1979) conceptualize the process of experience as an involvement of the total person: a living through activity. They propose a hierarchy of behavior which connotes various progressive stages the learner goes through in meeting the goal of learning from the experience. The categories are:

1. Exposure: consciousness of the experience
2. Participation: decision on basis of data already received to become physically a part of the experience

3. Identification: union of learner with what is to be learned in an organizational, emotional, and intellectual context for purposes of achieving objectives.
4. Reinforcement: experience incorporated and fitting into other aspects of a person's life.
5. Dissemination: experience extends inwardly and outwardly with the learner in more control than previously.

This structural format for viewing experience in the teaching and learning situation serves to guide the teacher toward appropriate activities which facilitate the learner's progress.

Experiential learning is the essence of clinical practice and as such must be conceptualized thoughtfully within the total teaching-learning framework used by the teacher. Many factors influence the selection of types of experiential learning in professional programs. These might include the degree of the teacher's rigidity or creativity, student resources and needs, the goal of the experience, resources available for teaching, time allocation for the experience, and the agency and school controls. Schön (1987) feels that a significant factor in selecting experiential learning activities is related to the teacher's perception of professional knowledge. Professional knowledge perceived to be facts, rules and procedures applied non-problematically to instrumental problems is a technical training. Professional knowledge perceived as evolving, uncertain, and limited in its problem-solving potential addressed to some of the complex practice problems is a reflection-in-action experience where new problem statements, methods of reasoning, and strategies of action are developed through experience. In many situations, both types of problem-solving experiences are needed.

Learning and Perception

The concept of the individual as an open-ended system in continuous, simultaneous interaction with the internal and external environment suggests that there is in each person's environment a perceptual field or life-space which is unique. This life-space is the internal environment which contains the cognitive structures, feelings, and potentials of the individual. Learning involves the interaction between both the inner and outer world so that new learnings can be incorporated within the life-space.

Human science theorists recognize the perceptual field phenomenon but approach the learning process from different perspectives. Gestalt and cognitive field theorists relate learning to perception and consider learning to be a reorganization of the perceptual field. The notion of the reorganization process suggests that the human has the ability to organize in a meaningful way the events and experiences that are accepted into the field. The perceptual field is more than the sum of its parts, for the process of organization establishes meaning which is not inherent in any of the elements. The process by which sensory data are organized into meaningful patterns is attributed by field theorists to brain function, genetically determined, so that there is a state of isomorphism between psychological experience and processes that exist in the brain. The perceptual field is a dynamic, continually changing, interrelated system of elements, with each element affecting every other element as well as the total field.

The stimulus to learning occurs when an individual is confronted with a problem and a state of cognitive disequilibrium results until there is a resolution. The origin of the problem may arise from factors in the outer environment or from problems of inner needs often related to self-actualization. The law of Pragnaz states that cognitive balance is more satisfying than cognitive disequilibrium. Therefore, the learner seeks a resolution of the state of disequilibrium through a problem-solving process aimed at bringing order to the field.

Problem solving requires the interpretation and analysis of the meaning of the problem so as to gain appropriate insights for problem solution. Insight development requires change in perception of the problem. Three processes are involved in changing perceptions:

Grouping: categorization of facts

Recentering: focus on an aspect

Reorganizing: from insight and figure background, focus on something that was in the background

Wertheimer, in his book, *Productive Thinking*, (1945, p. 190), used the Gauss problem to explain this phenomenon:

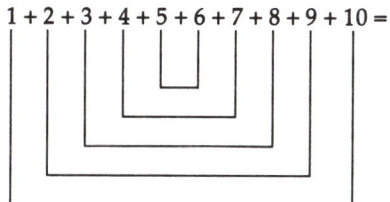

At first view, the problem appears to be a series of discrete numbers. A further analysis of the problem results in a different perspective of the problem.

Grouping: numbers can be categorized into multiples of 11
Recentering: 11 as the figure in the background
Reorganizing: 5 multiples of 11: solution = $11 \times 5 = 55$.

The change in the perception of the problem enabled the problem solver to gain insight into its meaning and, thus, solve the problem. The problem supports the notion that the solution of a problem lies within the problem (multiples of 11 were already present).

Insight, as noted by Gestalt and cognitive field theorists, is a deliberative approach to problem solving whereby the inner relations or basic principles are sought instead of using trial and error. Insightful learning may involve a total pattern or a partial feel for the pattern. Hergenhahn (1982) cites four characteristics of insightful learning:

1. Transition from pre-solution to a solution is sudden and complete.
2. Performance based upon solutions gained by insight is usually smooth and free of errors.
3. Solution of a problem gained by insight is retained for a considerable length of time.
4. Principles gained by insight are easily applied to other problems; a process of transposition. (p. 26)

Once the new insight is gained, it forms a new cognitive structure and causes a reorganization of the perceptual field. Learning, then, is not an additive process, but rather an integrative one.

Concepts, as such, facilitate the efficient use of experience through the identification and classification of objects and the use of symbolic responses which are known.

Bruner (1963) considers the act of learning as involving three almost simultaneous processes:

1. Acquisition of new information: refinement of previous knowledge.
2. Transformation: way of dealing information to go beyond it.
3. Evaluation: check on pertinence and adequacy of knowledge to task at hand. Judgment of knowledge's plausibility. (pp. 92–93)

Carl Rogers (1983) supports the notion of learning through insight, a process by which perceptual relationships in the field are identified. He particularly emphasizes the learning behavior that affects the component of the field which relates to the "self," the particular meanings and values which are identified with self-actualization. His phenomenologic perspective of learning states: "Significant learning combines the logical *and* the intuitive, the intellect *and* the feelings, the concept *and* the experience, the idea *and* the meaning" (p. 20).

Learning as conceptualized by these theorists is a holistic process involving perceptions, meanings, principles, and relationships resulting in new cognitive structures which are incorporated in the perceptual field. New learnings are accepted when related to present content of the perceptual field and result in a reorganization of the field. Its paradigm is stimulus-organism-response (S→O→R), which notes the role of the organism, (individual) in interpreting the stimulus and determining the response.

Learning and Thinking

The fundamental process in cognitive learning is reflective thinking, that which occurs in an experience when an organism meets, recognizes, and solves a problem. Wertheimer (1945) differentiates productive thinking from blind, habitual, mechanical thinking when he says, "Productive thinking consists in envisaging, realizing structural features and structural requirements; proceeding in accordance with and determined by these requirements" (p. 190). Meyers (1986) also differentiates between productive and reproductive thinking relative to learning critical thinking skills. Reflective thinking fosters divergent thinking, the derivation of more than one solution to a problem. Divergent thinking is a creative process, essential for effective problem solving; it is productive thinking. Convergent thinking, derivation of only one solution, is reproductive thinking, often resulting from rote or memorization.

Both types of productive thinking, creative and critical, are relevant to decision-making particularly in the practice domain. Critical thinking is an analytical process which not only addresses problem solving, but also concerns the ability to raise relevant questions and critique solutions without necessarily posing alternatives (Meyers, 1986). It is a complex process requiring an openness on the part of the students and a readiness for new experiences, new views, and new organization of meanings. Mahdi (1987) refers to innovative learning as sometimes a process of unlearning. Cognitive disequilibrium is often the result. Meyers (1986) states that this disequilibrium may be a function of the structure of thoughts as being more than a dispassionate cognition. "They are highly personal and emotional, involving cherished values and beliefs. Personal beliefs and values serve as a perceptual grid through which experience is screened" (p. 14).

Although the analytic process in productive thinking is stressed, Bruner (1963) is concerned that intuitive thinking, the process of arriving at plausible but tentative formulation without going through the analytic process, is neglected in educational practices. He says: "The shrewd guess, the fertile hypothesis, the courageous leap to a tentative conclusion—these are the most valuable coin of the thinker at work, whatever the line of work" (p. 13). Carl Rogers concurs with Bruner on this point and recognizes the significance of intuitive thinking in problem solving. Intuitive thinking, although not based on a rational thinking process, is not an irrational process, for it depends upon the existence of previous experience in the perceptual field which can be applicable to solving the new problem.

Rew (1988) in the study of nurses' use of intuition in decision making found that intuition is very much a part of practice, even though use of objective data as bases for decisions is emphasized in education and practice. Benner (1984) found that intuition, often derived from previous experience, becomes increasingly evident as the nurse develops toward expert practitioner.

Types of knowing, thought processes that require little analysis but lead to definitive actions, have been noted in the literature. Schön (1987) and Schultz and Meleis (1988) refer to this action knowledge as tacit knowledge, while Meyers (1986) refers to it as implicit knowledge. Regardless of the name, this type of knowing is readily recalled and so automatic and internalized that it does not lend itself to explanation. It is a type of knowing that is prevalent in professional practitioners. Schön (1987) refers to this knowing in action as professional artistry, "kinds of competence practitioners sometimes display in unique, uncertain and conflicted situations of practice" (p. 22).

Transfer of Learning

Compatible with the beliefs of the theorists relative to significance of the development of insight through perception change and the search for meaning and order in the new learning task, transfer of that learning is dependent upon the understanding of the meaning of the task. Bruner (1963) sees a relationship between the nature of the learning and the transfer. "Massive general transfer can be achieved by appropriate learning, even to the degree that learning properly under conditions (optimum) leads one to learn how to learn" (pp. 6-7). He emphasizes that learning the structure of a subject, the understanding of it in a way that permits many other things to be related to it meaningfully, is the "center of the problem of transfer."

Cognitive theorists relate transfer of learning to the significance of perceptions in noting similarities in situations, i.e., meanings, generalizations, concepts, or insights gained in previous learning experiences. Transfer is not simply related to mastery of facts and techniques and their applicability to the new situation. The transfer requires that the individual grasp the nature of the phenomenon to be transferred so that its applicability can be determined.

Learning and Knowledge

A concept of learning must not only incorporate the process but must also consider the scope of learning and the meaning of knowledge. Perry

(1970) addresses the intellectual and ethical development of students relative to the nature of knowledge, truth, values, and the meaning of commitment. His schema, representing four general categories (dualism, multiplicity, relativism and commitment), describes the development of students from a "simplistic categorical view of the world to a realization of contingent nature of knowledge, relative values, and affirmation of own commitment" (pp. 57–58).

This schema addresses the ability of students to deal with knowledge outside the perspective of absolutism. It is the discriminating use of knowledge and the potential for seeing various meanings of knowledge in a broader context that leads the learner to creative, reflective thinking in problem solving. The dualistic thinker is a convergent thinker unable to relate to a world of uncertainty.

Whitehead (1967) is also concerned about what individuals do with knowledge when he refers to "'inert ideas,' those ideas merely received into the mind without being utilized or tested or thrown into fresh combinations" (p. 1). Both Dewey and Whitehead see knowledge as the greatest freedom. Whitehead (1967) relates knowledge to "wisdom which concerns handling of knowledge, its selection for the determination of relevant issues, its employment to add value to an immediate experience" (p. 32). Knowledge, as perceived by Nelms (1991), differs from the notion of content or subject matter. It is, in essence, highly personal, contextual in nature, and derived from the individual's own experiences, interpretive meanings, and perceived relevancy.

Learning and Processing of Information

In addition to the cognitive process of learning, two factors concerning the handling of information are significant to teaching clinical practice skills. One factor refers to the cognitive style of the learner and the other relates to cultural patterns of learning accepted by various groups.

Cognitive Styles

Recent research is suggesting that there are different cognitive styles that relate to the way individuals process information. Cognitive style is not related to intelligence, skill performance, or cognitive performance or the *what* of learning, but rather, it addresses the process of data handling, i.e., the *how* of learning, namely perceiving, thinking, problem solving, and interactions with others. Cognitive style is a habitual mode of information processing which, as heretofore supported in research, is not amenable to major change.

Several theories of cognitive learning styles are found in the literature. The three most often studied in nursing are: (a) field-independent and field-dependent model (Witkin, Moor, Goodenough, & Cox, 1977), (b) four style model: concrete sequential, concrete random, abstract sequential, abstract random (Gregoric, 1982), and (c) four dominant style model: converger, diverger, assimilator, and accommodator (Kolb, 1985). The Gregoric and Kolb models present a range from concrete to abstract learning styles.

Many studies of cognitive styles of students in nursing have been reported in the literature. The majority of students and graduates studied have a defined cognitive style of learning with preference directed toward the concrete model. Laschinger and Boss (1989) express the belief that with a professional discipline, learning styles of members are compatible with the demands of the discipline, i.e., the structure of professional knowledge determines the competencies to be achieved. Concrete thinking is congruent with professional knowledge that reflects technical rationality.

Messick (1976) clarifies the difference between ability and cognitive styles by presenting the characteristics of each. Table 2-1 is extracted from his discussion.

The work of Witkin et al. (1977) is directed toward two different styles of habitual information processing and interacting: field independence and field dependence. Table 2-2 identifies the characteristics of individuals representing the two different cognitive styles.

This classification and the defined characteristics are helpful in understanding a process by which some learners handle information in their learning behavior pattern. The field independent-field dependent classification is one of several ways of approaching this important dimension of learning.

Knowledge of the cognitive learning styles of students is of particular significance in promoting transformational learning experiences in the

Table 2-1
Comparison of Characteristics of Cognitive Style and Ability

Cognitive Style	Ability
1. Addresses question of *how*	1. Addresses question of *what*
2. Measurement of characteristic modes in terms of typical performance—emphasis on process	2. Measurement of capacities in terms of maximal performance—emphasis on level of accomplishment
3. Bipolar—dynamic gestalt pits one syndrome or complex of interacting characteristics against contrasting complex at opposite end of pole	3. Unipolar—the top is significant
4. Range from one extreme to another. Each end has different implication for education	4. Range from zero to higher denotes greater facility
5. Value differentiated—each pole has adaptive value in different circumstances	5. Value directional—more is better
6. Neither end is more adaptive—it is a function of the situation	6. The higher the value, the more adaptive
7. Cuts across all domains	7. Usually delineates a basic dimension underlying a fairly limited area specific to a particular domain of content or function
8. Roots in study of perception and personality—close ties with laboratory or clinic	8. Measurement—roots in mental test theory in schools

clinical setting. This concern is expressed by Wells and Higgs (1990). When problems arise in faculty-student communication or when thought processes of students are not clearly identified, an assessment of the learning style may well indicate that a difference exists between the student and teacher's perception and processes used. Different learning and teaching strategies may be in order.

Table 2-2
Characteristics of Different Cognitive Styles

Field-Independent	Field-Dependent
1. Perception of figures more or less separate from surrounding field	1. Perception dominated by perceptual field
2. Able to dissemble a salient element from background	2. Difficulty in dissembling elements because of global view of the field
3. High in cognitive restructuring skills	3. Low in cognitive restructuring skills
4. Impersonal orientation—low in social skills	4. Social orientation—high in social skills
5. Preference—domains featuring analysis of items within the field	5. Preference—domains featuring interpersonal relationships and day-to-day work with people
6. High in analytic and differentiation skills	6. Low in analytic and differentiation skills
7. Hypothesis testing approach in concept formation	7. Spectator approach in concept formation—trial and error
8. Adept at learning material with natural science content	8. Adept at learning and memorizing material with social content
9. Intrinsic motivation for learning	9. Extrinsic motivation for learning—social group
10. Unstructured innner-directed environment	10. Structured outer-directed environment
11. Capacity to be self-referent for self-definition	11. Rely on external referent, particularly by authority, for self-definition
12. Autonomous	12. Low in personal autonomy
13. Low response to personal criticism	13. High response to criticism, positive or negative
14. Performs best when own strategies developed	14. Needs more explicit instruction and more exact definition of performance outcome

Cultural Determinants

The second factor that influences learning behavior is the influence of culture on learning. Cultural determinants are significant in any concept of learning, for they denote the structure of knowledge, its meaning and relationships, and the process by which members of a culture learn. Hall (1961) sees learning as an adaptive mechanism used by the culture as an agent of acculturation of its members as well as a mechanism for its continuance. Since people in various cultures learn to learn differently, a pattern not readily alterable, responses to learning situations will also vary. Differences occur in temporal and spatial dimensions as well as content and meaning. American culture values active involvement (the "doing," during the learning experience), rewards rapidity in grasping the learning task, and accepts the notion of pressure as an ingredient of the learning process. Other cultures may value the skill of memory or rote learning and reward correct learning regardless of the time needed so that the time pressure is not a factor.

Hall proposes three models of learning: formal, informal, and technical. Formal learning, the result of precept or admonition, establishes patterns by mistakes. It is a dualistic approach, emphasizing right/wrong or yes/no, and is suffused with emotion. Informal learning occurs as a result of identification with a model, often an "out of awareness" phenomenon. The learner asks no questions but follows the behavior pattern of the model. Technical learning results from the transmission of information, often after a mistake has been made. In contrast to the normal learning pattern, the learner in this pattern is supported and receives clarification and correction in a facilitative tone.

Because anthropology is concerned with the meanings of knowledge and behavior from a societal perspective, it is concerned with the influence of a group's perception or response to a learning event. Mead (1955) recognizes the difference in what a society accepts as proper reward or praise behavior, its notion of dualism and competition, and the content it deems to be acceptable in a teaching situation.

Crick (1982) raises questions about the notion of an anthropology of knowledge which would address meanings, cognitive knowledge, and how different cultures think. He notes that if the aim of anthropology is to make social life intelligible and knowledgeable, it can be assumed that knowledge must be seen in a social context. Accepting the notion of an early development in the domain of anthropology of knowledge, Crick raises questions that anthropology must answer. These questions are: Does language represent knowledge, or is there a linguistic language and a cultural language? How are ritual and knowledge related? How are knowledge and power related in a society? As the anthropology of knowledge is explored and articulated, the impact of culture in influencing meanings and learning styles will become even more significant to a framework of the learning phenomenon. Cultural influence on learning cannot be ignored.

CONCEPT OF TEACHING

Relationship to Concept of Learning

The concept of learning presented as relevant to teaching in the clinical field includes significant concepts that influence the process of teaching, for the two processes must be interrelated. Learning is an individual process; it is active, experiential; it is holistic, involving the total being and the environment. It emphasizes meanings, principles and relationships among phenomena, and it is concerned with perception, insight, and cognitive structure formation. It is an integrative process through which new learnings are incorporated into a perceptual field, thus causing a reorganization of the field; and it provides for transfer of knowledge or skill when there is relevance in meaning between previous experience and the new one. Learning is often precipitated by cognitive disequilibrium requiring problem solving based on reflective thinking for solutions, although in some instances intuitive thinking (and knowing-in-action) are effective. Learning is influenced by the cognitive style of the learner and the cultural pattern of learning adopted by the learner's referent group. Learning is perceived from a cognitive perspective because knowledge and its use is basic to all other domains of learning inherent in professional practice.

What process of teaching is most compatible with the above description of learning? It is certain that the notion of teaching as "telling" through which information is dispensed is not appropriate. Teaching is the facilitation of learning, which involves a sharing and mutual experience of learning on the part of both teacher and learner. It is a sharing of the perceptual field of both participants toward a goal-directed encounter with new experiences.

Teaching seeks to assist students in developing a sense of excitement, curiosity, and discovery about the world. It asks for involvement of the learner, not passivity, and provides the supportive environment required. It provides for experience in problem solving and accommodates reflective and intuitive thinking. It assists students in the pursuit of new knowledge and the skills in utilizing that knowledge in practice within a humanistic context. It includes the total learner in the experience, guarding against overemphasis on one domain, such as cognitive, to the exclusion of other domains, particularly the affective domain which provides the value base for use of new knowledges and skills.

Teaching: A Diagnostic and Intervention Process

Teaching, like other service professions, is a helping field which addresses the growth and developmental needs of individuals. It is a diagnostic and intervention process similar in structure to the nursing process. A comparison of these two processes is shown in Table 2-3.

The diagnostic process in teaching involves assessment of the individual's resources and limitations to enter into the task as well as the nature of the learning required for its attainment. The diagnostic dimension of teaching begins with the learner, the primary focus of the educational endeavor. Knowledge of students, their capabilities, interests, motivations, and readiness for the learning task at the point of entry is essential if the growth of the student is to be fostered. The heterogeneity of the student groups, the varied and complex motivations represented, and the differing cognitive learning styles are essential data as indicated by research of students in the context of their learning. Emphasis on fads in teaching could result in dysfunctional learning if the relevancy of the method to the student's learning potential is not ascertained (Reilly & Oermann, 1990).

Bloom (1982) believes that the history of the student is the core of learning and is vital information in predicting and recognizing the student's response to a learning experience. His research into entry behaviors, cognitive and affective, and the quality of the instruction suggest

Table 2-3
Comparison of Nursing Process and Teaching Process

Nursing	Teaching
Goal:	*Goal:*
Change in behavior—coping with health/illness	Change in behavior—new learning
Assessment:	*Assessment:*
Client needs—health	Client needs—learning
Nature of problem	Nature of problem
Health deficiency	Learning deficiency
Health maintenance	Learning continuance
Health promotion	Learning promotion
Priority based on nursing diagnosis	Priority based on diagnosis of learning needs
Planning:	*Planning:*
Determine short- and long-term goals with client	Determine short- and long-term goals with student
Establish pertinent objectives	Establish pertinent objectives
Select intervention strategies to meet objectives	Select intervention strategies to meet objectives
Intervention:	*Intervention:*
Supplemental	Supplemental
Supportive	Supportive
Curative	Alternate pacing
Educational	Alternate experience
Evaluation:	*Evaluation:*
Outcome—goals of health status	Performance—goals of learning
Process—means by which outcome was obtained	Process—means by which learning experience outcome was obtained

that they are significant factors in accounting for success or failure in learning. Diagnostic teaching addresses the alterable variables, available time vs. time on task, abilities and knowledge, evaluation and feedback, and quality of teaching which can be manipulated. Learning style behaviors influence learner responses to a learning experience and may call for variation in teaching strategies.

Witkin et al. (1977) suggest teaching strategies that are appropriate to different types of cognitive styles of learning. Field-dependent learners, with their inclination toward global perceptions of the field and domains that feature interpersonal relations, respond best to teaching methods that entail group interaction with responsibility shared by the teachers and students. Because they do not readily use a hypothesis-testing approach to problem solving and concept formation, they require more specific instruction and more exact definition of performance expectation. They are dependent upon salient cues for learning, and because of their use of the social group as a self-referral, they are more responsive to criticism of their performance, whether positive or negative.

The field-independent learners seek teaching strategies that stimulate analytic skills, and they prefer lecture and discovery methods. Their predilection for examining elements in a field and their interrelationships support a hypothesis-testing approach to problem solving and concept formation. They rely less on structure or cue saliency. With an internalized frame of reference and self-defined goals, they are minimally affected by criticism of their performance.

Another entry factor that influences student response to a learning experience is the role that grades play as motivators of students. Research by Milton, Pollio, and Eison (1986) resulted in two major classifications of students, high learning orientation and high grade orientation, as well as identification of characteristics of each group. In general, high learning-orientation represents inner locus of control, motivation toward pursuit of educational enrichment and personal growth, greater abstract reasoning, higher levels of sensitivity, and low tension. These learners are intellectually and emotionally able, willing and interested. High grade-orientation represents outer locus of control and all aspects of the learning experience are viewed within the context of grades. These learners exhibit a high degree of tension and endure self pressure to do the right thing and act in conventional ways. Their study habits tend to be poor and they approach learning experiences concretely.

Mastery of learning theory which Bloom (1982) based on Carroll's Model of School Learning provides five variables that can be used in diagnosing learner needs: aptitude for a particular learning task, quality of instruction, ability to understand the nature of the task to be learned, perseverance, and time period allowed for learning to occur.

Intervention addresses strategies for assisting the learner to achieve educational goals. The expediting or retarding of the pace of learning may be relevant for the learner with temporal needs for grasping the meaning of new learnings. Use of resources (teacher as well as library, field, or outside experts) is an important teaching strategy. Modifications in or use of alternative teaching methodologies compatible with the goals of the learning task are useful in broadening the experience of some students or helping to clarify new learnings for other students.

In the process of accommodating learning expectations and teaching strategies to meet the various needs of students, Bruner (1963) cautions us about the tendency in teaching groups of students to "unequalize" learning expectations. He states:

> *The pursuit of excellence must not be limited to the gifted student. But the idea that teaching should be aimed at the average student in order to provide something for everyone is an equally inadequate formula. The quest is to devise material which will challenge the superior student, while not destroying the confidence and will to learn of those who are less fortunate. (p. 70)*

Teaching and the Teacher

In the dynamic phenomenon of teaching and learning, it is the teacher who must assume the primary responsibility for the quality of the learning environment relative to the prevailing climate, availability of resources, and process of goal-directed learning. The climate is supportive to learning; it reflects caring about and liking students; it is generated by the teacher's enthusiasm for teaching; it accepts the involvement of the total learner in the process, regardless of the nature of the learning task.

Bloom (1980) states that educational research is moving from a study of the characteristics of teachers and students to direct observation of learning taking place in the interactions between students and teachers. This position is supported in the literature as the interactional process in the teaching-learning dynamic. Educationists, such as Meyers (1986), Clayton and Murray (1989), Eble (1988), Reilly and Oermann (1990) and Schön (1987) emphasize the importance of the interaction of the teacher and learner in a transformational process so that meanings of experiences can be searched, identified, and explained. Schön (1987) refers to the role of the teacher in this process as coach and describes an environment where coaching artistry can facilitate the learner's development of professional artistry. It promotes learning through participation that is relatively risk-free and provides coaches who can initiate learners into the traditions of the discipline while enabling them to explore for themselves the essence and meanings in the experience.

A transformational learning experience strategy that highlights an atmosphere of freedom promoting significant learning and stresses the learner's attitude toward and use of the experience differs markedly from a traditional model where emphasis is on content, often at the exclusion of inquiry, in a structured and formal setting. The skills of thinking and inquiry are critical ones if the professional practitioner is to fulfill the responsibilities inherent in the profession. The teaching of critical thinking involves challenging the implicit theories of the learner and helping the individual to gain new perspectives for interpreting the new experience. Jacobs-Kraemer and Huether (1988) caution teachers that students tend to believe that all problems can be solved by scientific approach and result in single answers. The charge to teachers is to help students deal with the reality of practice concerns and recognize that there may be multiple answers to one problem, varied views of reality, and some problems that are not readily solved empirically. This charge relates to the swampy lowland problems to which Schön (1983) referred.

The teacher recognizes variability in learner response to the learning task, sometimes due to differences in aptitude, preference, experience, or motivation relative to task achievement. Although motivation lies within the province of the learner, the teacher seeks to help the learner find meaning and relevance to the new experience. The teacher recognizes the role that biases, prejudices, and fear of change or self-encounter play in preventing the learner from entering new experiences which result in new insights and behavior change, and develops strategies that will assist the learner in becoming open.

The climate is a humanistic one which is authentic, supportive, and caring. However, the charge for learning to occur requires that it be stimulating, provocative, and disciplined in the pursuit of new learnings. Sensitivity and caring about learner needs does not mean lessening of acceptable performance; it means consideration of strategies directed toward helping the learner attain the desired goals. It means enhancing the learner's perspective so that learning does not become viewed as a personal possession, but rather it becomes a way of relating to the world at large, that is, the student's world and the outside world are an integral part of learning.

The teacher most effective in functioning within a humanistic climate is described by Eble (1988) as wiser, less judgmental; more generous, less arrogant yet more confident; more honest with self, students and subject matter; more willing to take risks; more willing to show forth without showing off; and impatient with ignorance, but not appalled by it.

The teacher is a vital link in the teaching-learning dynamic. Expertise in subject matter and teaching are basic requirements, inclusive of the human qualities that make the total experience stimulating, developmental, and fulfilling for both the teacher and the learner. It is the teacher, through the use of a theoretically based concept of the teacher-learning process, that sets the tone and provides for smooth functioning of the total endeavor.

THE DYNAMIC: TEACHING AND LEARNING

Teaching and learning, two discrete processes, are interrelated so as to form a gestalt that reflects a dynamic process. Congruency in the fundamental constructs of each provides a consistent pattern which unites the two processes. The dynamic which has been presented is eclectic, reflecting concepts and theories of theorists who view learning from the perspective of human science rather than natural science. It is an interactional phenomenon whereby the fields of the participants, teacher, and learner intersect and are open to new experiences. Total beings are involved in this interaction and learning occurs in all three domains: cognitive, affective, and psychomotor. The dynamic requires giving and receiving by both parties as each pursues the continuous search for knowledge, self identity, and living within the reality of one's own existence.

In a professional field, the participants in the process are not equal, for the field requires a distinct repertoire of skill and knowledge for its practice. The "knower" (the teacher) guides the "uninformed" (the student) through the learning process in pursuit of the requisite competencies for practice. Because of the continuous introduction of the "new" into the realm of practice, the teacher often becomes a learner when engaged in the dynamic and the learner may become the teacher as his or her own experiences elucidate practice behavior and provide data which contribute to the development of new insights. Diekelmann (1989) describes this process, "The teacher moves from being an information giver and facilitator to the explorer of meanings with students—their understandings of the experience" (p. 37). The total process, then, reflects the goals, experiences, and values of the participants at any point in time.

Learning can occur without teaching. Teaching can occur without learning as a result. In the educational field, however, the two ought to be interactive in accord with specifically defined goals appropriate to the parties involved. When the gestalt is perceived, there is greater attention to the congruency of the two processes, so that the outcome can be achieved with greater efficiency and the evaluation can be concerned with both the outcome (learning) in terms of desired goals and the process (teaching) by which it was guided.

RELEVANCE OF CONCEPTUAL FRAMEWORK OF THE TEACHING-LEARNING PROCESS TO TEACHING IN THE CLINICAL SETTING

As stated earlier, each teacher develops his or her own conceptual framework which can be operationalized in all decisions pertinent to curriculum matters. The framework presented represents concepts and theories deemed relevant to the educational experience that occurs in the clinical practice component of a nursing program. The framework recognizes that the three domains of learning, i.e., cognitive, affective, and psychomotor, occur within the clinical setting, but it also emphasizes the cognitive processes of learning as the principal element. This choice was made because nursing involves cognitive skills in all dimensions of its practice: clinical judgments inherent in its problem-solving process of care and the delivery of care; choice in the selection and use of intervention strategies and their alternatives necessitated by individual response; and moral reasoning essential for determining human actions in a complex field of practice. Nurses "do," but behind all actions are cognitive processes, even though some are primarily carried out as knowing-in-action—an automatic response which results from previous cognitive experience.

A framework which supports problem solving, experiential learning, and human caring is particularly relevant to teaching nursing practice competencies in a clinical setting, since they are the three processes that dominate the experience. The problem-solving activity is not only essential for individualizing client care, but it is also a means by which the learner develops skill in discrimination when ambiguous choices are encountered, broadens perspectives so that alternative responses or actions are evident in practice, and learns how to learn so that a questioning posture may be established, thus enabling continuous evaluation of new and continuing practice modes.

Caring, an inherent part of nursing, is becoming an overt rather than tacit critical element in education of students for humanistic professional practice. At one time, relegated to the process of imitation or expectation, it is now approached with the same pedagogic vigor as cognitive and psychomotor skills. Educational theories from the humanistic sciences, theories of ethics, and theories and models of the phenomenon of caring are now cognitively studied and incorporated into the problem solving and experiential components of learning. Thus, both the science and the art of nursing are learned within the context of patient care in the clinical area.

Experiential learning is essential in a practice discipline and provides opportunities for problem-solving practice with real clients and problems in the setting, hands-on experience in ministrations of care, and moral or ethical decision making relative to client, setting, or self. The knowledge of field-independent and field-dependent cognitive styles of processing information is particularly relevant here. Nursing is a people-oriented field and the practice setting provides the opportunity to work with people. The environment is well-suited to the field-dependent individual, but what can the teacher expect from the field-independent learner?

Nursing today requires the cognitive skills of analysis and hypothesis testing (field independent) and personal interaction skills (field dependent). Both types of behaviors are goals of clinical practice. How do we accommodate the predilections of each group and yet require both cognitive and social skill? The recognition of the cognitive style phenomenon enables teachers to foster the preferences of each type of learner and devise strategies for developing the opposite skill so that achievement can be attained.

Theorists who emphasize problem solving, experiencing, and the caring process as teaching modalities highlight the role of perception, insight, and general principles in the transfer of learning. The stress on meanings and the connections between previous experience and new learning highlight the importance in developing the understanding which underlies all nursing actions and not the "doing" of the action itself.

Teaching in the clinical field according to this teaching-learning concept is concerned with a learning climate that supports the activities of the learners in a situation where the learner is most vulnerable. Diagnostic and intervention components of teaching facilitate both teaching and learning activities. Consideration is given to providing sufficient time for problem solving and the carrying out of nursing ministrations, supporting creative proposals made by the learner, and accepting the potential of mistakes as an inherent part of any learning experience. The learner is not a practitioner; yet, in the clinical field where experienced practitioners are engaged in their respective activities, expectations of acceptable performances by the learner are often judged on the basis of what is observed in practice.

Opportunities to use knowledge under various circumstances foster the ability to transfer learnings by finding new meanings and relationships. The accumulation of learning culminates in a repertoire of related knowledge which comprises the basis of nursing practice.

SUMMARY

Knowledge, skill, and value commitment are the outcomes of clinical practice experience. All can be achieved in the practice setting if the teacher has a theoretically based conceptual framework of the teaching-learning process used in making all decisions relative to goals of the experience, diagnosis of learner needs, selection of learning and teaching strategies, management of learner responses during the experience, and use of self as a facilitator. The framework, proposed as appropriate for teaching in the clinical field, is derived from cognitive field theory and the ideas of others who perceive learning from a human science point of view.

Cognitive field theory, which stresses reflective divergent thinking in problem solving and decision making, is the focus because cognition is a critical competency in nursing. The role of perception, insight, meanings, relationships, and principles in learning and the transfer of learning is the essence of learning. Dewey's theory of experiential learning provides criteria for determining the educational value of the clinical experience. Bruner's stress on the importance of teaching the structure of knowledge (its meaningfulness and its relatedness) suggests the approach to teaching nursing's body of knowledge. Carl Rogers' concern about the role of education in moving people toward self-actualization provides the stimulus to support the growth and development of the person who is to be the nurse. Perry's thesis about the need for education to move individuals from dualistic thinking to relativistic thinking and commitment challenges nursing teachers to enable students to deal with the uncertainties of a field which is an inexact science. Schön's thesis that problem-solving learning extends to those problems not readily addressed empirically but still frequent patterns in a professional practice broadens the scope of nursing and health care concerns which faculty can and must select for inclusion in the educational experiences within the program. Witkin's work on the significance of cognitive style in learning behavior provides another basis for understanding learner needs and responses in the clinical practice site while Hall's and Mead's theses about cultural influences on the learning process provide new insight into a dimension of learning which has had little emphasis heretofore.

Teaching is a facilitative, supportive process; it is humanistic, but demanding of acceptable performance on the part of the teacher and the learner, which is compatible with an articulated concept of learning. It is a diagnostic and intervention process. Bloom's contribution to the teaching field in the development of the mastery of learning mode and the present research into teaching with a focus on alterable variables has major implications for the teacher or students engaged in multiple learning tasks in a multipurpose environment.

Teaching and learning is a dynamic which is mutually interactive and needs to be viewed as such by the teacher in the clinical setting. This perspective enables learners and teachers to engage in a sharing experience which highlights problem solving, experiential learning, and caring actions; is appropriate for meeting the multiple goals of clinical practice in the nursing program; and forms the basis for the learners eventual development of their own theory of practice.

REFERENCES

Benner, P. (1984). *From novice to expert: Excellence and power in clinical nursing practice.* Menlo Park, CA: Addison-Wesley.
Bloom, B. S. (1980). The new directions in educational research: Alterable variables. *Phi Delta Kappa, 61,* 382-85.
Bloom, B. S. (1982). *Human characteristics and school learning.* New York: McGraw-Hill.
Bruner, J. S. (1963). *The process of education.* New York: Vintage Books.
Chickering, A. W. (1976). The double bind of field dependence/independence in program alternatives for educational development. In S. Messick & Associates, *Individuality in learning.* San Francisco: Jossey-Bass.
Clayton, G., & Murray, J. (1989). Faculty-student relationships: Catalytic connection. In National League for Nursing, *Curriculum revolution: Reconceptualizing nursing education* (pp. 43-53). New York: National League for Nursing.
Crick, M. (1982). Anthropology of knowledge. *Annual Review of Anthropology, 11,* 287-313.
Dewey, J. (1963). *Experience in education.* New York: Collier Books.
Diekelmann, N. (1989). The nursing curriculum: Lived experiences of students. In National League for Nursing, *Curriculum revolution: Reconceptualizing nursing education* (pp. 25-41). New York: National League for Nursing.
Dubos, R. (1981). *Celebrations of life.* New York: McGraw-Hill.
Eble, K. (1988). *The craft of teaching* (2nd ed.). San Francisco, CA: Jossey-Bass.
Gregoric, A. F. (1982). *An adult's guide to style.* Maynard, MA: Gabriel.
Hall, E. (1961). *Silent language.* New York: Premier Books.
Hergenhahn, B. (1982). An introduction to theories of learning, 2nd ed., Englewood Cliffs, NJ: Prentice-Hall.
Jacobs-Kraemer, M., & Huether, S. (1988). Curricular consideration for teaching nursing theory. *Journal of Professional Nursing, 4*(5), 373-380.
Kolb, D. (1985). *Learning style inventory 1985: Technical specifications.* Boston: McBee.

Laschinger, H., & Boss, M. (1989). Learning styles of B.S. nursing students and attitudes toward theory-based nursing. *Journal of Professional Nursing,* 5(4), 215–223.

Mahdi, E. (1987). Learning needs in a changing world. *The Futurist, 21*(2), 60.

Mead, M. (1955). *Cultural patterns and technical change.* New York: Menton.

Messick, S. (1976). Personality competencies in cognition and creativity. In S. Messick & Associates, *Individuality in learning.* San Francisco: Jossey-Bass.

Meyers, C. (1986). *Teaching students to think critically.* San Francisco, CA: Jossey-Bass.

Milhollan, F., & Forisha, B. (1972). *From Skinner to Rogers.* Lincoln, NE: Professional Publications, Inc.

Milton, O., Pollio, H., & Eison, J. (1986). *Making sense of college grades.* San Francisco, CA: Jossey-Bass.

Nelms, T. (1991). Has the curriculum revolution revolutionalized the definition of curriculum? *Journal of Nursing Education, 30*(1), 5–8.

Perry, W. G., Jr. (1970). *Forms of intellectual and ethical development in the college years.* New York: Holt, Rinehart & Winston.

Reilly, D., & Oermann, M. (1990). *Behavioral objectives: Evaluation in nursing* (3rd ed.). New York: National League for Nursing.

Rew, L. (1988). Intuition in decision-making. *Image: Journal of Nursing Scholarship, 20*(3), 150–154.

Rogers, C. (1983). *Freedom to learn in the 80's.* Columbus, OH: Charles E. Merrill.

Schön, D. (1983). *The reflective practitioner: How professionals think in practice.* San Francisco, CA: Jossey-Bass.

Schön, D. (1987). *Educating the reflective practitioner.* San Francisco, CA: Jossey-Bass.

Schultz, P., & Meleis, A. (1988). Nursing epistemology: Traditions, insights and questions. *Image: Journal of Nursing of Scholarship, 20*(4), 217–222.

Steinaker, N. B., & Bell, M. R. (1979). *The experiential taxonomy: A new approach to teaching and learning.* New York: Academic Press.

Wells, D., & Higgs, Z. (1990). Learning styles and learning preferences of 1st and 4th semester baccalaureate nursing students. *Journal of Nursing Education, 29*(6), 385–390.

Wertheimer, M. (1945). *Productive thinking.* New York: Harper.

Whitehead, A. N. (1967). *The aims of education.* New York: Free Press.

Witkin, H. A., Moore, C. A., Goodenough, D. R., & Cox, P. W. (1977). Field-dependent and field-independent cognitive styles and their educational implications. *Review of Educational Research, 47,* 1–64.

BIBLIOGRAPHY

Agon, P. (1987). Intuitive knowing as a dimension of nursing. *Advances in Nursing Science, 10*(1), 63-70.

Allen, D. (1985). Nursing research and social control: Alternative models of science that emphasize understanding and emancipation. *Image: Journal of Nursing Scholarship, 17*(1), 58-64.

Bandura, A. (1977). *Social learning theory.* Englewood Cliffs, NJ: Prentice-Hall.

Bigge, M. (1982). *Learning theories for teachers* (4th ed.). New York: Harper & Row.

Benoliel, J. (1988). Some reflections in learning and teaching. *Journal of Nursing Education, 27,* 340-347.

Bruner, J. S. (1966). *Toward a theory of instruction.* Cambridge, MA: Belknap Press of Harvard University Press.

Cooper, L. N. (1980). Sources and limits of human intellect. *Daedalus, 109*(2), 1-17.

Cross, K. P. (1981). *Adults as learners.* San Francisco: Jossey-Bass.

DeBack, V. (1987). National commission on nursing implementation project. *Journal of Professional Nursing, 3*(4), 226-229.

DeCoux, V. (1990). Kolb's learning style inventory: A review of its application in nursing research. *Journal of Nursing Education, 29,* 202-207.

Derry, S., & Murphy, D. (1986). Designing systems that train learning ability: From theory to practice. *Review of Educational Research, 56,* 1-39.

Diekelmann, N. (1990). Nursing education: Caring, dialogue, and practice. *Journal of Nursing Education, 29,* 300-308.

Dressel, P. (1980). Models for evaluating individual achievement. *Journal of Higher Education, 51,* 194-206.

Frisch, N. (1987). Cognitive maturity of nursing students. *Image: Journal of Nursing Scholarship, 19*(1), 25-27.

Hammock, F. M. (1982). Education for nursing: Problems and prospects. *New York Educational Quarterly, 13*(2), 8-14.

Hodson, K. (1985). Cognitive styles and the behavioral differences in nursing students in the clinical setting. *Journal of Nursing Education, 24,* 58-62.

Intellect and imagination: The limits and presuppositions of intellect. (1980). *Daedalus, 109*(2).

James, W. (1962). *Talks to teachers.* New York: Dover.

Kitchner, K. S. (1983). Educational goals and reflective thinking. *Educational Forum, 47*(5), 75-79.

Knowles, M., & Associates. (1984). *Andrology in action: Applying modern principles of adult learning.* San Francisco: Jossey-Bass.

Laschinger, H., & Boss, M. (1984). Learning styles of nursing students and career choices. *Journal of Advanced Nursing, 13,* 341–344.

Marchione, J., & Stearns, S. (1990). Ethnic power perspective for nursing. *Nursing & Health Care, 11*(4), 296–300.

Meleis, A., & Price, M. (1988). Strategies and conditions for teaching theoretical nursing from an international perspective. *Journal of Advanced Nursing, 10,* 417–427.

Merritt, S. L. (1983). Learning style preferences of baccalaureate nursing students. *Nursing Research, 32,* 367–72.

Merritt, S. L. (1991). The abilities and aptitudes of students must be considered in program design. *Nursing & Health Care, 12*(6), 240–242.

Norris, J. (1986). Teaching communication skills: Effects of two methods of instruction on selected learner characteristics. *Journal of Nursing Education, 25,* 102–106.

Nuernberger, P. (1984). Mastering the creative process. *The Futurist, 18*(4), 30–32.

Parnes, S. J. (1984). Learning creative behavior. *The Futurist, 18*(4), 30–34.

Russell, J. (1990). Relationships among preferences for educational structure, self-directed learning, instructional methods, and achievement. *Journal of Professional Nursing, 6,* 86–93.

Seidl, A., & Sauter, D. (1990). The new non-traditional student in nursing. *Journal of Nursing Education, 29,* 13–19.

Steinberg, R. (1985). *Human abilities: An information processing approach.* New York: W. H. Freeman & Co.

Stevenson, J., & Tripp-Reimer, T. (Eds.). (1990). *Knowledge about care and caring; State of the art and future developments.* Proceedings of the Wingspread Conference. Kansas, MO: American Academy of Nursing.

Valiga, T. M. (1983). Cognitive development: A critical component of baccalaureate nursing education. *Image: Journal of Nursing Scholarship, 15*(4), 115–23.

Wolfgard, M. E., & Dowling, W. D. (1981). Differences in motivation of adult and younger undergraduates. *Journal of Higher Education, 52,* 640–48.

Worrell, P. (1990). Metacognition: Implications for instruction in nursing education. *Journal of Nursing Education, 29,* 170–175.

Younger, J. (1990). Literary works as a mode of knowing. *Image: Journal of Nursing Scholarship, 22*(1), 39–43.

3

Nursing Process: A Practice Modality

The term *nursing process* is very much in the nursing literature. However, this inclusiveness does not necessarily imply that it is accepted as an integral part of practice or, indeed, even understood by many nurses practicing in the field in spite of the literature which addresses the nature of the process and its use in meeting clients' health care needs. Nursing process is the *methodology* of nursing practice. As such, it is learned in the clinical field through continuous practice. The concern of this book is the teaching of the process in the clinical setting, for nursing has many excellent authorities, such as Yura and Walsh (1988), Marriner (1983), Carpenito (1989), Ziegler, Vaughan-Wrobel & Erlen (1986), and Carnevali (1983), who address the process from the theoretical and practice perspective.

A CONCEPT OF NURSING PROCESS

Nursing process is a systematic series of sequential, but interrelated interdependent nursing actions with the ultimate goal of meeting a client's health need to the level of optimum wellness for that client. The client may be an individual, family, or community. The nursing process is primarily a cognitive activity, although the actions inherent in the process represent all three domains: cognitive, psychomotor, affective. According to Reilly and Oermann (1990), the process involves:

1. Intellectual operations, such as problem solving, concept formalization, inference reasoning, judgment, and decision making, and the application of theories, ideas, and concepts.
2. Value judgments based on the respect of the dignity and worth of human beings.
3. Psychomotor skills, both for assessment and intervention. (p. 194)

The potential variability of nursing activities ranging from simple to complex, which are inherent in the process, provide the nurse with a framework for individualizing client nursing care in terms of implicit and explicit needs determined by both the nurse and the client. The process sequence, defined by its four phases (assessment, planning, implementation, and evaluation), facilitates a systematic, logical approach to addressing real needs of clients. As with any process, it is a dynamic series of activities directed toward change. It is a process of care action with its own conceptual base. It is *not* a theory of nursing.

DERIVATION OF THE NURSING PROCESS

Florence Nightingale delineated nursing actions from physician actions, particularly in the realm of environmental and supportive measures to ease the discomfort and to facilitate the recovery of the patient. However, in the early years of nursing, most nursing and physician activities were palliative, for there was a limited knowledge base for intervening in the course of the disease. Patient care was shared by the two disciplines. With the advent of the germ theory and other scientific developments, an increasing array of intervention activities became available. Physician education moved into the university setting to receive the benefits of the knowledge gleaned from the developing scientific community. Nursing education, however, remained in the hospital setting, continuing to emphasize palliative and environmental measures with little impact from the scientific revolution that was occurring.

The separation of physician and nurse became increasingly more marked as scientific knowledge altered the delivery of care to the patient. Physicians could now intervene in the disease process, and because of the nurse's lack of scientific knowledge, the nurse began to see the patient through the "physician's eyes," and a pattern of nursing care developed which was composed primarily of delegated tasks. Nurses tended to patients in terms of designated medical intervention.

The movement of nurses into institutions of higher learning, especially after World War II which brought about the G.I. Bill, enabled nurses to obtain the critical biologic, behavioral scientific knowledge and began the evolution of a patient care modality in which nurses saw the patient through "their own eyes." This evolutionary movement has now reached the point where nursing research is addressing nursing's own science.

Nursing process has been one result of this evolutionary movement. The "seeing of the patient through one's own eyes" demanded a system of relating these observations to a method of nursing intervention in the patient's health problem. Yura and Walsh (1988) note that prior to the 1960s, the term nursing process was seldom seen in the nursing literature, although references to a process inherent in nursing practice was reported by Peplau (1952), Hall (1955), Johnson (1959) and in the early sixties by Orlando (1961) and Wiedenbach (1964). Nursing process is acknowledged as the mode of nursing practice, and nursing theorists have incorporated the essence of process into their theory development. In the nineties, precision in identifying nursing diagnoses, the last phase of the assessment process, has become the concern of nursing researchers and practitioners, for it is the nursing diagnosis that states the problem and directs all actions of the nurse toward meeting client needs.

Chinn and Jacobs (1985) see that the nursing process "has developed from a skeleton description of actions that were intended to replace rule-oriented and principle-oriented approaches to nursing with a more detailed description of the components of thought and action that constitute effective practice" (p. 29). Nursing practice viewed from the "nurse's eyes" now requires a more deliberative, thoughtful systematic activity that reflects judgment and creativity.

The evolution of nursing process as a systematic method has been influenced by the advent of systems theory which addresses whole phenomena and the dynamic interaction of its parts toward a clearly defined goal. The nature of wholeness is acknowledged in the nursing process, as all phenomena acting upon an individual in the health-illness spectrum is of concern to the nurse throughout the total process. Nursing process, defined as a sequential series of operations toward the goal attainment of optimal health for a particular client, reflects the nature of any system that synthesizes the actions of each part into a unified, goal-directed function.

Issues Surrounding Nursing Process

In the 90s as more philosophical discussions about nursing's essence and practice are occurring, questions relative to the appropriateness of nursing process as a methodology of nursing practice are being posed. The focus of some of the current dialogue relates to the philosophic base of the process itself. Nursing is viewed in accord with the philosophy of holism; the concern of nursing is the total human being as the primary focus of nursing actions whereby the individual is perceived from a unitary view, rather than the sum of its parts. Nursing process, the selected method of practice, is described within the context of a series of systematic phases which can suggest a linear, reductionist process. The inconsistency between the philosophic basis of the holism view of nursing and that of the perceived part vs whole approach in nursing process concern some nursing leaders such as Kobert and Folan (1990), Barnum (1987) and Fuller (1987).

Much of the concern centers around the incompatibility between nursing care based on the uniqueness and individuality of the total person and a process of care which consists of specifically designed phases that suggest rigidity and an unalterable sequence of actions. Barnum (1987) proposes that a problem-solving methodology would be more congruent with the holism view of nursing; yet, when nursing process was first proposed as a method of practice, it was perceived to be a problem-solving rather than a task-oriented method. Perhaps the current difficulty has not been so much with the process itself, but rather the way it has been interpreted, taught, and used in practice.

The definition of the process in terms of steps could readily lead to a sequence of concrete actions, rather than a dynamic flow of goal-directed actions. A defensive posture in accounting for each item in each step, particularly from a scientific context, leaves little opportunity for other ways of knowing in nursing, such as intuition and tacit knowing-in-action. Henderson (1982) questions whether nursing process is the right title, for it implies that it is the only approach to problem-solving, ignoring the role of intuition.

Nursing process, like the problem-solving method, does have a logical framework: recognition of cues to suggest the existence of a problem, delineation of the problem and strategies for solution, and evaluation of the outcome in terms of the stated problem. This sequencing does not suggest a rigid, linear, mechanistic pattern of actions, for closure of one of the phases is not a criterion for the onset of the next major series of actions. The interaction among the various phases is dynamic which accommodates new cues, new insights, new meanings. Formative evaluation is an inherent element in nursing actions, whether specific or tacit, and guides the practitioner toward the appropriate action within the total process.

Each of the phases in the process is composed of many other actions. Studies of nurses' approach to problem-solving indicate a proclivity toward concreteness derived from an empirical basis. This tendency to concreteness has impeded the use of nursing process as a true problem-solving process. Terms are used that reflect this concreteness, i.e., steps in the process, and when a holistic term, such as assessment, is used it is classified in several concrete terms. Assessment implies a decision, a value, derived from a certain data base. However, often in the literature or in practice, it is referred to as a concrete act of data gathering, requiring no interpretation or decision-making. Thus interpretation with the ultimate diagnosis or statement of the problem are considered to be sequential to the assessment process rather than an integral part of the process.

Several trends in the health care practice area portend some changes in the delivery of health care and the philosophic bases underlying the practice. Economic issues relative to the disbursement of money for health care are resulting in changing patterns that provide limited contact between the client and care-giver, such as ambulatory one day surgery, and limitations on time allocated in clinics for client's visit. These short-time contacts with little follow through will require more focused attention to the overt problems at hand and keener assessment skills on the part of the nurse to detect and interpret less obvious cues.

Computers using nursing information systems (NIS) are being introduced into the practice setting. Such systems directed toward patient care provide varied patterns of assessment data, data bases for facilitating the nurse's decision-making and various standardized nursing care plans. Brown (1991) sees these expert systems in nursing as contributing to the quality and efficiency of nursing care delivery. The inclusion of typical patterns of assessment and standardized care plans, however, have the potential for minimizing holistic care of clients. The possibility exists that nurses may accept the programs as projected and fail to pursue a more indepth study of the client from a holistic framework, thereby failing to make the appropriate alterations to accommodate the unity and uniqueness of the client.

Nursing process is a problem-solving activity within a logical framework which can be relevant to holistic nursing when viewed within both concrete and abstract contexts. The scope within which this process occurs will be affected significantly by the economic patterns for health care, needs of the client and the competencies of the nurse. In the following discussions, the various nursing actions in the process are explored with no intent of implying that the sequential actions must be viewed from a linear perspective. The nursing actions are presented as discrete items to identify the complexity of the actions that constitute each one.

NATURE OF NURSING PROCESS

Nursing process is a series of sequential interrelated phases in a goal-directed delivery of nursing care; yet the sequence is not inviolate, and there can be movement among the different phases. Various proposals have been made for the desired number of phases in the process, but there is general agreement that four steps comprise the essence of the process. The four steps and their operations are:

1. Assessment — Problem recognition
Data gathering
Data analysis
Nursing diagnosis
2. Planning — Desired goal setting
Priority setting
Selection of intervention measures
3. Implementation — Carrying out of nursing actions
Formative evaluation of actions
Change as indicated
4. Evaluation — Relationship of outcome to defined goals
Consistency of actions in process phases with pre-determined criteria and standards of care
Influence of structural variables on outcome and process (environment, agency policies and procedures, staffing in relation to quality and quantity)

These operations are reflected in the American Nurses Association (ANA) Standards of Nursing Care (1973) which serves as a valuable resource in process evaluation.

The sequence of the phases in the nursing process is comparable to that in the problem-solving process, but there are other significant processes involved. It is the development of these processes and their synthesis into a unified whole of action for delivering nursing care that is of concern to the teacher in the clinical field, since it is in this setting that actual delivery of care occurs. An examination of the various operations in the total process and each of the phases signals the charge to the nursing instructor.

Assessment

Assessment is an interactive process involving the nurse, client, family, and significant others in defining the health problem(s) to be addressed.

Skills in all three domains are involved. Cognitive skills in problem solving, concept formation, inference reasoning, critical thinking, decision making, and judgment are used. Intuition and knowing-in-action are other cognitive processes significant in this aspect of the process. Psychomotor skills which determine anatomic and physiologic functioning status provide critical data. Skills in valuing individual's rights to self-personhood and to be a participant in the assessment process as a primary source, when possible, are essential if data supplied are to meet the criterion of reality and human caring.

There are four parts to this phase: problem recognition, data gathering, data analysis, and nursing diagnosis. The term nursing diagnosis is here referred to as the use of categories in naming the health problem, but in reality all steps in the assessment process can be recognized as the *process* of nursing diagnosis.

Problem Recognition. This action is a function of the nurse's knowledge by which the nurse recognizes an implicit or explicit potential health problem which requires delineation of nursing actions. The stimulus may arise from the client, significant others, nurse, or other caregivers.

Data Gathering. Reflective of a holistic perspective of nursing, data are gathered on major matters related to clients' health. Client responses to occurring phenomena provide cues to the client's health status in relation to assets and deficits for handling the health problem and to the potential level of wellness if needs are met. Perception is a critical factor here, for data must reflect the client's or significant other's perception of events that are occurring as well as those of the caregivers. Knowledge of the anticipated pattern in relation to the suspected health problem direct the nurse in data gathering, but data must be within the context of other knowledge, which also influences client responses. Such knowledge includes cultural, social, interpersonal, systems, and patterns of communication. Gordon (1987) suggests important cues for data gathering which contribute to the nursing diagnosis:

1. Change in a client's usual pattern that is unexplained by expected norms of growth and development. (Change may be either positive or negative).
2. Deviation from an appropriate population norm.

3. Behavior that is nonproductive in the whole-person context.
4. That which indicates pattern development. (p. 191)

Cognitive skills of observation, communication, perception, and interviewing in concert with physical assessment skills provide the means for obtaining data. Basic to these skills is the nurse's repertoire of knowledge for appropriate retrieval.

Data Analysis. Cognitive functioning is the critical process in this activity, for more is involved than interpreting each discrete item of data on the basis of biologic or behavioral science principle. Analysis calls for information-processing strategies that depict the relationship among data, discriminate data cues suggestive of a real or potential problem from those that are reflective of wellness, and provide a basis for designating health problem(s) for which a course of nursing action is to be prescribed. Clinical knowledge recall, perceptual skills for seeing relationships among cues in the data field, and inferential reasoning are the significant intellectual operations during this stage. The significance of inference as a cognitive skill in data analysis is well recognized as the means by which the nurse is able to expand the boundaries of the data interpretation from a known data base to the unknown where explanations and predictions also can be derived from intuition and knowing-in-action. The judgment the nurse makes at this juncture to attest the relationship among data cues enables the nurse to cluster discrete data cues with common properties into cue sets or groups. Gordon suggests three possible errors in data clustering:

1. Premature closing—inadequate supporting data
2. Incorrect clustering—inadequate knowledge of critical signs and symptoms.
3. Not synthesizing—leads to error of omission. (pp. 290-291)

The clustering activity prepares the way for the final activity in the assessment step of the process. This activity is the identification of the nursing diagnosis.

Nursing Diagnosis. At the point at which the cue sets are identified, a concept of the health problem is ready to be stated as a nursing diagnosis. Lack of clarity and inconsistency still characterize the definition of nursing diagnosis. Gordon (1987) perceives nursing diagnosis as an actual or potential health problem amenable to nursing therapy. Carpenito

(1987) describes nursing diagnosis as a statement which notes the health state in an actual or potential alteration in one's processes. Shoemaker (1984) views nursing diagnosis as a clinical judgment of an individual, family, or community which has been derived from a systematic data collection and analysis. Carroll-Johnson (1990) cites the definition approved by the North American Nursing Diagnosis Association (NANDA) at the ninth general assembly in March 1990.

> A nursing diagnosis is a clinical judgment about individual family, or community responses to actual or potential health problems/life processes. Nursing diagnosis provides the basis for selection of nursing interventions to achieve nursing outcomes for which the nurse is accountable. (p. 50)

The general theme of these definitions is that a nursing diagnosis delineates the health status of a client. Two notions of the term, nursing diagnosis, are evident. The above definitions reflect nursing diagnosis as an outcome of a deliberate and systematic process of data collection and analysis. The term, nursing diagnosis, can also refer to the process itself. Weber (1991) describes this diagnostic process as she relates nursing diagnosis to nursing process within the reality of patient care.

The concept attainment reflected in the diagnostic category represents a clinical judgment, a decision on the part of the nurse which was derived from all activities in the assessment process. It is, however, a probabilistic statement, for clinical data are subject to differing perceptual interpretation on the part of the client and caregiver. Reliable and valid data arise from rigorous scientific investigation.

The categorization of health problems into nursing diagnoses is the most significant component of the nursing process, for it provides the focus for determining goals of care, the derivation of an appropriate realistic plan of care, the selection and use of pertinent nursing actions of intervention, and the evaluative judgments pertinent to the client's progress toward goal attainment. In other words, all therapeutic activities of the nurse involving the client arise from nursing diagnosis. It is a problem statement; not one of need or a way of meeting the need. It is important to emphasize that the diagnostic process and the resultant categorization are functions of nursing and its domains of practice and do not involve the diagnostic process of other health caregivers. A diagnosis of ineffective breathing patterns is a nursing diagnosis; a diagnosis of emphysema is a medical diagnosis.

The statement of a nursing diagnosis includes two major concerns: the substance of the statement and the classification system for selecting a diagnosis. Gordon (1987, p. 8) proposes three essential components in a statement of a nursing diagnosis, which she refers to as PES format:

P—*Health Problem* or health state of client stated in clear, concise words.

E—*Etiologic Factors*: the probable factors causing or maintaining the client's health problem; behaviors of client, factors in the environment, interaction of both.

S—*Defining signs and symptoms*: a cluster of critical defining signs and symptoms which permit discrimination among health problems. It is a subcategory of the diagnostic category.

In the 1990s the process of categorization of nursing diagnosis is an activity engaging many nurses at both the theoretical and empirical levels. This activity is a critical one, for any science must have a classification system which serves as a communication avenue among its practitioners and directs the activities of the group. In nursing it is an outgrowth of nurses seeing "the patient through one's own eyes."

Abdellah's 21 nursing problems (1960), McCain's schema of assessment in 13 problem areas (1965), and Henderson's 14 basic needs (1966) were early movements toward giving nursing its unique focus, different from that designated by the medical profession. In 1973, the First National Conference in Classification of Nursing Diagnosis was held in an attempt to define nursing's own classification system.

The first conference approached the task from an inductive methodology, which involves proceeding from the particular to the general. Nurses in practice described client health problems with which they were concerned during the course of their practice as a participant observer or through recall of previous experiences. Other nurse scholars, such as Campbell (1978), also used nurses in practice in their pursuit of nursing diagnoses labels.

By the third conference in 1978, a need for a conceptual framework was recognized, for there was no system by which data could be organized and classified. The use of a conceptual framework signifies a deductive approach, the movement from the general to the particular. It is apparent that both deductive and inductive methodologies will be used in the search for a classification system.

In 1986, Taxonomy I Revised was endorsed as a means of systematizing nursing diagnoses. Nine major categories that represent central human response patterns included in the taxonomy are:

1. Exchanging: mutual giving and receiving
2. Communicating: sending messages
3. Relating: establishing bonds
4. Valuing: assigning relative worth
5. Choosing: selection of alternatives
6. Moving: activity
7. Perceiving: reception of information
8. Knowing: meaning associated with information
9. Feeling: subjective awareness of information.

(NANDA, 1986)

Accepted diagnoses are subcategories of these patterns. A list of the NANDA approved nursing diagnostic categories (1990) are presented in Table 3-1.

A clinical validation of the diagnoses is the approach of the 90s with the ultimate goal of standardizing definitions and terms from an empirical basis. Two determinates from research are identified by Werley and Fitzpatrick (1985) as essential for declaring a diagnostic concept to be reliable:

a. Consistency of application to the same clinical data, across clients by one diagnostician.
b. Agreement in application across diagnosticians exposed to same clinical data.

Whatever system is eventually developed, it is essential that diagnoses are clear, concise statements acceptable to and understood by practitioners as well as investigators. Once categories are identified, they need to be validated; i.e., reliable indicators for each category must be determined before the classification can be standardized and incorporated into a nursing diagnosis taxonomy.

Table 3-1
List of Approved Nursing Diagnostic Categories (1990)

Activity Intolerance
Activity Intolerance, Potential
Adjustment, Impaired
Airway Clearance, Ineffective
Anxiety
Aspiration, Potential for
Body Image Disturbance
Body Temperature, Potential Altered
Breastfeeding, Effective
Breastfeeding, Ineffective
Breathing Pattern, Ineffective
Communication, Impaired Verbal
Constipation
Constipation, Colonic
Constipation, Perceived
Decisional Conflict (Specify)
Decreased Cardiac Output
Defensive Coping
Denial, Ineffective
Diarrhea
Disuse Syndrome, Potential for
Diversional Activity Deficit
Dysreflexia
Family Coping: Compromised, Ineffective
Family Coping: Disabling, Ineffective
Family Coping: Potential for Growth
Family Processes, Altered
Fatigue
Fear
Fluid Volume Deficit
Fluid Volume Deficit, Potential
Fluid Volume Excess
Gas Exchange, Impaired
Grieving, Anticipatory
Grieving, Dysfunctional
Growth and Development, Altered
Health Maintenance, Altered
Health Seeking Behaviors (Specify)
Home Maintenance Management, Impaired
Hopelessness
Hyperthermia
Hypothermia

Table 3-1 *(Continued)*

Incontinence, Bowel
Incontinence, Functional
Incontinence, Reflex
Incontinence, Stress
Incontinence, Total
Incontinence, Urge
Individual Coping, Ineffective
Infection, Potential for
Injury, Potential for
Knowledge Deficit (Specify)
Noncompliance (Specify)
Nutrition: Less than Body Requirements, Altered
Nutrition: More than Body Requirements, Altered
Nutrition: Potential for More than Body Requirements, Altered
Oral Mucous Membrane, Altered
Pain
Pain, Chronic
Parental Role Conflict
Parenting, Altered
Parenting, Potential Altered
Personal Identity Disturbance
Physical Mobility, Impaired
Poisoning, Potential for
Post-Trauma Response
Powerlessness
Protection, Altered
Rape-Trauma Syndrome
Rape-Trauma Syndrome: Compound Reaction
Rape-Trauma Syndrome: Silent Reaction
Role Performance, Altered
Self Care Deficit
   Bathing/Hygiene
   Feeding
   Dressing/Grooming
   Toileting
Self Esteem, Chronic Low
Self Esteem, Situational Low
Self Esteem Disturbance
Sensory/Perceptual Alterations (Specify)
   (visual, auditory, kinesthetic, gustatory, tactile, olfactory)
Sexual Dysfunction
Sexuality Patterns, Altered
Skin Integrity, Impaired

Table 3-1 *(Continued)*

Skin Integrity, Potential Impaired
Sleep Pattern Disturbance
Social Interaction, Impaired
Social Isolation
Spiritual Distress
Suffocation, Potential for
Swallowing, Impaired
Thermoregulation, Ineffective
Thought Processes, Altered
Tissue Perfusion, Altered (Specify Type)
   (renal, cerebral, cardiopulmonary, gastrointestinal, peripheral)
Trauma, Potential for
Unilateral Neglect
Urinary Elimination, Altered
Urinary Retention
Violence, Potential for: Self-Directed or Directed at Others

(From North American Nursing Diagnosis Association. St. Louis, MO)

Search for nursing theory is proceeding on many fronts in the eighties, all of which have an impact on the nature of the classification system. Although classifications arise from specific knowledge, values, and philosophies, in nursing there are diverse philosophies reflected in the notions of nursing as a science and practice discipline by the various theorists. The concepts of nursing diagnosis held by King, Neuman, Orem, Rogers and Roy are noted later in this chapter in Table 3-2; each suggests a different perspective and approach to problem solution. Can a classification system be developed that is understood by all nurses, yet accommodate to differing philosophies of nursing?

The notion of patterning as a function of nursing assessment appears in the nursing literature relative to nursing diagnosis. In an effort to address the diversity in perspective of nursing theorists yet recognizing the need for some unity in nursing practice for standardizing the assessment process, Gordon (1987) has proposed a typology of assessment areas, functional health patterns common to all clients. This typology attempts to provide unification of structural areas while leaving the approach to assessment and analysis of data to the domain of each of the theorists.

The 11 functional health patterns proposed by Gordon (1987) are:

1. *Health-perception–health-management pattern.* Describes client's perceived pattern of health and well-being and how health is managed.
2. *Nutritional-metabolic pattern.* Describes pattern of food and fluid consumption relative to metabolic need and pattern indicators of local nutrient supply.
3. *Elimination pattern.* Describes patterns of excretory function (bowel, bladder, and skin).
4. *Activity-exercise pattern.* Describes pattern of exercise, activity, leisure, and recreation.
5. *Cognitive-perceptual pattern.* Describes sensory-perceptual and cognitive pattern.
6. *Sleep-rest pattern.* Describes patterns of sleep, rest, and relaxation.
7. *Self-perception–self-concept pattern.* Describes self-concept pattern and perceptions of self (e.g., body comfort, body image, feeling state).
8. *Role-relationship pattern.* Describes pattern of role engagements and relationships.
9. *Sexuality-reproductive pattern.* Describes client's patterns of satisfaction and dissatisfaction with sexuality pattern; reproductive patterns.
10. *Coping-stress-tolerance pattern.* Describes general coping patterns and effectiveness of the pattern in terms of stress tolerance.
11. *Value-belief pattern.* Describes patterns of values, beliefs (including spiritual), or goals that guide choices or decisions. (pp. 431–434)

Issues Relating to Nursing Diagnosis

As nurses pursue the evolution of a valid and reliable categorical listing of nursing diagnoses, questions are being raised relative to the meaning of diagnoses within the phenomenon of nursing care. Those individuals in nursing who challenge the notion of nursing process relative to holism philosophy of nursing care see the incompatibility of nursing diagnosis to that philosophy of care. Nursing diagnosis as proposed by NANDA is perceived to be antithetical to holism by Ziegler et al. (1986) because of the restrictions it places on care of an individual to limited areas which are only addressed by nursing intervention. The question is being raised as to the scope of nursing diagnosis, i.e., should diagnosis include those matters which are under the purview of nursing, or should diagnosis also include health states (primarily physiological) which are concerns of other health care providers and require nursing referral? This approach is referred to as collaborative nursing diagnosis and is seen by Roberts (1987) as appropriate for critical care nursing where both medical and nursing interventions are required.

Porter (1986) questions the appropriateness of the use of a taxonomy to categorize nursing diagnoses, for the two criteria of a taxonomy, having an organizing principle which specified how the entities are classified and hierarchical in nature, are not in evidence.

Other concerns relate to the selection of nursing diagnoses on the basis of human responses. Human responses are often complex and defy a simple interpretation, thus acceptance of a behavioral diagnosis without further exploration could lead to inaccurate perceptions and actions. Several authors, Jenny (1987), Porkony (1985), and Dennison and Keeling, (1989) challenge the designation of knowledge deficit as a diagnostic category. Such a diagnosis implies need for promoting knowledge (teaching) when in fact, the deficit may reflect other behavioral problems related to fear, anxiety, dependency or cultural pattern. As of this writing, knowledge deficit as a nursing diagnosis is being questioned, but it still appears in the 1990 NANDA list. There is further concern that the diagnostic list will be used at face value and the deliberative process of reaching a nursing diagnosis will not be pursued.

Geissler (1991) notes the deficiency in the present NANDA listing of diagnostic categories which do not reflect cultural characteristics and factors antecedent to nursing diagnosis. The universality of nursing must be viewed within a transcultural context and human responses interpreted thusly. Ethical issues in the use of nursing diagnoses are the concern of Mitchell (1991) and Hagey and McDonough (1989). The use of labels to refer to or to identify patients' problems runs the risk of violating the principle of "to do no harm." Mitchell notes the serious consequences of labeling which can result in suffering and stereotyping when the personal meanings of human experiences are ignored. When there is incongruency between the nurse's and client's perspective of an experience or problem, there is a tendency to label the client as uncooperative or noncompliant. This latter word should not appear in the nursing language for clients have the right to choose or reject a course of action. Labeling narrows the problem and when applied to a client response, it can excuse the client or care-giver from pursuing any further therapeutic action.

Suffice to say, nursing diagnosis is a critical component of the nursing process. The standardization of the classification system is the province of nurse theorists, researchers, and practitioners, a task deemed necessary if nursing practice is to have a scientifically determined, goal-directed, orderly process for meeting health care needs of clients. Knowledge has advanced sufficiently at this time to enable nurses to accept the notion of nursing diagnosis and to develop practice modes in accordance with this notion, while still realizing that there is a probabilistic dimension to nursing diagnosis.

Planning

Nursing diagnosis sets the stage for the second step of the nursing process: the design for nursing care which addresses the client's health problem. Nursing literature includes much recent discussion concerning this step in the process by such authorities as Yura and Walsh (1988), Marriner (1983), Carnevali (1983), Bower (1982), and Carpenito (1987). Of particular concern in this book is the identification of the critical elements in this step that are significant to the teacher in the clinical field. Planning is an intellectual and ethical operation involving decision making, critical thinking, and value choice making. It calls upon the nurse to activate the problem statement into a process by which the solution is pursued. Bower (1982) notes three ethical issues which are of concern to nurses in planning care:

1. What is best for the client in order for maximum benefits to occur.

2. Whether the client's rights were protected when decisions were made about the plan.
3. Whether there has been justice in the way materials, resources, and time have been allocated to the client. (p. 134)

Goal Setting. The use of nursing diagnosis, a reflection of a clustering of signs and symptoms, rather than the use of each sign and symptom as a discrete item, enables the nurse to direct nursing actions in a holistic manner toward resolution of the total problem. The nursing diagnosis directs the nurse in the determination of goals, the desired outcome of care. These goals refer to the desired level of wellness/health status appropriate for the client and describe a state, condition, or behavior. The goals specified must be congruent with the goals of other caregivers for the concern is a unified approach in the management of the total needs of the client.

Goals are designated as either short-term or long-term, for the time variable is an important dimension. Short-term goals are noted in times of urgency or as interim steps toward a goal requiring a greater time span for achievement. Long-term goals recognize the health problem as an episodic event in the life activities of the client whose management greatly influences the quality of the total life span. Immediate short-term resolution is not an end in itself but must be viewed within the context of the client's total existence.

Participation of the client or significant others in the assessment process continues in this step of the nursing process, as goals must be mutually met by all concerned. It is imperative that both the caregiver and the client have the same perception of the desired goals so that there is a complementary and supportive interaction in problem resolution. Goal setting is a function of the nurse's knowledge and the client's acceptance.

Priority Setting. Often, multiple diagnoses are developed for an individual client and the nurse is called upon to determine a priority among the various goals since all goals cannot, or in all probability should not, be addressed at the same time. This process entails the establishment of a preferential order of goals which provides direction for nursing actions. Priority setting entails skills in decision making and judgment, drawing upon the nurse's repertoire of knowledge and the ensuing nursing action required.

Bower (1982) suggests ==three criteria for determining a hierarchy of importance of problems for priority setting==:

1. Those which threaten the life, dignity, and integrity of the individual, family, or community.
2. Those which threaten to change destructively the individual, family, or community.
3. Those which affect the normal developmental growth of the individual, family, or community. (pp. 22-23)

In addition to the criteria stated above which relate to the nature of the health problem, other factors may be considered in establishing priorities. In some instances, the treatments the client receives may have a high priority because of their impact on promoting or maintaining the integrity of the individual's functioning. Treatments may be those prescribed by nurses or by other caregivers, such as physicians or specialty therapists. The relationship of nursing actions to those of other caregivers must be considered in any priority setting for there must be coordination of all actions involving the client. Factors such as availability of time for goal attainment, resources (finances, facilities, services, people) essential for therapeutic management, and the social, cultural, psychologic and spiritual meanings of events are important in the ordering of goals in those instances where the criterion of urgency does not apply. Priority setting requires skill in discriminating among various goals so that planning for care is congruent with the needs of the client and proceeds according to the range of intensity of these needs.

Selection of Intervention Strategies. The designation of a goal signals the need to determine strategies by which the nurse can intervene for purposes of resolving or ameliorating disturbances in response patterns and lead a client to the desired state of health as specified in the goals. As with the other parts of the planning process, the client or significant others are participants in the decisions.

Intervention modalities are directed toward the etiology factor, which is noted in the statement of the nursing diagnosis. Some selections are the result of convergent thinking, since therapeutic measures have been specifically identified as prescriptions for particular types of responses. However, in many situations, nursing prescriptions are not readily available and the need for divergent thinking resulting in creative management strategies is paramount. The nurse needs to be prepared to consider alternatives for intervention and should be willing to be a risk taker when proposing new strategies whose outcome is uncertain. A careful examination of the potential consequences of the action enables the nurse to anticipate the degree of risk involved and reach the decision as to whether or not to proceed with the action.

Although nursing does have some prescriptive actions for certain diagnoses which can be incorporated in a plan of care, many times even the prescription has to be evaluated in terms of its appropriateness to a particular client. Gordon (1987) suggests six areas of information that are essential in individualizing interventions for a particular client:

1. Personal client factors—unique characteristics.
2. Client's perception—particularly any misconceptions related to etiology.
3. Current level of compensation—resources, strengths.
4. Problem magnitude and urgency—type and timing of nursing actions.
5. Extended effects—influence on other areas of client's life.
6. Cost-benefit factors—financial, social and psychologic. (pp. 313–314)

Individualization in the selection of nursing intervention actions calls upon, once more, the nurse's ability to be creative in the selection of alternatives, each of which has the capability to address the health problem.

Nursing practice includes a repertoire of intervention modalities available to the nurse. Three different forms of nursing action are proposed by the Nursing Theories Conference Group (1980):

1. Assuming responsibility for a person until he or she is able to be responsible for self.
2. Changing (manipulating) environment to facilitate health.
3. Helping person toward some goal. (p. 216)

Therapeutic communication skills of listening, observing, interacting, and transacting with clients are important methods by which the nurses use themselves in the process of care. Teaching is a communication skill which is a significant intervention strategy, ranging from information sharing to assisting the client in developing new patterns of functioning. Teaching is a function of nursing, and its substance for any particular client is derived from the assessment process, inclusive of the diagnostic statement which delineates the knowledge status of the client. Teaching selected for a care plan addresses knowledges the client needs to cope with a real or potential disturbed health state and to partake in one's own care during the illness episode and that which is essential for promoting or maintaining an optimum level of wellness.

The development of a protocol for teaching a client is the prerogative of the nurse functioning in accord with the stated nursing standards. Nurses who rely on physician approval for the plan and its implementation view teaching as a delegated function rather than a nursing function. Protocols for teaching clients in a health care setting need to be reviewed and approved by a nursing board, not a medical board, as happens in some settings. Teaching methods selected for the plan relate to the goals to be achieved, the ability and resources of the learner, and the nature of the material to be learned.

Psychomotor skills represent many intervention strategies, which may be either for restorative or supportive purposes. Their selection is determined by the problem to be addressed, and their actions may be carried out solely by the nurse, solely by the client, or by both. The range of skill involved varies from the simple to the complex, which calls upon more than one psychomotor skill for the total operation. The selection of the appropriate skill is a judgment decision on the part of the nurse; however, the client is afforded the opportunity to be a part of the decision-making process and to be fully informed as to the procedure and what is entailed in the skill.

The American Nurses Association Social Policy Statement (1980) indicates that the aims of nursing actions are to ameliorate, improve, or correct conditions to which those practices are directed to prevent illness and promote health. The planning for all actions recognizes the integrity of the individual as a total phenomenon.

The selection of intervention strategies may be prescriptive or it may be exploratory requiring validation. Regardless of the derivation of the strategy, the nurse must be able to predict the probability that such a measure will be effective in meeting the desired outcome of care. The prediction is a function of the nurse's knowledge about nursing actions and their relationship to various health–illness phenomena.

Implementation

This is the action phase of the process and represents the implementation of the nursing plan. It demands not only skill in performance of the activities, but the process of perception and observation in the continuous appraisal of the actions as they occur. It requires critiquing skills as the actions are viewed in terms of goals to be achieved and the original data base on which they were based. Nursing judgments are made and decisions are often arrived at to modify actions or to obtain other types of data when there is a suggestion that the client is not being moved toward the desired goal. Judgments are also made about the interrelationship of nursing interventions and those of other caregivers who are also ministering to the client. The interventions of all concerned must be complimentary and directed toward the desired health status goal.

Nursing textbooks contain detailed information of various intervention modalities which nurses use for designated purposes. It is sufficient here to acknowledge that this phase includes the "doing" for, about, or with the client and the use of feedback to ascertain the effectiveness of the "doing" or the need for alternative approaches when intervention is not achieving the desired result.

Evaluation

The fourth phase in the nursing process, evaluation, is concerned with the quality dimension of care. It answers such questions as: Were client outcomes achieved? If not, why not? How was the process executed? What events in the setting influenced positively or negatively the outcome and the process? Answers to these questions rely upon professional judgment based on skills of perception, analysis, and knowledge retrieval.

Most references to this phase in the process include the evaluation of process and outcome. Little emphasis is placed on the role assumed by characteristics of and events in the setting in influencing both process and outcome. Donabedian (1969) refers to three components in assessing the quality of health care: structure in which health care occurs, process of care, and the outcomes of care.

Outcome, the health characteristics, behavior, and states which were specified as goals following the diagnostic process, are the foci of the nurse's evaluation efforts in terms of the effectiveness of care. They are assumed to be the result of interventions, although such a causal relationship is difficult to ascertain because of the inexactness of predictability. The outcomes are client centered, i.e., what happened to the client; not caregiver centered in terms of the quality of the performance.

Process is another focus of evaluation of the nursing process. Phaneuf (1976) describes the actions involved:

Evaluation of process of care entails appraisal of all major or minor steps taken in the care of the patient with attention to the nature of the rationale for, and the sequence of the steps and the degree to which they help the patient reach specified and attainable therapeutic goals. (p. 21)

Evaluation questions address the comprehensiveness and accuracy of the assessment, the precision of the inferences and resulting diagnosis, the relevance of the goals of care to the stated diagnosis, the appropriateness of the plan components, and the effectiveness of the implementation activities.

The American Nurses Association Standards of Nursing Care (1973) provides a framework for this activity, for the standards are described from a nursing process perspective. Generic standards and specialty standards are available. The nursing audit is another means for evaluating the process of care.

Structural variables are significant in their impact on both process and outcome, yet they are seldom incorporated in the evaluation protocol of direct care. They are more likely to appear in quality assurance programs of a total health care delivery service. The beliefs, values, policies, and procedures of an agency; the quantity and quality of the staff of nursing and other caregivers and support services; the availability of resources needed for care; the financial resources of the institution; the interpersonal interaction patterns; and the management style with particular emphasis on locus of decision making all influence the ability of the nurse to carry out the nursing process. An evaluation of care without consideration of the role played by some of the variables mentioned above can often produce spurious results.

Evaluation is a critical activity in the nursing process. At this stage, it is a summative evaluation, a declaration of *what is* in contrast to formative evaluation which is ongoing in the previous steps, particularly in implementation, which states *what is and what can be*. Appraisal of client outcome in relation to the total effect and the structural variables' influences on the process and its outcome constitutes an effective framework for professional judgment as to the quality of nursing care.

Data dealing with outcome collected at this time are valuable resources for determining the effectiveness of nursing's impact in the health care delivery system. Compilation of outcome data and their interpretation related to cost factors, decrease in recidivism, and effective use of time and resources would be most influential in portraying the real significance of the nurse as a health care provider.

NURSING PROCESS—NURSING FRAMEWORKS

Earlier, the nursing process was identified as the methodology of nursing, the means by which the delivery of nursing care is administered to clients. The substance of that delivery system is determined by the framework of nursing beliefs accepted by an individual nurse, a nursing service, or a school of nursing. It is the belief about nursing that gives direction to the activities inherent in the nursing process. It is generally accepted that professionals go to the theory base of their discipline to obtain the basis for curriculum and program development, research, and practice. The very fact that the discipline exists provides the source of authority for its practitioners (Reilly, 1975).

Nursing is in pursuit of its own science as various theorists in nursing propose their philosophic notions of nursing and the relevant elements and their relationships which characterize the practice. (See Table 3-2; text continues on page 94.) Some theorists have operationalized their beliefs into a pattern of practice, while others have described

Table 3-2
Nursing Process According to Five Nursing Theorists

	King*	Neuman*
Definition of Nursing	Nursing is a helping profession involving a process of action, reaction, interaction and transaction whereby nurse and client share their perceptions in the nursing situation through: purposeful communication; identify specific goals, problems, or concerns; explore means to achieve a goal; agree to means to the goal; and both move toward goal attainment.	Nursing is a unique, wholistic profession concerned with all variables affecting a client(s)' response to environmental stressors. Nursing actions are appropriate to the total needs of the client on his/her own wellness/illness continuum toward providing optimum client/client system stability or wellness.
Goal of Nursing	Promote health: i.e., help individuals and groups attain, maintain, and restore health and if not possible,	Promote client/client system integrity through retention, attainment, and/or maintenance of an optimal

* Updated by theorists, 1991.

(Continued on page 82)

Orem*	Rogers*	Roy
Nursing is a human service whose concern is the individual's need for self-care and the provision and management of it on a continuous basis in order to sustain life and health, recover from disease or injury and to cope with their effects. Conditions that validate the existence of requirement for nursing as an adult are the absence of ability to maintain continuously that amount and quality of self-care which is therapeutic in sustaining life and health, in recovery from disease or injury or in coping with their effects. In children, the condition is the inability of parent (or guardian) to maintain continuously for the child, the amount and quality of care that is therapeutic.	Nursing (nursing science) is the science of irreducible human and environmental energy fields arrived at by a synthesis of facts and ideas commensurate with a new world view; an organized system of abstract knowledge; a new product. The practice of nursing is the imaginative and creative use of nursing knowledge for human betterment. The science of irreducible human beings basic to nursing requires a new world view and an abstract system specific to nursing's phenomenon of concern. People and their environments are perceived as irreducible, pandimensional energy fields integral with one another and continuously creative in their evolution. It is postulated that people have the capacity to participate knowingly in the process of change.	Nursing is a scientific way of providing care for the ill or potentially ill person which acts through nursing process to promote adaptation in each of the four modes of adaptation in situations of health and illness.
Dependent upon the therapeutic self-care demand and self-care deficit, goals are to	Promotion of optimum well-being within the potential of individuals and groups through	Promotion of a person's adaptation in physiologic needs, self-concept, role function,

(Continued on page 83)

Table 3-2 *(Continued)*

	King*	Neuman*
	help individuals die with dignity.	functional or wellness level for the client.
Concept of Nursing Process	Nursing is a process of human interaction leading to goal attainment. It is a process of action, reaction, interaction, and transaction where nurse/patient share mutually set goals and move toward goal attainment. Nursing process is the standard method used in most nursing situations which has identified some of the essential functions of the nurse: assessment of patient's health, formulation of a plan on the basis of information gathered, implementation of a plan of care, and evaluation of its effectiveness.	Nursing process is systemized into the following three categories: Nursing diagnosis—Accomplished by acquisition of comprehensive appropriate data base and synthesis of theory for determining variance from wellness from which hypothetical interventions can be made to reach the desired client/client system stability or wellness level. Nursing Goals—Arrived at by data related to theory and client negotiations for prescriptive change which form the bases for nursing intervention strategies and are postulated to retain, attain and/or maintain client/client system stability. Nursing Outcomes—Affected by use of one or more prevention as intervention modes (primary, secondary, and/or tertiary) to confirm client prescriptive change. Short-term goal

(Continued on page 84)

Orem*	Rogers*	Roy
(1) protect or promote the individual's capabilities for rendering care to self, (2) meet the person's therapeutic self-care demand, (3) promote the capabilities of the dependent care agent for rendering care to patient.	use of descriptive, exploratory principles distinctive of this organized abstract system. Nurses are concerned with all people whomever they are and whether they may be deemed well or sick.	and relations of interdependence in situations of health and illness.
Consciously selected activities directed by the nurse toward accomplishing nursing goals within a health care situation which involves 3 steps: (1) determination of why a patient needs nursing care, (2) design of a nursing system specific to the patient's needs, (3) initiation, conduction, and control of assisting actions addressed to meeting the therapeutic self-care demand or to regulate the exercise in development of self-care agency or dependent care agency.	The application of the science of unitary human beings in continuously innovative ways through evaluative and noninvasive modalities directed toward actualizing optimum well-being for the individual, family and society.	A problem-solving approach required by client-centered goal of nursing and the need to verify the service the nurse provides which includes diagnosing patient adaptation problems and planning, carrying out and evaluating care.

(Continued on page 85)

Table 3-2 *(Continued)*

	King*	Neuman*
		outcome influences intermediate and long-term goal setting and possibility of reformulation of short-term goals.
Assessment Basis	Extent to which client is able to perform daily activities, cope with health and illness, and function in social role.	Extent to which there is actual or potential penetration of normal line of defense of usual wellness condition of the client by stressors which may be intra, inter, or extrapersonal in nature.
Data	Personal System *Perception:* Patient's perception of the event, sensory system integrity, chronologic age, developmental level, sex, educational level, nurse's perception of patient's perceptions *Stress:* Patient's stress and nurse's stress, potential anxiety, positive force in life, energy use, interference with perceptual system, drug and diet history *Self:* Client's perception of self, current health status, body image	Client/Client System *Stressors:* Identification of actual and/or potential environmental stressors, intra, inter and extrapersonal in nature *Client/Client System:* Basic structure factors, energy resources, flexible line of defense, normal line of defense, lines of resistance, potential for reconstitution *Client/Client System Stability:* Past, present and future life process factors, coping patterns, expectations *Client/Environment Interactions:* Intrapersonal, interpersonal

(Continued on page 86)

Orem*	Rogers*	Roy
Features that identify why a person requires nursing in relation to therapeutic self-care demand: capabilities and limitations for engaging in self-care, potential for further development of self-care capabilities and quality and quantity of self-care deficit in relation to therapeutic self-care demand.	Appraisal of the nature of human and environmental fields as manifest in field patterning. The integrality of human and environmental fields is a basic premise. Pattern manifestation appraisal is relative, continuously innovative, and characterized by non-repeating rhythmicities.	Extent to which the patient has achieved an adaptive state within four adaptive modes and cognator/regulator effectiveness in bringing about that adaptation.
Therapeutic Self-Care Demand: Particularization of each existent requisite, selection of method, and identification of care measured. *Universal Self-Care Requisites:* Adequacy of air intake, adequacy of water intake, adequacy of food intake, elimination and excretion processes, balance-rest and activity, balance-solitude and social interaction, existence and potential hazards to human life functioning and well-	*Manifestations of Field Patterning:* Change from: Lesser diversity to greater diversity; longer rhythms to shorter rhythms to rhythms that seem continuous; slower motion to faster motion to motion that seems continuous; time experienced as slower to times experienced as faster to timelessness; pragmatic to imaginative to visionary; longer sleeping to longer waking to beyond waking	First Level Adaptive Modes: Identification of patient behaviors in each adaptive mode and recognition of person's position on health-illness continuum *Basic Physiology Needs:* Nutrition, elimination, fluid and electrolyte, oxygen, circulation, regulation, exercise and rest *Self-Concept:* Physical self, personal self, interpersonal self Role Function: Role conflict, role

(Continued on page 87)

Table 3-2 *(Continued)*

King*	Neuman*
Growth and Development Status: Client's background, ability to carry out developmental tasks, ability to carry out activities of daily living	and extrapersonal environmental interactions are influenced by the five variables of man: physiologic, psychologic, sociocultural, developmental and spiritual
Body Image: Client's perception, influence of body image on lifestyle, family members' perception of body image	*Resources:* Internal, external system strength
Space: Perception of personal space, cultural interpretation of space and use of space as a form of nonverbal communication	*Perceptions:* Caregiver, Client assessed differences in perception must be negotiated.
Time: Perception of chronological and experiential time, altered perception of time	
Interpersonal Systems	
Communication: Patterns, communication between client, family, and caregiver; relevance of nonverbal communication	
Interaction: Purposeful, information component of interactions	
Transaction: Value component of interactions, perceptions of client and nurse; goal setting, and agree to means to attain goals	
Role: Perception of role of nurse, client, other professionals	

(Continued on page 88)

Orem*	Rogers*	Roy
being, evidence of need for action to protect normal functioning *Developmental Self-Care Requisites:* Living conditions: supportive, nonsupportive of life processes; conditions that promote, interfere with developmental processes; deleterious effects of conditions that affect human life and development *Health Deviation Self-Care Requisites:* Evidence of need to seek appropriate medical assistance, effects and results of pathologic conditions and status that set up requirements for care, effects and results of medically prescribed diagnostic, therapeutic and rehabilitation measures, evidence of discomforting or deleterious effects of medical measures, evidence of ability to accept self in a particular state of health or with specific forms of treatment, evidence of maintaining a lifestyle which	*Principles of Homeodynamics:* *Principle of Resonancy:* Continuous change from lower to higher frequency wave patterns in human and environmental fields *Principle of Helicy:* Continuous innovative, unpredictable, increasing diversity of human and environmental field patterns *Principles of Integrality:* Continuous mutual human field and environmental field process	failure, role mastery Interdependence: Need for affiliation, need for achievement, independency/dependency *Second Level:* Identification of focal, contextual, and residual stimuli relative to ineffective response behavior or client *Focal Stimuli:* Degree of change, stimulus is cause *Contextual Stimuli:* All other stimuli which contribute to behavior *Residual Stimuli:* Stimuli having an undetermined effect on behavior.

(Continued on page 89)

Table 3-2 *(Continued)*

	King*	Neuman*
	Stress: Environmental, present disturbance, past experience, coping mechanism	
	Social System–Environment: One of client/caregiver, concepts of organization, power, authority and decision making understanding of background of nurse/client demographic variables.	
	Social environment in which individuals grow, develop and perform activities of daily living.	
Nursing Diagnosis	Disturbance in health status resulting from interferences in the client's personal, interpersonal, and social systems.	Consists of variances from wellness as determined by analysis of a comprehensive, wholistic client/client system data base and theoretical considerations.
		Hypothetical interventions are postulated to reach the desired client stability or wellness level.

(Continued on page 90)

Orem*	Rogers*	Roy
promotes continued personal development		
Self-Care Agency and Potential for its Development: Repertoire of self-care practices, usual components of patient's self-care system, abilities and limitations for deliberate actions, knowledge, skills, and motivation to meet each particularized self-care requisite; what patient is able to do and does do to meet prescribed care/ measures of the therapeutic self-care demand; what patient should do, should not do, is willing to do, in meeting prescribed therapeutic self-care demands; potential for future exercise of self-care agency and its continued development.		
Existence of or potential self-care deficits by associated factors or combinations of factors with limitations for performing self-care operations specific to knowing and meeting a prescribed therapeutic self-care demand	Rather than diagnosis, descriptive statements based on principles of homeodynamics summarize manifest variations in rhythms, pattern, diversity and other mutual human and environmental field processes.	A statement of the client's adaptive behavior with the most relevant influencing factors as determined from the assessed data base.

(Continued on page 91)

Table 3-2 *(Continued)*

	King*	Neuman*
Planning	Setting of mutual goals between client and caregiver when possible, to move the individual toward health in the social system and joint planning on how the goals can be reached together. Interactions are critical in making transactions that lead to goal attainment; goals are influenced by client's and nurses' perceptions, backgrounds, values and health status. Priority setting is carried out mutually whenever possible.	Negotiation with the client for desired prescriptive change to correct variances from wellness, inherent in classified needs and resources identified in the nursing diagnosis. Appropriate nursing (action) intervention strategies are postulated for retention, attainment, and/or maintenance of client/client system stability or desired outcome goals.
Implementation	A Transaction *Personal:* Help patient maintain self-esteem and interact in ways that give patient choices to exert some control over environment; control environment and protect against too much intrusion on patient's personal space; schedule activities to meet the needs of the individual; control environment to limit unnecessary disruption in Circadian rhythms	One or more of three prevention as intervention modes are used to confirm prescriptive change for the client as follows: *Primary Prevention:* Action required to retain client/client system stability, i.e., maintain the integrity of the flexible line of defense by strengthening resistance to stressors *Secondary Prevention:* Action required to attain client/client system

(Continued on page 92)

Orem*	Rogers*	Roy
Based on why person needs nursing and the nurse's judgment about the kind and amount of nursing required. Contains details regarding time, place, and roles of nurse and patient. Designation of a system of nursing assistance based on patient defined self-care deficit: wholly compensatory; partly compensatory; and supportive-educative. Goal of action-compensate for patient self-care limitations to insure that self-care is given and is therapeutic and to enable patient to regulate the exercise or development of self-care capabilities.	Developed on the basis of pattern manifestation appraisal with evaluative and non-invasive modalities used to attain optimum well-being for the individual and group. Deliberative mutual patterning is predicated upon irreducible wholeness of the human being and derives its safety and effectiveness from the integral nature of change. Planning encompasses both preservation and enhancement of a meaningful life and meaningful transitions from living through dying. Individual and groups knowingly participate in the planning.	Setting goals determined by relative importance of the problem with intent of changing ineffective adaptive response to adaptive behavior or of reinforcing adaptive behavior. Intervention actions are selected on the basis of influencing stimuli that can be managed. To effect change and stabilize adaptation, possible approaches are listed with the highest probability of achieving the goal selected.
Modes of helping are: acting for, teaching, guiding and directing, supporting (physical and psychological), providing developmental environment, initiation, conduction, and control of assisting actions to achieve nursing results that are related to identified therapeutic self-care measures and to self-care limitations and capabilities.	Based on principles of homeodynamics and theories distinctive of this organized abstract system. It includes individualization of services coupled with creativity in integrating nursing knowledge for continuously innovative use of evaluative and non-invasive modalities. Tools of practice require intellectual skill for their safe and competent	Intervention attempts to manage the environment by removing, increasing, decreasing, and/or altering stimuli related to ineffective response. When possible, focal stimulus is channeled first. Nurse is the external regulatory force to modify stimuli affecting adaptation on the part of the patient.

(Continued on page 93)

Table 3-2 *(Continued)*

	King*	Neuman*
	Interaction: Goal-oriented interaction, move toward reciprocally contingent interaction, decrease stressors on patient and family, provide information, assist patient to verbalize concerns and expectations, minimize stress when carrying out procedures.	stability, i.e., mobilize client's internal and external resources to reduce reactions to stressors *Tertiary Prevention:* Action required to maintain client/client system stability, i.e., mobilize and utilize client internal and external resources to maintain the highest possible level of well-being following secondary prevention as intervention.
Evaluation	Identified goals and attainment of goals provides a measure of effectiveness of care. Client's perception in evaluating effects. Nurse's perception of changes. Goal-oriented nursing record is an information system that if implemented provides a permanent record for research studies and documents care to measure effectiveness. Goal attainment = outcome.	Client outcome following nursing intervention reflects the degree of confirmation of prescriptive change. For example, nursing goals, designed in the planning phase, are measurable in terms of increased resistance to stressors, decreased degree of reaction and maintenance of a desired level of wellness following intervention because of a reaction. Evaluation of nursing outcome following intervention (action) confirms the degree of goal attainment. Reformulation or further goal planning may be desirable for subsequent nursing intervention. Client outcome thus validates the nursing process and the model from which it was derived.

Orem*	Rogers*	Roy
According to nursing system: compensate for patient's self-care limitations, overcome when possible self-care limitations of patient and family so future short-term and long-term therapeutic self-care requisites can be met effectively, foster and protect patient self-care abilities and prevent development of new self-care limitations.	identification and use. Tools include technical and manual skills, therapeutic touch, humor, imagery, meditation and multiple other means. Modalities based on motion, light, sound, and color are particularly useful.	
Can patient realize self-management and provide continuing therapeutic self-care? Do self-care limitations decrease? Do capabilities increase? What evidence of personal development and human well-being? Use evidence in evaluating results achieved against results specified in the nursing system design.	Appraisal is continuous, dynamic and reflects the nature and direction of change in irreducible human beings and their environments as manifested in field patterning. Client knowing participation is also essential in evaluating the effectiveness of nursing modalities.	Effectiveness of nursing intervention in client goal achievement; behavior-adaptive, movement toward peak health, individual needs of biologic, social, and psychologic integrity are met. Basis of judging effectiveness by result that nursing approach had regarding the client's adaptive behavior. If behavior still ineffective adaptation, reassess influencing stimuli to see if nursing approach should be modified by managing another stimuli.

their theory in abstract terms. Nursing literature is replete with data which describe the various frameworks of nursing, the ongoing research related to each, and the critiques, both positive and negative. All frameworks are abstractions, but some are postulated as theories, while others are referred to as conceptual representations. Reilly (1975) differentiates between these two frameworks:

> A conceptual model (framework) provides a perspective, a way of looking at nursing. It is a representation of reality since it is derived from and pertains to reality, but it does not constitute reality. A theoretical model (framework), on the other hand, does constitute reality since it has a scientifically accepted base. (p. 567)

Some nursing educational programs and nursing care settings have adopted a particular nursing theorist's framework or have developed an eclectic framework reflective of components from several theories, nursing and other disciplines. All such frameworks acknowledge the nursing process as the means by which nursing care is delivered to clients. In situations where no nursing framework exists, nursing process may or may not be the accepted mode. Orb and Reilly (1991) describe the process of a faculty in developing an eclectic model of nursing based on the interaction in the nurse-client-environment. This model is then described in a nursing process protocol, so there is consistency between the concept of nursing taught and the process by which nursing care is delivered.

Fawcett (1989) recognizes the role of conceptual models of nursing as a guideline for all aspects of practice. She concludes: "the model tells the clinician what to look at when interacting with clients and how to interpret observations. It also tells the clinician how to plan interventions in a general manner and provides beginning criteria for evaluation of intervention outcomes" (p. 30).

Gordon (1987) emphasizes the significance of a nursing model "because nursing diagnosis cannot be done without a *nursing model* that provides clear guidelines for the collection of clinical information. It is the model that delineates the data to be assessed, their rationale and the resultant nursing diagnosis" (p. 28). It is because at this time there is not one nursing theory or nursing science that Gordon proposes the use of functional health patterns, described earlier as a framework for assessment, so that there may be some consistency in the type of data collected. The meaning and interpretation of data remain within the realm of the nursing framework chosen by the individual nurse or the agency.

Table 3-2 depicts the nature of nursing process within the concept of nursing as described by five theorists. The theorists selected are not meant to be inclusive of all nursing theories, but are selected because they are at this time generally recognized in the nursing community and they reflect different levels of theory development. Their inclusion in this chapter is an attempt to emphasize that nursing process is not a suitable conceptual framework, as perceived in some schools of nursing and health care settings, but is in reality the means of operationalizing nursing as conceptualized in a framework.

TEACHING THE NURSING PROCESS IN THE CLINICAL SETTING

Because the nursing process is a practice model, the teaching for competency can only be obtained in a practice setting where students care for real clients with real or potential health problems. Attainment of competency requires a progression of experiences reflecting increasing complexity over a period of time which, although variable in accord with individual differences, is sufficient for development to occur.

A Holistic Process

The teaching of the nursing process must respect its holistic nature—four phases discrete in themselves but interrelated into a total phenomenon. It is the interrelationship among the phases that provides the essence of the process. Although, as noted earlier, each phase has its own goal, purpose and specialized tasks, its significance in patient care is only in terms of its relationship to the goals, purposes and tasks of the other phases. Data obtained in assessment are of little value if they are not formulated into a plan of care which denotes intervention strategies which are implemented and evaluated. Likewise, a technically developed plan of care not based on nursing diagnoses derived from comprehensive and accurate data, has no meaning for a particular client.

Bruner's notion of teaching the *structure* of a subject is particularly relevant to the teaching of nursing process, for it provides the student very quickly with a sense of the essence of nursing practice. Bruner (1963) states: "Grasping the structure of a subject is understanding it in a way that permits many other things to be related to it meaningfully. To learn structure, in short, is to learn how things are related" (p. 7). The ability to transfer knowledge of the subject to a more complex phenomenon is a function of the individual's ability to know the structure of the subject. Bruner suggests the notion of a spiral curriculum whereby the structure of the subject once learned, is related to increasing complex phenomena.

Nursing process needs to be introduced conceptually to students early in the educational program in terms of its structure as a holistic, interrelated activity which addresses simple to complex health problems. The repertoire of knowledge and skills inherent in each phase increases in complexity as the student carries out the process with increasing numbers or complexity of variables. The skill of the process remains constant; it is the different parameters with which the process is used that are the changeable element. The tendency to emphasize the complexity of the substance and of the skills of each phase as discrete items separate from the total process destroys the integrity of the process and precludes the ability of the student to see the unitary nature of the process. The tendency to view nursing process primarily in terms of complex variables negates the essence of the process and interferes with the student's ability to see its interrelationships.

The following vignette describes the experience of a student in her beginning clinical practical experience:

I noticed that my patient was sad, for she was very quiet and did not want to see anyone. When I questioned her about her sad expression, she told me that she was embarrassed at the way she looked. Usually she went to the hairdresser weekly, but she had been in the hospital over a week and she knew she looked terrible. I asked her if she would like to learn to set her hair while in the hospital so that she could do it at night and her hair would look nice in the daytime. She expressed interest, so I bought some curlers and showed her how to use them. The next day when I went into her room, I saw her smiling and she commented on how proud she was of her new accomplishment.

Did the student experience the nursing process?

1. Assessment

    Data gathering:

    Client quiet; did not want to see anyone; stated distress over appearance of hair.

    Hospitalization interfered with pattern for hair care.

    Interpretation:

    Failure to maintain usual hair care resulted in lessening of self-image.

    Nursing diagnosis:

    Withdrawal from interaction with others because of poor self-image due to inability to provide for usual hair care.

2. Planning

    Goal:

    Meet client's need for hair care.

    Interventions:

    Mutually agreed to by nurse and client.

    Teach client to set her own hair.

3. Implementation

    Curlers purchased.

    Client taught to set her own hair.

4. Evaluation

    Client's self-image regained.

    Greeted student with a smile.

    Expressed pride in new skill.

This simple example is developed to emphasize the point that the teaching of nursing process in its entirety is not dependent upon a vast array of knowledge and skills. There are many opportunities to assist the beginning student to care for a client in terms of the nursing process so that the interrelationships among the phases can be perceived before more complex judgments and decisions are involved. That is, the structure of the process and its relationship to the practice of nursing must be taught early in the first clinical experience. As the parameters with which the process is used increase, so do the cognitive, psychomotor, and affective skills to carry out the process. Regardless of the character of the parameters, the integrity of the nursing process as a holistic activity is maintained in the teaching.

Skills in Nursing Process. As noted in the discussion thus far, nursing process entails multiple and diverse skills in the three domains of learning, namely cognitive, psychomotor, and affective. The charge to teachers of clinical nursing is that each of the relevant skills are mastered so that they can be synthesized into this critical process for delivery of nursing care. Subsequent chapters address the teaching of these skills within the clinical setting which are relevant not only to nursing process, but to the other dimensions of roles that nurses assume within the practitioner role.

Cognitive Skills in Nursing Process. Because nursing process is itself a cognitive activity which addresses not only what nurses do, but how they arrive at what they do, special consideration is given here to the issues in teaching cognitive skills that are directly related to nursing process, particularly in the crucial step of making a nursing diagnosis. As the process of categorizing nursing diagnosis proceeds in professional arenas, the process by which nurses make nursing diagnoses for clients has become of concern to nursing educators, practitioners, and researchers.

Skill in diagnosing requires more than data collection and a decision for action. It requires the ability to attach meaning to the data, not each datum as an entity in itself, but rather, meaning to the conglomerate of data obtained so that some sense of the client's health status is determined. Diagnosing is an abstract concept which entails cognitive information processing skills, and involves clustering of cues and making inferences so that a valid meaning is established. Concept formation in nursing diagnosis is a complex process, for it is a disjunctive concept attainment task. This task, as described by Bruner, Goodnow, and Austin (1956), entails analysis of cues, not all of which are related. That is, a diagnosis that is made does not preclude the notion that other diagnoses also must be made. In working with client data in nursing, more than one diagnosis is the usual rather than the unusual. This activity contrasts with the conjunctive concept attainment task where all data are related to each other and one diagnosis is possible.

It is the process between data collection and action that the instructor must stress, for studies at this time suggest that nurses are not engaging in a theoretical process of diagnosing. DeBack (1982) studied senior nursing students' ability to make nursing diagnoses from a case history. Three criteria were used in evaluating the diagnosis skill:

1. Client rather than disease centered.
2. Stated in terms of client concerns and level of competence in dysfunction.
3. Statement of client concerns, competence in dysfunction that can be altered or maintained through nursing action. (pp. 29-30)

Results of the 200 analyses suggest there is much work to be done in teaching diagnostic skill. While 56 percent of respondents could meet the first criterion, only 34 percent could meet the second criterion. It is this criterion that is especially critical, for it directs the intensity and strategy selection for nursing care. It also requires skills of concept formation, inferential reasoning, and knowledge recall. The third criterion was obtained by less than half (49 percent) of the respondents. While one may accept the notion that some of the difficulty is a function of the state of the art in nursing diagnosis, data from the study suggest more emphasis on management of client data is in order.

Cognitive skill development is essential for nursing diagnosis and, thus, must be of considerable concern to the instructor because of the role nursing diagnosis assumes in directing client care. The nursing instructor needs to reckon with what the student does with the data as well as what data were collected. Acknowledgement of the impact of one's own biases, preconceived ideas, and knowledge limitations is essential in helping students examine data. Simon (1947) speaks of "bounded rationality" as limiting the ability to make accurate decisions. This concept refers to the limitation of completely objective rationality. Of particular note is the danger of limitation on data collection and cue interpretation when students have preconceived notions of what ought to be the cues that accompany certain dysfunctional states.

Putzier et al. (1985), in their study of the thinking strategies of practicing nurses and nursing students relative to a diagnostic reasoning model, support this concern. Data suggest that the clinicians and novices develop mindset toward favored hypotheses resulting in underutilization of disconforming data and over estimate the value of the information concerned with the favored hypotheses. Premature acceptance and rejection of cues results in failure to gather sufficient information, therefore the diagnosis is often inaccurate or limited. This difficulty may in part be a function of the nurse's tendency to think in concrete terms, i.e., approach cues as discrete data rather than think in abstract terms which generates multiple cues for discrimination as to significance and fosters the development of interrelationship among relevant cues.

In addition to concern about the data themselves and the way they are interpreted is the process by which they are clustered and inferences made. It is the information processing skills that are often lacking in the educational process. Many nursing care plans which are developed as learning experiences, in contrast to those used in practice, do not provide for demonstrating cue clustering and inferential reasoning. Data are presented as discrete items, each described and interpreted from some scientific perspective. A quantum leap is then required to state a nursing diagnosis (although even this step is often omitted) and to design plans of action, often related to each datum collected. The critical step which demonstrates the information-processing behavior before nursing diagnosis or action is seldom seen in such a plan. Nursing plans of this type foster the notion of nurses as "doers" who respond to what they see without the deliberative processes that provide a reasonable validation of clients' needs on the basis of accurate and relevant data.

Cognitive skills are the baseline for competency in using the nursing process. Of particular concern in this chapter are the information processing skills that are essential if a valid nursing diagnosis is to be made. The process of teaching these cognitive skills within the clinical setting is described in Chapter 7.

CONCERNS REGARDING THE TEACHING OF NURSING PROCESS

Although nursing process has been an integral part of many nursing curricula during the past decade, its success in practice has been varied. Some of the issues to explore in this matter relate to question, by whom, for what purpose, and how has this aspect of nursing been taught?

Teachers of nursing, whether in the academic or clinical environment, have been charged to assist learners develop mastery of this practice skill. The belief systems of the teachers in terms of the nature of nursing process and its role in the delivery of nursing care greatly influence the quality of the outcome of the teaching. Is the process viewed and therefore taught as a problem-solving process? Or is it viewed as a procedure rather than a goal-directed dynamic process, thus being taught from a routinized, mechanistic, linear perspective? A further question relates to the teachers' understanding of the theoretical basis of nursing process so that they can conceptualize the process within the context of nursing's accountability to provide quality care to the clients. Nursing process is *action*. It results in an outcome. Confusion as to the nature of nursing process is evident in some expressions and activities of teachers and practitioners. One hears reference to application of nursing process. A process is an action in itself; it cannot be applied, it can be used. Some student assignments request a written nursing process. Since process is action; it cannot be written. Some parts of the process can be written, i.e., assessment, planning, and evaluation, but the intervention actions must be carried out in practice.

A major concern in teaching nursing process is the teacher's perception of the process relative to its wholeness or to its parts. A procedural approach emphasizes parts in a rigid sequence and each is treated as a discrete entity. A problem-solving approach emphasizes the total process where parts are not discrete in themselves but are interwoven into the whole and seen within the context of the whole. The whole is a gestalt in itself, not reflecting the addition of the parts.

Teaching of nursing process must acknowledge its dynamic nature and assure that as the various skills inherent in the process are taught, they are seen within the context of the whole. The role of formative evaluation as the process proceeds is well recognized. Evaluation data obtained through this process may alter the planned course of action at any point, which may mean that more data or data analysis are required or other intervention strategies are in order.

Two activities that are prevalent in many nursing curricula reflect this tendency to see a part of the process as an end in itself. Nursing care plans are important learning experiences within the nursing process. However, they are often overly emphasized in some programs as written assignments, and since they are not necessarily carried through to practice they may be seen as outside the nursing process. The excess use of this experience beyond its value to student learning often is perceived as busy work by students. Reilly and Oermann (1990) recommend that the use and frequency of this learning strategy is justified in terms of its educational value, and students need to be moved as quickly as possible into the mode of planning in the clinical setting. The nursing care plan is to be seen within the context of the total nursing process and not outside of it.

Another learning experience within nursing process that has the potential of being seen as an entity outside the process is the development of a teaching plan for a client. This does not refer to group instructional programs designed for clients with similar needs. It does refer to the development of a teaching plan for a client which is separate from the nursing plan. Learning needs are an essential component of assessment, and after careful data analysis the specific learning need is identified and stated. The plan of care incorporates the provisions for addressing the needs and they are met within the total intervention protocol. Evaluation is then carried out and decisions are made. Teaching is one of the important intervention strategies of nurses and must be used under the same principles relating to use of other strategies. It needs to be seen as integral to the total nursing process. When planning for teaching is separated from the total process, it is often viewed as outside the realm of the usual nursing actions and may become a victim of time pressures.

Because nursing process is the mode of nursing care delivery, it is essential that it not become a classroom entity but that it become an integral part of nursing behavior in the practice setting. The learner needs to be assisted in seeing how the new skills being learned relate to the total process of client care. The student also needs help in problem-solving thinking about client concerns. Peer reviews at clinical conferences where students present the processes they went through in meeting client needs are helpful in enabling students to engage vicariously in the client care being presented and determine the logic and relevance of the presenter's actions. Emphasis in such seminars and other activities is placed on the whole process, not any one part. The dynamic nature of nursing process as it is being used with various clients is the critical dimension of teaching, not the rigidity of a sequence of steps.

SUMMARY

Nursing process is a methodology of practice. It is the mode through which a theory or concept of nursing is operationalized into the delivery of nursing care. Because it is a practice modality, its mastery is attainable in the clinical setting where the learner is a participant in the care of real clients with real or potential health problems. The client may be an individual, a family, a group, or a community.

Nursing process is primarily a cognitive activity encompassing cognitive, psychomotor, and affective skills. Each of its four phases (assessment, planning, implementation, and evaluation) has its own constellation of skills that must be learned and synthesized into the total process.

The teaching of the nursing process requires the need to protect the integrity of the total process so that its phases are not viewed as separate phenomena, but rather as interrelated activities producing a whole. Introduction to nursing process early in the education program emphasizes its structure, its relationship to other dimensions of nursing. The principle of teaching from simple to complex is relevant as the student learns to use the process with increasingly complex variables necessitating increasingly complex skills.

The movement of the profession toward establishing a nursing diagnosis classification system places a particular challenge to instructors in the clinical setting to facilitate the learner's development of cognitive skills essential for handling client data so that valid nursing diagnoses can be made and the planning and delivery of care is congruent with the diagnoses. Nursing process addresses not only doing for or with the client, but also the means by which the nurse arrives at the decisions to take a particular course of action.

REFERENCES

Abdellah, F. G., Beland, I., Martin, A., & Matheny, R. (1960). *Patient centered approaches to nursing*. New York: MacMillan.

American Nurses Association. (1973). *Standards of nursing practice*. Kansas City, MO: Author.

American Nurses Association. (1980). *Nursing, A social policy statement*. Kansas City, MO: Author.

Barnum, B. (1987). Holistic nursing and nursing process. *Holistic Nursing Practice, 1*, 27-35.

Bower, F. (1982). *The process of planning nursing care* (3rd ed.). St. Louis: C.V. Mosby.

Brown, P. (1991). Computers in nursing practice. In M. Oermann, *Professional nursing practice: A conceptual approach* (pp. 197-215). Philadelphia: J.B. Lippincott.

Bruner, J. S. (1963). *The process of education*. New York: Vintage Books.

Bruner, J. S., Goodnow, J., & Austin, G. (1956). *Study of thinking*. New York: Wiley.

Campbell, C. (1978). *Nursing diagnosis and intervention in practice*. New York: Wiley.

Carnevali, D. (1983). *Nursing care planning: Diagnosis and management* (3rd ed.). Philadelphia: Lippincott.

Carpenito, L. (1989). *Nursing diagnosis: Application to clinical practice* (2nd ed.). Philadelphia: Lippincott.

Carroll-Johnson, R. (1990). Reflections on the ninth biennial conference. *Nursing Diagnosis, 1*, 50.

Chinn, P. L., & Jacobs, M. (1983). *Theory and nursing*. St. Louis: C.V. Mosby.

DeBack, V. (1982). The relationship between senior nursing students' ability to formulate nursing diagnosis and the curriculum model. In B.J. Brown, & P.L. Chinn (Eds.), *Nursing education: Practical methods and models* (pp. 21-36). Rockville, MD: Aspen Systems.

Dennison, P., & Keeling, A. (1989). Clinical support for eliminating the nursing diagnosis of knowledge deficit. *Image: Journal of Nursing Scholarship, 21*(3), 142-144.

Donabedian, A. (1969). Medical care appraisal—quality and utilization. In *Guide to medical care administration*, vol. 2. (pp. 2-96). New York: American Public Health Assoc.

Fawcett, J. (1989). *Analysis and evaluation of conceptual models of nursing* (2nd ed.). Philadelphia: F. A. Davis.

Fuller, S. (1987). Holistic man and the science and practice of nursing. *Nursing Outlook, 36*, 700-774.

Geissler, E. (1991). Transcultural nursing and nursing diagnosis. *Nursing and Health Care, 12*(4), 190-192, 203.

Gordon, M. (1987). *Nursing diagnosis; Process and application* (2nd ed.). New York: McGraw-Hill.

Hagey, R., & McDonough, P. (1989). The problem of professional labeling. *Nursing Outlook, 32*(3), 151-157.

Hall, L. (1955). Quality of nursing care. *Public Health News*. New Jersey State Department of Health.
Henderson, V. (1966). *The nature of nursing*. New York: MacMillan.
Henderson, V. (1982). The nursing process—is the title right? *Journal of Advanced Nursing, 7*, 103–116.
Jenny, J. (1987). Knowledge deficit: Not a nursing diagnosis. *Image: Journal of Nursing Scholarship, 19*(4), 184–185.
Johnson, D. (1959). The philosophy of nursing. *Nursing Outlook, 7*, 198–200.
King, I. (1981). *A theory for nursing: Systems, concepts, process*. New York: John Wiley & Sons.
Kobert, L., & Folan, M. (1990). Coming of age in nursing: Rethinking philosophies behind holism and nursing process. *Nursing & Health Care, 11*(6), 308–312.
Marriner, A. (1983). *The nursing process* (3rd ed.). St. Louis, MO: C.V. Mosby.
McCain, R. (1965). Nursing by assessment—not by intuition. *American Journal of Nursing, 65*(4), 82–84.
Mitchell, C. (1991). Nursing diagnosis: An ethical analysis. *Image: Journal of Nursing Scholarship, 23*(2), 99–103.
Neuman, B. (1989). *The Neuman's systems model* (2nd ed.). Norwalk, CT: Appleton-Century-Crofts.
North American Nursing Diagnosis Association. (1986). 21 new diagnoses and a taxonomy. *American Journal of Nursing, 86* (12), 1414–1418.
Nursing Theories Conference Group. (1980). *Nursing theories: The basis for nursing practice*. Englewood Cliffs, NJ: Prentice Hall.
Orb, A., & Reilly, D. (1991). Changing to a conceptual base curriculum. *International Nursing Review, 38*(2), 56–60.
Orem, D. (1991). *Nursing concepts of practice* (4th ed.). New York: McGraw-Hill.
Orlando, I. J. (1961). *The dynamic nurse patient relationship*. New York: Putnam.
Peplau, H. (1952). *Interpersonal relationships in nursing*. New York: Putnam.
Phaneuf, M. (1976). *The nursing audit: Self regulation in nursing practice* (2nd ed.). New York: Appleton-Century-Crofts.
Porkony, B. (1985). Validating a diagnostic label: Knowledge deficit. *Nursing Clinics of North America*.
Porter, E. (1986). Critical analysis of NANDA nursing diagnosis taxonomy I. *Image: Journal of Nursing Scholarship, 18*(4), 136–139.
Putzier, D., Padrick, K., Westfall, U., & Tanner, C. (1985). Diagnostic reasoning in critical care nursing. *Heart & Lung, 14*(5), 430–435.
Reilly, D. (1975). Why a conceptual framework? *Nursing Outlook, 23*, 566–569.
Reilly, D., & Oermann, M. (1990). *Behavioral objectives: Evaluation in nursing* (3rd ed.). New York: National League for Nursing.

Roberts, S. (1987). The role of collaborative nursing diagnosis in critical care. *Critical Care Nurse, 9*(4), 81–86.
Rogers, M. (1970). *An introduction to the theoretical basis of nursing*. Philadelphia: F. A. Davis.
Roy, C., & Andrews, H. A. (1991). *Roy adaptation model: A definitive statement*. Norwalk, CT: Appleton & Lange.
Shoemaker, J. (1984). Essential features of a nursing diagnosis. In M. Kim, A. McFarland, & A. McLane (Eds.), *Classification of Nursing Diagnosis Procedures of the Fifth National Conference*. St. Louis, MO: C.V. Mosby.
Simon, H. (1947). *Administrative behavior*. New York: MacMillan.
Weber, G. (1991). Making nursing diagnosis work for you and your client: A step-by-step approach. *Nursing & Health Care, 12*(8), 424–430.
Werley, H., & Fitzpatrick, J. (Eds.). (1985). *Annual review of nursing research*. New York: Springer 3, 127–146.
Wiedenbach, E. (1964). *Clinical nursing: A helping art*. New York: Springer.
Yura, H., & Walsh, M. (1988). *The nursing process* (5th ed.). New York: Appleton-Century-Crofts.
Ziegler, S., Vaughan-Wrobel, B., & Erlen, J. (1986). *Nursing process, nursing diagnosis, nursing knowledge*. Norwalk, CT: Appleton-Century-Crofts.

BIBLIOGRAPHY

Alfaro, R. (1986). *Application of nursing process*. Philadelphia: J.B. Lippincott.
Anderson, J., & Briggs, L. (1988). Nursing diagnosis: A study of quality and supportive evidence. *Image: Journal of Nursing Scholarship, 20*(3), 141–145.
Andrews, H., & Roy, C. (1986). *Essentials of Roy adaptation model*. Norwalk, CT: Appleton-Century-Crofts.
Bailey, D. (1988). Computer applications in nursing: A prototypical model for planning nursing care. *Computer Nursing, 6*(5), 199–203.
Barrett, E. A. (1989). (Ed.). *Visions of Rogers science-based nursing*. New York: National League for Nursing.
Baumann, A., & Deber, R. (1989). Limits of decision analysis for rapid decision making in ICU nursing. *Image: Journal of Nursing Scholarship, 21*(2), 69–71.
Becker, A. (1987). Nursing diagnosis: The past with NANDA. In K. Hannah, M. Reimer, W. Mills, & S. Letourneau (Eds.), *Clinical judgment and decision making: The future with nursing diagnosis* (pp. 89–93). New York: J. Wiley & Sons.

Donnelly, G. (1987). The promise of nursing process: An evaluation. *Holistic Nursing Practice, 1*(3), 1-6.

England, M. (1989). Nursing diagnosis, a conceptual framework. In J. Fitzpatrick, & A. Whall, *Conceptual models of nursing* (2nd ed.), (pp. 347-369). Englewood Cliffs, NJ: Appleton-Lange.

Field, P. (1967). The impact of nursing theory in clinical decision-making process. *Journal of Advanced Nursing, 12,* 563-571.

Gordon, M. (1991). *Manual of nursing diagnosis, 1991-1992.* St. Louis, MO: C.V. Mosby.

Jenny, J. (1989). Classifying nursing diagnoses: A self care approach. *Nursing & Health Care, 10*(12), 82-89.

Jenny, J. (1991). Self care deficit theory and nursing diagnosis: A test of conceptual fit. *Journal of Nursing Education, 30* (95), 227-232.

Jones, J. (1988). Clinical reasoning in nursing. *Journal of Advanced Nursing, 13,* 185-192.

Kritek, P. (1985). Nursing diagnosis in perspective: Response to a critique. *Image, Journal of Nursing Scholarship, 17*(1), 3-8.

Kritek, P. (1986). Diagnostics: The struggle to classify our diagnoses. *American Journal of Nursing, 86*(6), 722-723.

Levine, M. (1989). The ethics of nursing theoretic. *Image: Journal of Nursing Scholarship, 21*(1), 4-6.

Lindquist, G. (1990). Integration of international and transcultural content in nursing curricula: A process for change. *Journal of Professional Nursing, 6*(5), 272-279.

MacLane, A. (1987). Measurement and validation of diagnostic concepts. *Heart & Lung, 16*(1), 616-624.

Mitchell, P., Gallucci, B., & Fought, S. (1991). Perspectives on human response to health and illness. *Nursing Outlook, 39*(4), 154-157.

Moccia, P. (1988). A critique of compromise: Beyond the methods debate. *Advances in Nursing Science, 10*(4), 1-9.

Mollick, M. (1983). Nursing diagnosis and the novice student. *Nursing & Health Care, 4*(11), 455-59.

Neziolek, C., & Shaw, S. (1991). Professional practice: Whose plan-whose care. *Journal of Professional Nursing, 7*(3), 145.

Parker, M. (1991). (Ed.). *Nursing theories in practice.* New York: National League for Nursing.

Parsi, R. (1987). *Nursing science: Major paradox, theories, and critiques.* Philadelphia: Saunders.

Rasch, R. (1987). The nature of taxonomy. *Image: Journal of Nursing Scholarship, 19*(3), 147-149.

Riehl-Sisca, J. (1989). *Conceptual models for nursing practice* (3rd ed.). Norwalk, CT: Appleton & Lange.

Rios, H., Delaney, C., Kouckeberg, T., Younghae, C., & Mehment, P. (1991). Validation of defining characteristics of four nursing diagnoses using a computerized data base. *Journal of Professional Nursing, 7*(5), 293-299.

Roberts, S. (1987). The future marriage between diagnoses related groups and nursing diagnoses related groups. *Critical Care Nursing Quarterly, 9*(4), 70-81.

Roy, C., & Roberts, S. (1981). *Theory construction in nursing: An adaptation model.* Englewood Cliffs, NJ: Prentice-Hall.

Ryan, N. (1990). A nursing process methodology. *Nursing Outlook, 38*(4), 194-197.

Scahill, L. (1991). Nursing diagnosis vs goal-directed treatment planning in inpatient child psychiatry. *Image: Journal of Nursing Scholarship, 23*(2), 95-97.

Shanskey, S., & Yanni, C. (1983). In opposition to nursing diagnosis: A minority opinion. *Image: Journal of Nursing Scholarship, 15*(2), 47-50.

Sohn, K. (1991). One method for comparing different nursing models. *Nursing & Health Care, 12*(8), 410-413.

Stevens, B. (1984). *Nursing theory: Analysis, application,* evaluation (2nd ed.). Boston: Little Brown.

Taylor, F. (1988). Nursing theory and nursing process: Orem's theory in practice. *Nursing Science Quarterly, 1,* 111-119.

Turkos, B. (1988). Nursing diagnosis in print, 1950-1985. *Nursing Outlook, 36*(3), 142-144.

Turner, S. J. (1991). Nursing process, nursing diagnoses, and care plans in a clinical setting. *Journal of Nursing Staff Development, 7*(5), 239-243.

Vinvent, K., & Coler, M. (1990). A unified nursing diagnostic model. *Image: Journal of Nursing Scholarship, 22*(2), 93-95.

Walker, L. (1986). Nursing diagnosis and intervention: New tools to define nursing's unique role. *Nursing & Health Care, 7*(6), 7-18.

Watson, J. (1985). *Nursing: Human science and human care.* Norwalk, CT: Appleton-Century-Crofts.

Weber, G. (1991). Nursing diagnosis: A comparison of nursing textbook approaches. *Nursing Educator, 16*(2), 22-26.

Woodtle, A. (1988). Identification of nursing diagnoses and defining characteristics: Two research models. *Research in Nursing & Health, 11*(6), 399-406.

Yeo, M. (1989). Integration of nursing theory and nursing ethics. *Advances in Nursing Science, 11*(3), 33-42.

4

Clinical Practice Setting: A Learning Environment

Teaching is an interactive process which requires involvement of the teacher and learner in a supportive and facilitative learning environment. The psychosocial climate in which the teaching and learning take place is a major contributing factor to the learning responses of students and ability of the teacher to carry out the educational responsibilities. The climate for learning may support these individuals, impede them, or limit options for learning. A supportive learning environment is characterized by valuing learning; exhibiting a caring relationship for all concerned; providing for student freedom within structure for exploring, questioning, and trying out different approaches; accepting differences in others; and fostering the development of each individual.

In a profession like nursing, the learning environment provides for the development of new patterns of thinking, feeling, and doing that serve not only the individual but also the greater society. New knowledge is meant to be used by the nurse for the benefit of others. It is in the practice setting where the student develops knowledge and learns how to use it in service for others. In order for the reality of practice to be experienced by students, learning occurs in clinical settings which have goals other than educational. Service goals and learning goals may or may not be in competition, but their relationship greatly influences the character of the environment in which the student and faculty function.

CLINICAL SETTINGS FOR NURSING EDUCATION

In the clinical setting, the student learns to apply theories of action to real clinical problems, learns how to learn, develops skill in handling ambiguity, and becomes socialized into the profession. These purposes of clinical practice can be achieved in any setting where the student is involved in the practice of nursing.

Types of Clinical Settings

While clinical practice in nursing programs occurred traditionally in hospitals and public health agencies, more recently a wide range of clinical settings have come into use. The present scope of nursing practice and that projected for the future have resulted in different types of settings appropriate for use in a nursing education program.

The patterns of delivery of health care suggest that hospitals will continue to be centers for highly acute and critical care. Student experience in critical care nursing prepares learners for practice in these settings and for care of acutely ill patients in other areas of the hospital and in the home (Oermann, 1991). In a survey of baccalaureate nursing programs, Tanner, Hartshorn, and Rosenfeld (1989) reported that 95.2 percent of 371 schools surveyed offered content and learning experiences in critical care, including a clinical component with opportunities for direct patient care.

With the goal of preparing students for care of the elderly, clinical settings which serve the aged, whether healthy or ill, provide important experiences for learners. Reinardy and Quam (1989) described the use of senior high rises as a site for clinical experience in a nursing program. In this setting senior nursing students provided health care to elderly residents in the apartments. For two mornings per week, students staffed an office in the high rise buildings for walk-in residents and, in addition, delivered health care to referrals within the setting. Health promotion/support groups also were planned and implemented by the students. A faculty member from the school was available on-site with the students.

Other clinical settings devoted to health promotion and care of the elderly also have been recommended as possible sites for nursing student experiences. Lyles, Larisey, and Morrill (1988) reported on the development of a health promotion center for the aged established jointly by faculty and students of a BSN completion program and the local housing authority. A campus wellness vacation for elderly persons was developed to provide experiences with the healthy aged for registered nurses enrolled in a baccalaureate program (Feeley, 1991). Vacationers were senior citizens who were healthy and willing to spend five days living on a college campus. Student experiences focused on health assessment, interventions to meet primary prevention needs, and other aspects of health promotion and maintenance.

With the increase in the number of aged persons and projection as to a continued growth in the nursing home population, experience in nursing homes and other long term care settings is important in preparing students for future practice. Tagliareni, Sherman, Waters, and Mengel (1991) describe the effort among associate degree programs involved in the W.K. Kellogg Foundation Community College-Nursing Home Project to influence present and future care in nursing homes. Students have clinical experience in settings with the well elderly in the beginning part of the nursing curriculum; second year students have clinical experience in a nursing home. The outcome of this experience is to teach the student about care of the frail elderly and "empower students to provide new ways of caring" (Tagliareni et al., 1991, p. 250). Senior citizens programs and day care centers for the aged are other clinical settings which are appropriate for use in an educational program.

In nursing centers faculty and students provide direct patient care through the center which is under the direction of the nursing program. Barger and Crumpton (1991) describe a nursing center operated by a college of nursing, health district, and health department. The center provides learning experiences for students, a practice setting for faculty, opportunities for research, and nursing services to the community. Higgs (1988) reported that 65 schools of nursing had an academic nurse-managed center and 12 more planned on developing one. Clinical experiences through these centers "provide students with the opportunity to observe faculty members as clinical role models in control of their practice arena" (Higgs, 1988, p. 425). Development of skill in the delivery of primary care services is also facilitated in a nursing center. Some nursing centers provide experiences with specific client populations, such as centers devoted to services for children (Barger, 1988).

Nursing will be called upon increasingly to provide health education and promotion at the work place. Nursing services to keep people healthy and on the job are needed now and will be in the future. Clinical experience in occupational health settings provides a means of preparing students for future roles in these settings and other areas of practice with a focus on health promotion. Craig (1991) described a practicum experience in a large electronic corporation she completed as a student. In this clinical setting she engaged in health teaching, delivery of care services, and other aspects of health promotion.

Home care and community agencies provide valuable experiences for students particularly as more and more care is provided outside of hospitals. Harrington (1991) recommends collaborative efforts between schools of nursing and home care sites to improve care delivery and provide clinical experiences for students. Forker (1988) describes the integration of psychiatric mental health and community health nursing experiences into one practicum. Students are assigned to existing community health facilities which include a county health department; a mental health, mental retardation, and substance abuse facility; outpatient clinics associated with a hospital; and an experience in community geriatric care.

Along with traditional public health and community agencies, there are many other types of settings within the community appropriate for student clinical experience. Outpatient facilities; day care, ambulatory care, and rehabilitation centers; offices of physicians and other practitioners; and agencies and organizations within the community with a primary or secondary health care focus are settings to be considered for student experience. Clinics are valuable in providing experience in the care of specific client populations such as patients with AIDS (Matocha, 1990). These experiences are important in sensitizing students to the problems faced by clients and their families and important dimensions of their care (Oermann & Gignac, 1991).

Shelters for the homeless provide experiences which prepare students to be responsive to changes in society and the health care needs of clients who are underserved. The problem of homelessness, for instance, has continued to grow. The homeless are often faced with chronic health problems and may be unable to find treatment when ill. Witt (1991) describes the Homeless Health Care Project which serves two purposes: to provide nursing care to the sheltered homeless and assist nursing students in financing their education. In this project, in exchange for an eight-hour clinical experience in the homeless shelter, students receive funding for their tuition and credit for clinical courses. An important benefit of this clinical experience in a shelter is the gaining of insight into the way the homeless perceive their lives (Witt, 1991).

Other clinical settings include shelters for battered women, schools, and even prisons (Fontes, 1991). Any setting in which the student is involved in health care, in concert with the objectives of the experience, is appropriate for use in a nursing education program.

Purposes of Clinical Settings

Clinical settings have their own purposes which may be delivery of health care and other services for selected populations, education for practitioners and students in different disciplines, and in many settings conduction of research. Each setting has its own priorities among these various purposes which, in turn, dictate the options available for learning. In some settings, such as schools, health care delivery is secondary to a product goal, i.e., education. Health care is viewed as having a supporting role toward the ultimate goal of the organization.

Nature of Clinical Setting

The multipurpose goals of clinical settings have much to do with the kinds of services provided in the agency and types of personnel functioning there. Although the ultimate goal of health care agencies is the welfare of the client served, there is much potential for dissonance and discord as each group of individuals seeks its own territory and method of operation. This is particularly true in health care settings where there are two types of authority: (1) administrative authority and (2) professional authority. Administrative authority includes responsibility for the organization and functioning of the institution in terms of institutional goals, such as delivery of a service, efficiency, and cost effectiveness. Professionals may have other goals such as developing their own knowledge, skills, and professional practice and contributing to the body of knowledge of their disciplines.

The authority of professionals is necessary for effective practice. Schön (1990) describes a professional as one who has extensive knowledge and as a result of this knowledge, is accorded a "relatively high degree of autonomy in the regulation of his practice" (p. 32). Professionals need autonomy to engage in innovative practice and try out new ideas and strategies for the delivery of care. Professionals act independently in the use of professional knowledge; their decisions are their own, not dictated by institutional authority. The authority of the professional is based on this knowledge. Independent judgments and adherence to a professional code of ethics that extends beyond the organizational structure are consistent with professional practice (Deremo, 1989). An organization, health care or otherwise, needs to make accommodations between competing goals of the institution and professionals who function within it. The environment for learning is influenced by this accommodation of goals.

Individuals meeting service goals of an institution represent various levels of practice and accountability, generally with reasonably defined functions and expectations. The relationships among individuals within any group, for example nurse assistants and registered nurses, and between groups, such as physicians and nurses, may interfere with effective functioning within the organization, particularly when responsibilities are perceived differently by the parties involved. Such conflicts often arise because of problems in communication and changing demands on a professional group by expanding knowledge and technology and political, social, and economic decisions.

Every clinical setting has its own cultural values, norms, and expected behaviors. This cultural dimension serves to control the behavior of various individuals in the setting and provides sanctions for those who deviate. The cultural norms are directed primarily toward those who are providers of service. New entrants, such as students and clients, need to learn the expected behaviors and accommodate accordingly if they are to be accepted in the organization.

The clinical setting in which learner and teacher are to enter is multigoal-directed and multidisciplinary. It has potential for competition and conflicting forces influencing its activity at any one moment.

Rationale for Use of Clinical Setting in Nursing Education

Clinical practice provides experiences with real clients and real problems which enable learners to use knowledge in practice, develop skill in problem solving and decision making, learn how to learn, and develop a commitment to be responsible for one's own actions. Only in the clinical setting are there experiences for applying theories of action to real problems. According to Argyris and Schön (1976), a theory of action has not been learned unless it can be put into practice. Concrete situations to which these theories correspond are available in the clinical setting.

The clinical setting, however, is more than a place to apply theory to practice. It provides opportunity for developing problem-solving and decision-making skills and for collaborating with other disciplines in finding solutions to clinical problems. Experiences in the clinical setting facilitate development of skill in divergent thinking and ability to deal with the ambiguities inherent in clinical practice. Unpredictability, multiple distractions and variable time demands, sometimes interfering with learning, help prepare the student for reality.

Experiences in the clinical setting initiate students into the practice world enabling them to learn the conventions, constraints, language, systematic knowledge, and patterns of knowing-in-action of the professional (Schön, 1990, pp. 36–37). In the clinical setting students are faced with problems of clients and staff which do not have one right answer and presented with clinical situations which are unique and sometimes conflicting. Schön (1990) suggests that through the practicum experiences students learn that existing professional knowledge does not fit every case; they are faced with the need to learn a reflection-in-action which goes beyond the stable rules.

Schön (1990) describes a reflective practicum aimed at assisting students to acquire the kinds of artistry essential to competent practice in "unique, uncertain, and conflicted situations of practice" (p. 22). Much of professional practice includes problems which defy technical rationality; they are in the indeterminate zones of practice. Schön (1990) believes that competent practitioners generate new forms of understanding and action through their reflection-in-action undertaken in these indeterminate zones of practice. In clinical practice the student has opportunity to learn reflection-in-action, reason from general rules to problematic cases, and then develop new ways of thinking and approaching problems and new actions where familiar ones fail (Schön, 1990, p. 40). The student learns through the clinical experience how to think about and handle such problems, problems which are not solved by technical rationality. In clinical practice students learn to think like professionals, an important outcome of a nursing education program.

In the clinical area, learners observe variations in the responses of clients and encounter situations that challenge them to develop their knowledge and skills further. The practice setting is a place to learn how to learn because it fosters independence with learning and self-reliance and provides opportunity for questioning and seeking new knowledge. Students are challenged to examine and try out new modalities of care with clients and families. In clinical practice students devise new methods of reasoning, test new categories of understanding, and develop new strategies of actions (Schön, 1990).

Clinical experiences also provide the means through which the student becomes socialized into the profession and its values and learns to accept the notion of professional responsibility. The student is "initiated into the traditions of a community of practitioners and the practice world they inhabit" (Schön, 1990, p. 36). From this clinical experience, learners acquire an understanding of the role and responsibilities of the nurse and the way in which they carry out these responsibilities in practice. There is a transition from the role of student in the classroom and laboratory setting to practitioner responsible for care of real clients and problems.

Clinical practice provides opportunity for the student to develop a commitment to be responsible for one's own actions. In any clinical setting, the learner must be willing to accept responsibility for his or her own actions and for fulfilling commitments relative to practice. Even with beginning practice, it is important for the student to be accountable for identifying where further learning and guidance are needed and for carrying out the clinical activities for which responsibility was given and accepted. The development of a commitment to be responsible for one's own actions occurs most effectively through the student's clinical experience because the learner is faced with real clients and problems needing resolution. It becomes the student's responsibility to work with others to meet the goals of care within a specified time frame. The clinical setting places demands on the student, both in terms of performance and accountability, which assist the learner in developing an understanding of the meaning of professional responsibility.

DEVELOPMENT OF LEARNING ENVIRONMENT

A clinical setting rich in learning experiences but lacking a supportive environment discourages learners in seeking experiences and results in the loss of many opportunities for growth. Likewise, a setting with potentially limited experiences but rich in a supportive environment may provide opportunity for students to examine new health care needs and ways of addressing them. Regardless of the setting for clinical practice, the climate for learning is a factor in determining student achievement and satisfaction with the learning experience. The teacher and agency personnel influence the nature of this climate and degree to which it supports learning.

Faculty Responsibilities

Development of a climate for learning requires a teacher who is knowledgeable, clinically competent, skillful as a teacher, and committed to clinical teaching. It is important for faculty to examine their own beliefs and values about teaching and learning, their role in promoting learning, and the role of the student, for these influence how the instructional process is carried out and also the quality of the climate for learning. The teacher's attitudes toward students and staff affect interactions and the type of relationships established in the setting.

In a supportive learning environment, the teacher encourages independence with learning and self-reliance rather than fostering dependence and reliance on the teacher for sanctions, information needed for practice, solutions to problems, and evaluation of learning. With this independence the student learns how to learn.

In the clinical setting, students need freedom to explore, question, and dissent because without this, critical thinking is inhibited. In clinical practice the student can experiment in applying concepts and theories to practice, solving problems, and evolving new modes of care. To foster such experimentation, the learner needs freedom to try out different approaches with clients and staff. Taking calculated risks means that the decision to try a different approach was carefully made after considering the consequences. Teachers may not be sure enough of themselves to encourage such experimentation and thus may stifle the innovative potential of students. Teachers as advocates of students often must intervene with staff to facilitate student opportunities for trying out the "new."

Fear of making an error limits student development and willingness to experiment with care. Teachers, fearful themselves of student mistakes, often place unrealistic demands on learners for perfect practice. Mistakes are an inherent part of the learning process and in most clinical situations there is room for error. It is the faculty's responsibility to intervene in the decision-making process and in delivery of care to minimize the chance of the student making an error that would result in harm to the client. Errors are expected in beginning practice of new behaviors and skills regardless of the level of the learner. The climate for learning needs to be one in which teacher and student together examine failures and learn from them. Unless failures and mistakes are valued, there will be no learning from the experience. For the student to admit error, seek guidance from faculty, and value the feedback given, the relationship between teacher and student is characterized by trust and mutual respect.

In a supportive learning environment, the teacher accepts differences among students in their approaches to solving clinical problems and in the ways they analyze situations. Research suggests, for instance, that field-independent and -dependent learners vary in these approaches and style of interacting. Field-independent learners are high in analytical skills and favor tasks that require analysis rather than those that emphasize the interpersonal dimension. Field-dependent learners, in contrast, demonstrate less analytical skills and prefer situations involving interactions with others. Both types of competencies are needed in clinical practice.

In an environment which fosters independent learning, experimentation, and risk-taking behavior, students are still held accountable for their actions and for fulfilling commitments relative to practice. Learners in any clinical setting must assume responsibility for providing quality care, whatever the extent is of that care, and for carrying through with activities for which they accepted responsibility. Students must also be accountable for identifying their abilities and limitations in practice. It is important to emphasize that a supportive learning environment does not permit students to be free of responsibility.

The teacher is accountable for providing students with the clinical learning experiences needed to prepare them for practice. Lessner (1990) suggests three areas of legal concern to nurse educators: (a) issues related to student-university relationships, (b) tort liability, and (c) due process (p. 29). The university bulletin and other school documents, such as the student handbook, represent an agreement made between the students and university. These documents and the processes outlined in them are important for they guide the behavior of faculty and students in the clinical setting and have legal implications. Both teachers and students should be familiar with documents which describe the academic appeals process, ineligibility of a student to continue in the clinical setting, types of grades allowed for clinical practice, and other policies related to student experience in the clinical setting.

Lessner (1990) also emphasizes the need for an adequate data base when grading students in the clinical area, reflecting the requirements of the course and grading criteria (p. 30). This is important in justifying each student's grade so that no one is treated arbitrarily. Guidelines for evaluating clinical practice and grading the clinical experience are described in Chapters 11 and 12. The clinical objectives, requirements associated with the clinical experience, methods of clinical evaluation, and grading criteria should be written and distributed to students. Lessner (1990) recommends that educators keep anecdotal notes "which address the course requirements and the grading criteria" for each student in the clinical group (p. 30). Evaluative data and the progress of each student toward achieving the clinical objectives should be shared with the learner on a regular basis.

The second issue identified by Lessner (1990) relates to tort liability, including negligence and malpractice. An important principle in this area is that both faculty and students are held to the standard of care that a reasonable person would use in similar circumstances. Walker

(1989) describes this standard of care as that which "a reasonably prudent person with the same education and experience practicing in the same community would exercise under the same or similar circumstances" (p. 181). According to Lessner (1990), "a nursing instructor would not be considered vicariously liable for the negligent acts of his or her students" (p. 30). The teacher, however, would be responsible if she or he was negligent in supervising the student or assigned the student a task, procedure, or activity the teacher knew, or should have known, the learner was unable to perform (Lessner, 1990). Walker (1989) explains that "only an employer may be held liable for the negligent act of an employee" (p. 182); staff nurses, supervisors, and nurse educators are not employers. They are responsible, and subject to liability, for their own negligent acts, such as inadequate supervision of a student in the clinical setting. The teacher is responsible for facilitating students' learning in the clinical setting and adequately supervising their experience; students, in turn, have a responsibility for seeking guidance when unsure of nursing care.

The third area of importance to faculty teaching in the clinical setting is assuring that students have due process in disciplinary actions. This means that procedural requirements must be followed in situations such as ones involving academic appeal, lack of accountability and unacceptable behavior in the clinical setting, and plagiarism on clinical assignments. Lessner (1990) emphasizes that faculty should understand "which student issues require procedural due process action and what the appropriate action should be" (p. 31). The teacher in the clinical setting should be aware of the legal implications of statements in the university bulletin and school of nursing documents relevant to the teacher-student relationship, policies in the student handbook and other program documents related to clinical teaching, and the specific procedures to be followed in assuring due process for students.

Relationships with Agency Personnel

Development of a supportive climate for learning depends upon the relationships established between the teacher and agency personnel and between students and staff. These relationships influence the practice experience in terms of learning and the satisfaction of students, faculty, and staff with the experience. Development of collaborative relationships between faculty and agency personnel is essential for a supportive learning environment.

Collaboration is an ongoing interaction which occurs between professionals in which each person contributes from their own professional knowledge base to problem-solving. "Collaboration expresses the value that patient needs are multidimensional and should remain the focus of concern for all caregivers. Mutual respect among colleagues and open communication are the cornerstones of collaborative practice" (Dumont & Niziolek, 1991, p. 331).

Northouse (1991) suggests that collaboration "is a distribution of control or a give-and-take of control rather than a fixed dominance of one professional over another" (p. 190). Working relationships between faculty and agency staff are important in creating a positive environment for learning and taking advantage of the many opportunities available for student learning in the setting. Conflicts and misunderstanding among professionals interfere with positive working relationships. Northouse (1991) identifies three factors which promote effective interprofessional relationships: (1) clarifying roles in order for each professional to have an understanding of one another's roles, (2) sharing control in which faculty and agency personnel collaborate in planning student assignments and other experiences in the setting, and (3) maintaining contact through clear and continuous interactions between faculty and staff in the setting.

Knowledge of the objectives of clinical practice enables staff to assist faculty in identifying experiences available in the setting which might be appropriate. The teacher, in turn, is sensitive to requests of staff in relation to client care and other kinds of learning experiences. In many practice settings, staff has contact with students from various types of programs, including nursing and other health professions, who are at different levels of development, who have varying objectives to be achieved, and who engage in a wide range of learning experiences. It is no surprise that, at times, service personnel become weary regarding student experiences. Faculty should be sensitive to the purposes and priorities of the clinical setting and cognizant of the adaptations by staff necessary for implementing student experiences there. Agency personnel, in turn, need to recognize that because of varying clinical objectives and levels of students, the responsibilities of students and types of experiences in which they engage will differ.

There are a variety of efforts to blend education and practice in order to strengthen the ties between schools of nursing and clinical settings. The unification models at Rush University, University of Rochester, and Case Western Reserve University provide mechanisms for combining teaching, practice, and research. Although differences exist among these models, faculty has responsibility, in varying degrees, for teaching of students, client care, and research. Joint appointments with commitments to both education and service provide another means of enhancing the relationship between the two settings. With joint appointments faculty teach as well as provide a specific clinical service to the agency. Other strategies to strengthen the relationship between education and practice include models in which service personnel teach students in the role of adjunct and contracted faculty; programs in which faculty serve on agency committees and service personnel on school of nursing committees; collaborative financing of nursing education by hospitals and other clinical settings through the use of service-payback loans, scholarships, cooperative education programs, and externships; and preceptorships in which students have the opportunity to work closely with expert nurses in the clinical setting. The American Association of Colleges of Nursing established as one of its goals for schools of nursing to develop collaborative relationships with practice settings to advance the common goals in practice, education, and research (Hegyvary, 1991).

Regardless of the organizational relationship of faculty with the practice setting, the teacher is responsible for assisting students in working with staff. This requires clarifying the role and expectations of staff in relation to student learning and supervision in the clinical setting and establishing lines of communication among faculty, students, and agency personnel. The role of staff varies according to the objectives and type of experience. Preceptors, for instance, assume a different role with students than do staff nurses in a setting where the teacher provides on-site supervision.

Development of working relationships with agency personnel begins with the initial contacts made with the clinical setting and planning with agency staff for the practice experience. Initial meetings with agency representatives serve to clarify the nature of the practice experience, overall objectives to be achieved, and faculty role and responsibilities and provide opportunity for agency personnel to present requirements of the clinical setting and the agency's expectations of faculty and students. These meetings provide the basis for establishing a contract or formal agreement between the clinical setting and nursing program, usually negotiated by administrative personnel of both settings. Often, the nature of the practice experience influences whether a contract is necessary or if a letter of agreement is sufficient. A contract, usually stated in general terms, may be followed by a letter of agreement where the arrangements for the experience are detailed (Jones, 1983). A sample contract is shown in Table 4-1.

Subsequent planning conferences, involving the teacher and staff with whom the students will interact, are necessary to complete the arrangements and deal with the specifics of the experience. Orientation of staff to the objectives, student role and responsibilities, level of the learner, times in clinical setting and in contact with clients, faculty role, expectations of staff, and other details is accomplished in these planning meetings. The roles and responsibilities of the involved parties and specifics of the experience need to be mutually agreed upon and not dictated by either faculty or staff.

SELECTION OF CLINICAL SETTINGS

The clinical setting selected is important in achieving the objectives and purposes of clinical practice in a nursing education program. In some communities, selection of clinical sites is a difficult process because of competition among nursing programs for use of clinical settings, particularly hospitals and community health agencies. Access to patients has even become a problem in some ambulatory settings where nursing students compete for placement with medical, social work, and other students in the health professions (Jones, 1983).

Many of the settings traditionally used by nursing programs may not be appropriate for the diversity of objectives to be achieved in clinical practice, such as health promotion, care of families, and management of chronic health problems. Use of multiple sites for clinical practice is often needed to meet these program objectives and provide opportunity for the student to care for clients with varying health concerns and

Table 4-1

AGREEMENT[a]

XYZ   UNIVERSITY OF WASHINGTON
SCHOOL OF NURSING

The UNIVERSITY OF WASHINGTON SCHOOL OF NURSING, a public institution of higher education and XYZ, enter into the following cooperative agreement to provide educational experiences for students of the SCHOOL OF NURSING.

IT IS HEREBY AGREED:

1. The SCHOOL OF NURSING, through a designated faculty member for each student or group of students, will be responsible for instruction and administration of the students' educational program.

2. Within the scope of health care services provided by XYZ, the students will be given a desirable clinical learning experience. During this experience, the students shall in no sense be considered employees except if they are employed during time designated as not part of their educational program and will not be relied upon for patient care services to maintain the quality of patient care.

3. XYZ will retain full responsibility for the care of patients/clients and will provide administrative and professional supervision of the students insofar as their presence affects provision of health care services and/or the direct or indirect care of patients/clients. For placements under supervision of a preceptor, where the preceptor is an employee of XYZ, the XYZ shall retain full responsibility for administrative and professional supervision of the students while providing care for patients/clients.

4. The students and faculty of the SCHOOL OF NURSING will comply with the policies and procedures established by XYZ.

5. XYZ will make available to the students basic supplies and equipment necessary for the care of patients/clients and will make available, within the limitations of facilities, office and conference facilities for the students and, if applicable, faculty of the SCHOOL OF NURSING.

6. XYZ and the SCHOOL OF NURSING will plan jointly the evaluation of the students' learning experience.

7. The SCHOOL OF NURSING will require, at the beginning of each student's program, evidence of current immunizations against diphtheria, tetanus, poliomyelitis, measles, mumps, rubella (or have a positive rubella titer) and hepatitis B for students who will be engaged in the delivery of nursing care. Additionally, the SCHOOL OF NURSING requires routine (yearly) PPD testing *or* follow-up as recommended by Hall Health staff if the student is PPD positive or has had BCG.

Table 4-1 *(Continued)*

8. The University of Washington will hold harmless XYZ from any loss, claim, or damage arising out of the negligent acts or omissions of students or faculty associated with the educational programs of the University of Washington SCHOOL OF NURSING except for any such loss, claim, or damage arising out of the negligent acts or omissions taken, made, or occurring while under the administrative and professional supervision of XYZ pursuant to paragraph three above.

9. There will be no discrimination against any participant in the program covered by this agreement, or against any applicant for participation, because of race, religion, color, sex, handicap, age, or national origin, or status of disabled veteran or Vietnam era veteran, nor shall there be any such discrimination in the employment practices and personnel policies of either party.

10. This agreement will continue from year to year and will be reviewed at the request of either party. The SCHOOL OF NURSING and XYZ will jointly plan in advance student placement, taking into account the needs of the SCHOOL OF NURSING for clinical placements, maximum number of students for whom XYZ can provide educational experiences, and the needs of other disciplines or schools desiring clinical placements. This agreement may be canceled by written notice one year prior to termination.

OR

10. This agreement will continue from quarter to quarter and will be reviewed at the request of either party. Prior to each quarter student placements are to be made, the SCHOOL OF NURSING will provide a list of students and the name of the responsible faculty member to XYZ for concurrence. This agreement may be canceled by written notice one full academic quarter prior to termination.

OR

10. This agreement is to provide an educational experience for STUDENT for QQQ Quarter 199X and may be extended by letter to include additional student placements for subsequent quarters.

XYZ   UNIVERSITY OF WASHINGTON
                                       SCHOOL OF NURSING

BY: _____   BY: _____
    (Name of Administrator)   (Name of Administrator)

    _____   _____
    DATE   DATE

[a] This contract is from the School of Nursing at the University of Washington, Seattle, and has been reprinted here in its entirety with the permission of Dr. Sue Hegyvary, Dean.

participate with other disciplines in the provision of that care. Unfortunately, diversity places demands on faculty for expertise in practicing in different kinds of settings, for development of collaborative relationships with staff from multiple agencies, for obtaining information about the settings (their expectations and requirements, the availability of learning experiences and preceptors, and other specifics important in planning the experience), and for completion of arrangements with each agency. Use of multiple settings for clinical practice may also result in increased cost for the nursing program in terms of number of faculty, faculty time in planning for the clinical experiences, and travel time for faculty and students. Van Ort and Putt (1985) indicate that the cost of one hour of clinical instruction per student varies with each clinical setting, the number of students involved, and the faculty member's salary. It is important for faculty to weigh the benefits of using a large number of clinical settings with the associated demands on faculty and resources.

Criteria for Selection

The setting selected for clinical experience facilitates student achievement of the objectives and purposes of clinical practice in a nursing program. The selection of agencies depends primarily on the objectives for the specific course; other aspects to consider include the type of desired clinical experiences and level of the learner (de Tornyay & Thompson, 1987).

Several major criteria need to be considered in selecting settings for clinical practice. Critical in any setting is maintaining faculty responsibility for the practice experience. Hawkins (1981) reported this was one criterion faculty was not willing to compromise when choosing clinical agencies. The criteria are organized in four areas: (1) overall: setting and faculty, (2) clients, (3) staff, and (4) resources for students and faculty.

Overall: Setting and Faculty

1. Setting is licensed or accredited, as applicable
2. Administrative personnel and staff are flexible as to learning experiences, student time in agency, faculty role, on-site time of faculty, and other aspects of learning experience

3. Philosophy of clinical setting and nursing department is consistent with values and beliefs of faculty
4. Faculty is available to teach in setting
5. Faculty recognizes rights and responsibilities of setting
6. Evaluation of prior experience of faculty and students in setting reflects standards of nursing program
7. Costs associated with use of clinical setting are acceptable to nursing program

Clients

1. Client population is appropriate for objectives to be attained
2. Client population is sufficient in number for number of students to be placed in setting
3. Clients are present in setting an adequate amount of time for achievement of objectives
4. A range of learning experiences is available in setting
5. Nursing care practices are current
6. Nursing care reflects standards of practice and faculty values and beliefs
7. Resources (e.g., social service) for care of clients are available in setting and accessible to students
8. Client records are accessible to students and reflect current practices

Staff

1. Nursing staff is available to serve as preceptors, mentors, and in other roles, depending on the objectives
2. Staff collaborates with faculty and students in selection of learning experiences
3. Staff participates in orientation by faculty to experience and expectations and in evaluation of experience
4. Faculty and/or students are oriented by staff to clinical setting

Resources for Students and Faculty

1. Resources for student learning (e.g., staff development, library, reference materials) are available in setting
2. Space is provided for faculty and students to store personal belongings and have conferences
3. Setting includes dining facilities if none are available nearby.

Some criteria are of greater importance than others in relation to the objectives, and faculty makes this determination prior to reviewing potential settings. It may be necessary to add to the criteria presented here more specific ones depending on the philosophy of the nursing program, objectives to be attained in practice, and specific type of setting being considered. An instrument that incorporates the selection criteria and collects general information about the clinical setting as a whole, shown in Table 4-2, facilitates selection by providing a systematic way of reviewing potential sites and recording the data obtained.

Table 4-2
Instrument for Assessment of Clinical Setting

General Information:

Name of clinical setting _____

Location _____

Purpose _____

Contact persons (Name, title, and telephone number) _____

_____

_____

_____

_____

Type of setting _____

Client population (Describe) _____

_____

_____

_____

Table 4-2 *(Continued)*

Agency staff (Describe qualifications of staff with whom students would be working, include potential preceptors in setting)

_____
_____
_____
_____

Other disciplines practicing in setting _____

_____

Restrictions of setting (e.g., number of students, student time in setting, on-site time of faculty)

_____
_____
_____

Requirements for students and faculty (e.g., health screening, dress, name tags, list of students to be forwarded to setting)

_____
_____
_____
_____
_____

Resources for students and faculty (e.g., for learning, dining, parking)

_____
_____
_____

Contractual agreement: (1) Yes   (2) No   (3) Pending

Information given to clinical setting (e.g., school of nursing bulletin, course materials, clinical evaluation instrument)

_____
_____
_____
_____
_____

Table 4-2 (Continued)

	Yes	No	N/A[a]
Overall: Setting and Faculty:			
1. Is the clinical setting licensed or accredited, if relevant for this type of setting?			
2. Are administrative personnel and staff flexible as to learning experiences, student time in agency, faculty role, on-site time of faculty, and other aspects of the learning experience?			
3. Is the philosophy of the clinical setting and nursing department consistent with the values and beliefs of faculty?			
4. Is faculty available to teach in the clinical setting?			
5. Does faculty recognize the rights and responsibilities of persons in the setting?			
6. Do the evaluations of prior experience of faculty and students in the setting reflect standards of the nursing program?			
7. Are the costs associated with use of the clinical setting acceptable to the nursing program?			
Clients:			
1. Is the client population appropriate for the objectives to be attained?			
2. Is the client population sufficient in number for the number of students to be placed in the setting?			
3. Are clients present in the setting an adequate amount of time for student achievement of the objectives?			
4. Is there a range of learning experiences available in the setting?			
5. Are nursing care practices current?			
6. Does the nursing care reflect standards of practice and faculty values and beliefs?			

[a] Not applicable

Table 4–2 (*Continued*)

7. a. Are resources (e.g., social service) for the care of clients available in the setting? ____ ____ ____
   b. Are these resources accessible to students? ____ ____ ____
8. a. Do client records reflect current practices? ____ ____ ____
   b. Are client records accessible to students? ____ ____ ____

Staff:

1. Is nursing staff available to serve as preceptors, mentors, and in other roles, depending on the objectives? ____ ____ ____
2. Is the staff willing to collaborate with faculty and students in the selection of learning experiences? ____ ____ ____
3. Will the staff participate in orientation by faculty to the experience and expectations and in the evaluation of the experience? ____ ____ ____
4. Will the staff orient faculty and/or students to the clinical setting? ____ ____ ____

Resources for Students and Faculty:

1. Are there resources for student learning (e.g., staff development, library, reference materials) in the clinical setting? ____ ____ ____
2. Is there a place for faculty and students to store personal belongings and have conferences? ____ ____ ____
3. Are there dining facilities if none are available nearby? ____ ____ ____

Other:

1. ____ ____ ____
2. ____ ____ ____
3. ____ ____ ____
4. ____ ____ ____
5. ____ ____ ____

Evaluation of Clinical Setting

The decision to continue with use of a setting for clinical practice needs to be based on an evaluation of the setting and extent to which learners achieved the objectives for clinical practice. Criteria for the selection of clinical settings may be used for their evaluation. The identification of factors which promoted or impeded student learning provides a basis for modifying the practice experience if the decision is made to use the setting again.

Evaluation incorporates agency personnel, particularly staff most directly involved with the experience, and students. Inclusion of staff provides a means of identifying issues to be resolved and gives staff an opportunity to evaluate the experience and its role in it. Evaluation by learners of the clinical setting and of the experiences in which they engaged provides another source of data important in making the decision to continue or not with use of the setting. Sharing learner evaluations with members of the staff reinforces the importance of their role in the experience and assists them in modifying subsequent experiences. Evaluation by staff and students is particularly significant for those clinical settings in which there is minimal on-site faculty supervision, such as ones involving graduate students and preceptors.

When the setting no longer provides experiences for learners to attain the goals of clinical practice and when the objectives change and different characteristics of the practice setting become important, faculty needs to examine alternate sites for clinical practice. The decision to change clinical settings might also be based on continuing problems in the agency unable to be resolved by faculty, students, and staff.

The process of selecting a clinical agency and evaluating the experience may be viewed as a sequence of events, depicted in Figure 4-1, beginning with the objectives of the experience. An assessment of the setting determines its appropriateness for promoting attainment of these objectives and whether or not it meets other criteria for selecting clinical sites. Through collaborative efforts of faculty and staff, an environment for learning is established, and service and educational goals are both achieved. Formative evaluation carried out by faculty, students, and staff takes place throughout the clinical experience and provides continuous feedback to them. Formative evaluation is diagnostic in nature, informing faculty, students, and staff of problems

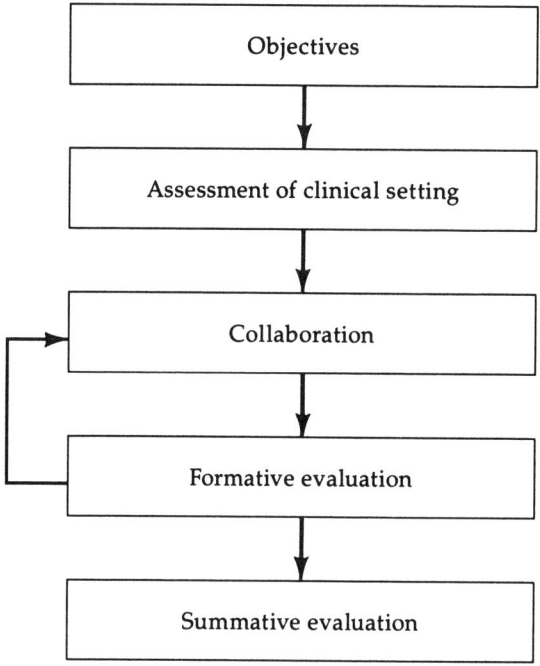

Figure 4-1
Selection and Evaluation of
Clinical Setting

with the practice experience needing resolution and confirming positive aspects. Summative evaluation, conducted periodically, serves to ascertain whether or not the clinical setting has provided the necessary experiences for achievement of the objectives and the impact on the agency of student experience there.

SUMMARY

Through experiences in the clinical setting, the learner acquires the knowledge, skills, and values necessary for professional practice and becomes socialized into the profession. In clinical practice, students apply theories of action to real problems, develop skill in problem solving and decision making, learn how to learn, and develop a commitment to be responsible for their own actions. Learning is enhanced in an environment which supports student independence and freedom to learn and provides opportunity for experimentation. The relationships established among faculty, students, and staff are important in creating a supportive climate for learning.

The purposes of clinical practice in a nursing program may be achieved in any setting in which the student is involved in the practice of nursing. There are many clinical settings appropriate for use in a nursing education program—hospitals, homes, community health agencies, schools, industry, ambulatory care centers, shelters, hospices, nursing homes, senior citizens programs, day care centers, and other agencies and community programs with a health focus. Since experiences in the clinical setting are critical in developing a practitioner capable of formulating a theory of practice, selection of clinical settings is a major faculty responsibility. Other responsibilities of the teacher in the setting involve development of collaborative relationships with agency personnel, planning with them for the practice experience, and periodic evaluation of the setting.

The practice setting is rich in learning experiences for students; granted a supportive environment, learners will be encouraged to engage in them. The teacher carries the major, but not the sole, responsibility for developing and maintaining this environment for learning.

REFERENCES

Argyris, C., & Schön, D. A. (1976). *Theory in practice: Increasing professional effectiveness.* San Francisco: Jossey-Bass.

Barger, S. E. (1988). Child development center—Nursing center partnership: A win-win arrangement. *Nursing & Health Care, 9*(3), 147-149.

Barger, S. E., & Crumpton, R. B. (1991). Public health nursing partnership: Agencies and academe. *Nurse Educator, 16*(4), 16-19.

Craig, C. A. (1991). Using unfamiliar clinical settings for RN students. *Nurse Educator, 16*(1), 18.

de Tornyay, R., & Thompson, M. A. (1987). *Strategies for teaching nursing* (3rd ed.). New York: John Wiley & Sons.

Deremo, D. E. (1989). Integrating professional values, quality practice, productivity, and reimbursement for nursing. *Nursing Administration Quarterly, 14*(1), 9-23.

Dumont, J., & Niziolek, C. (1991). The cornerstones of collaboration. *Journal of Professional Nursing, 7*(6), 331.

Feeley, E. M. (1991). Campus wellness vacation: A creative clinical experience with the elderly. *Nurse Educator, 16*(1), 16-21.

Fontes, H. C. (1991). Prisons: Logical, innovative clinical nursing laboratories. *Nursing & Health Care, 12*(6), 300-303.

Forker, J. E. (1988). The community as the site for psychiatric-mental health nursing clinical practicum. *Journal of Professional Nursing, 4*(6), 447-452.

Harrington, C. (1991). Why we need a teaching home care program. *Nursing Outlook, 39*(1), 10-29.

Hawkins, J. W. (1981). *Clinical experiences in collegiate nursing education*. New York: Springer.

Hegyvary, S. T. (1991). Collaborative relationships for education and practice. *Journal of Professional Nursing, 7*(3), 148.

Higgs, Z. R. (1988). The academic nurse-managed center movement: A survey report. *Journal of Professional Nursing, 4*(6), 422-429.

Jones, C. (1983). Negotiating student placements in ambulatory settings. *Journal of Nursing Education, 22*, 255-258.

Lessner, M. W. (1990). Avoiding student-faculty litigation. *Nurse Educator, 15*(6), 29-32.

Lyles, D. C., Larisey, M., & Morrill, L. S. (1988). Health promotion for the elderly: A student experience. *Nurse Educator, 13*(3), 23-26.

Matocha, L. K. (1990). Student clinical experience with persons who are HIV-positive or have ARC/AIDS: A model of success. *Journal of Nursing Education, 29*(2), 90-92.

Northouse, L. L. (1991). Communication and nursing practice. In M.H. Oermann, *Professional nursing practice: A conceptual approach*. Philadelphia: J.B. Lippincott.

Oermann, M. H. (1991). Effectiveness of a critical care nursing course: Preparing students for practice in critical care. *Heart & Lung, 20*(3), 278-283.

Oermann, M. H., & Gignac, D. A. (1991). Knowledge and attitudes about AIDS among Canadian nursing students: Educational implication. *Journal of Nursing Education, 30*(5), 217-221.

Reinardy, J. R., & Quam, J. (1989). Providing health services to elderly in public housing: A case for clinical experience. *Journal of Nursing Education, 28*(3), 127-132.

Schön, D. A. (1990). *Educating the reflective practitioner*. San Francisco: Jossey-Bass.

Tagliareni, E., Sherman, S., Waters, V., & Mengel, A. (1991). Participatory clinical education. *Nursing & Health Care, 12*(5), 248-250, 261-263.

Tanner, C. A., Hartshorn, J., & Rosenfeld, P. (1989). Critical care nursing in baccalaureate programs. *Nursing & Health Care, 10*(9), 483-488.

Van Ort, S. R., & Putt, A. M. (1985). *Teaching in collegiate schools of nursing.* Boston: Little, Brown.

Walker, D. J. (1989). Health care litigation: A case for professional liability coverage. In C. E. Lambert & V. A. Lambert (Eds.), *Perspectives in Nursing,* (pp. 176-195). East Norwalk, CT: Appleton & Lange.

Witt, B. S. (1991). The homeless shelter: An ideal clinical setting for RN/BSN students. *Nursing & Health Care, 12*(6), 304-307.

BIBLIOGRAPHY

Andrews, M. M. (1988). Educational preparation for international nursing. *Journal of Professional Nursing, 4*(6), 430-435.

Baker, C. M., Boyd, N. J., Stasiowski, S. A., & Simons, B. J. (1989). Interinstitutional collaboration for nursing excellence: Part 1, Creating the partnership. *JONA, 19*(2), 8-12.

Baker, C. M., Boyd, N. J., Stasiowski, S. A., & Simons, B. J. (1989). Interinstitutional collaboration for nursing excellence: Part 2, Testing the model. *JONA, 19*(3), 8-13.

Barger, S. E. (1991). The nursing center: A model for rural nursing practice. *Nursing & Health Care, 12*(6), 290-294.

Bevil, C. W., & Gross, L. (1981). Assessing the adequacy of clinical learning settings. *Nursing Outlook, 29,* 658-661.

Blazek, A. M., Selekman, J., Timpe, M., & Wolf, Z. R. (1982). Unification: Nursing education and nursing practice. *Nursing & Health Care, 3,* 18-24.

DeBack, V. (1991). The National Commission on Nursing Implementation Project. *Nursing Outlook, 39*(3), 124-127.

Eschbach, D. (1983). Role exchange: An exciting experiment. *Nursing Outlook, 31,* 164-167.

Gorman, M., & Morris, A. (1991). Developing clinical expertise in the care of addicted patients in acute care settings. *Journal of Professional Nursing, 7*(4), 246-254.

Haukenes, E., & Mundt, M. H. (1983). The selection of clinical learning experiences in the nursing curriculum. *Journal of Nursing Education, 22,* 372-375.

Hawken, P. L., & Hillestad, E. A. (1987). Weighing the costs and the benefits of student education to service agencies. *Nursing & Health Care, 8*(1), 223-227.

Klisch, M. L. (1990). The one-to-one relationship: An alternative to the psychiatric setting for baccalaureate students in psychosocial nursing. *Journal of Nursing Education, 29*(2), 92-94.

Lambert, C. E., & Lambert, V. A. (1988). Faculty practice: Unifier of nursing education and nursing service? *Journal of Professional Nursing, 4*(5), 345-355.

Neighbors, M., Eldred, E., & Sullivan, M. (1991). Nursing skills necessary for competency in the high-tech health care system. *Nursing & Health Care, 12*(2), 92-97.

Slimmer, L. W., Wendt, A., & Martinkus, D. (1990). Effect of psychiatric clinical learning site on nursing students' attitudes toward mental illness and psychiatric nursing. *Journal of Nursing Education, 29*(3), 127-133.

Sorensen, G., Gassman, A., & Walters, M. (1984). An experiment in a working relationship between nursing education and nursing service. *Journal of Nursing Education, 23,* 81-83.

Styles, M. M. (1984). Reflections on collaboration and unification. *Image, XVI,* 21-23.

Tu, K-S., Gay, J. T., McKay, J. (1991). Undergraduate clinical experience in health education. *Journal of Nursing Education, 30*(5), 235-237.

5

Student-Teacher Interactions Within the Clinical Practice Setting

Development of a climate for learning is concerned not only with the setting in which clinical practice takes place but also with the interpersonal relationship developed between the teacher and student and the way in which the teaching process is carried out in the clinical setting. Teaching is an interactional process; it is facilitating rather than controlling. Teaching "occurs within a climate of trust, authenticity, and caring where learners are supported as they enter into learning experiences which may involve risk and new use of self" (Reilly & Oermann, 1990, p. 29). Teaching, like nursing, is humanistic and caring, involving diagnosis of learning needs and interventions geared to developing the learner's knowledge and skills further. It reflects concern for the individual learner and learner's own goals.

In teaching in the clinical setting, there are many faculty behaviors and characteristics which promote learning—knowledge of nursing, clinical competence, interpersonal relations with students on a one-to-one basis and as a group, teaching practices and skill in the instructional process, availability to students, and personal characteristics such as enthusiasm. Lowman (1985) believes that teaching effectiveness is based on two dimensions: creating an intellectual environment for learning and developing positive rapport with students. The interpersonal dimension of teaching cannot be underestimated; it is a critical variable in the way the instruction is designed and carried out with students and in the process of learning and its outcomes. The teacher's relationship with learners influences to a great extent the psychosocial climate for learning in the clinical setting.

QUALITIES OF TEACHER IN CLINICAL SETTING

Much has been written about attributes which constitute effective and ineffective teaching. Certainly students are able to differentiate teachers who facilitated their learning with ones who inhibited it and related characteristics of those teachers. The teacher can promote learning in the clinical setting or can discourage it; the teacher, therefore, becomes a significant variable in establishing a learning environment in the clinical area.

Characteristics of an effective clinical teacher may be grouped into four areas: (1) knowledge and clinical competence, (2) teaching skill, (3) relationships with students, and (4) personal characteristics.

Knowledge and Clinical Competence

Knowledge of the subject matter pertains to the teacher's breadth and depth of understanding as it relates to the topic at hand but also to a larger sphere where that knowledge interfaces with other knowledges. Ability to analyze theories and synthesize from multiple sources, emphasis on promoting a conceptual understanding among learners, and willingness to examine different points of view are characteristics of a teacher who possesses this knowledge.

In Bergman and Gaitskill's (1990) study of effective clinical teachers, both faculty and students identified knowledge as an important characteristic. Windsor (1987) interviewed 19 senior nursing students at a large midwestern university. Students expressed the need for knowledgeable clinical instructors who were willing to share their knowledge and expertise. These findings are similar to other studies in higher education which have demonstrated that knowledge of the teacher and ability to communicate that knowledge to learners are important dimensions of teaching effectiveness.

Boyer (1990) describes the scholarship of teaching in which teaching "both educates and entices future scholars" (p. 23). He calls for teaching to be defined as scholarship. As such it begins with the teacher's knowledge of the subject. "Those who teach must, above all, be well informed, and steeped in the knowledge of their fields (Boyer, 1990, p. 23). The teacher is effective only when widely read and engaged intellectually in the teaching of nursing.

The teacher's theoretical and clinical knowledge used in the practice of nursing and attitude toward the profession influence teaching effectiveness. Nehring (1990) and Knox and Mogan (1987) referred to this theoretical and clinical knowledge as nursing competence. Findings of studies by them indicated that the best clinical teachers possess nursing competence and the worst lack such ability. The best clinical teachers were ones who enjoyed nursing, were good role models, demonstrated clinical skills and judgment, assumed responsibility for their own actions, and demonstrated a breadth of knowledge in nursing. In Bergman and Gaitskill's (1990) study, findings suggested that important dimensions of clinical teaching included ability to relate underlying theory to nursing practice, being well-informed, and ability to communicate knowledge to students. Bergman and Gaitskill (1990) recommend that "special attention should be given to developing a functional body of knowledge in the area of instruction and in communicating that knowledge to students" (p. 41).

Effective clinical teaching also requires competence in clinical nursing practice. Maintenance of clinical competence is essential in assisting students in development of knowledge and skill and providing expert supervision in the clinical setting. Nehring (1990) found, similar to an earlier study by Knox and Mogan (1987), that the best teachers were ones who demonstrated expert clinical skills and judgment. Ability to demonstrate the skills, attitudes, and values that are to be developed by the student in the clinical area and ability to stimulate the student to want to learn behaviors associated with professional competence also have been reported as important characteristics of an effective clinical teacher (Bergman & Gaitskill, 1990).

In an early study by Rauen (1974) of role characteristics of clinical nurse teachers, one of the highest ranking characteristics was the teacher's skill in demonstrating how to function in a real nursing situation. This skill is dependent upon maintaining clinical competence. Pugh (1988) also reported that the teacher's ability to demonstrate nursing care in a real situation was an important behavior in clinical teaching identified by students. The teacher serves as a role model for students in the clinical setting.

Teaching Skill

Teaching skill involves the ability to diagnose learning needs, plan instruction in terms of learner characteristics and goals to be achieved, supervise students, and evaluate learning. An effective teacher presents information in an organized manner, gives clear explanations and directions to students, answers questions clearly, and demonstrates procedures and other care practices effectively. Good teachers are masters of a subject, well organized, emphasize important points during teaching, clarify ideas and point out significant relationships, motivate students through their teaching practices, and pose and elicit useful questions (Eble, 1988).

In Pugh's (1988) study on clinical teaching effectiveness, many of the teaching behaviors rated by students as important pertained to teaching skill: ability of the teacher to correct and comment on written assignments, make specific suggestions for improvement of performance, plan assignments which assist in the transfer of theory to clinical and are based on course objectives, give encouragement and praise, suggest resources for learning, and assist the learner in preparing for difficult and new situations and in analyzing client data. Nehring (1990) found that the best clinical teachers enjoyed teaching and were well prepared for teaching in the clinical setting. In addition, faculty reported that skill in promoting student independence was also important.

The ability and practices of the teacher in evaluating learning in the clinical setting are important aspects of teaching effectiveness. Qualities in this area are ability of the teacher to provide useful feedback on student progress, exhibit fairness in the evaluation process (Bergman & Gaitskill, 1990), promote student independence through evaluative practices, correct student mistakes without belittling, and communicate clear expectations to students (Nehring, 1990). Flagler, Loper-Powers, and Spitzer (1988) found that giving positive feedback was most valuable in helping students develop self-confidence as a nurse; giving mostly negative feedback hindered students' development of self-confidence in clinical practice. Greer (1990) believes that honest praise generously given early in the semester "bolsters students' self-confidence" (p. 38).

Relationships with Students

The ability of the teacher to interact with students is another important teacher behavior. This skill involves interacting with the group of students as a whole and on a one-to-one basis and includes developing mutual respect and rapport between teacher and learner. Clayton and Murray (1989) emphasize the importance of this relationship in the teaching of nursing; this relationship represents a caring experience between teacher and student.

Bergman and Gaitskill (1990) found that the characteristics of effective clinical teachers in nursing could be grouped into three categories: (1) relationships with students, (2) professional competence, and (3) personal attributes. In their research, relationships with students were ranked as the most important characteristic. Other studies have confirmed the importance of the relationships established between teacher and students (Brown, 1981; Knox & Mogan, 1987; Nehring, 1990; Pugh, 1988). Earlier studies in nursing education revealed similar results—the interpersonal relationships established with students in the clinical setting were important in terms of promoting learning. These relationships are characterized by the teacher being approachable, encouraging mutual respect, providing support and encouragement, and listening attentively (Nehring, 1990). Edwards (1991) recommends using a variety of listening skills and techniques to facilitate communication, enhance the student-teacher relationship, reduce stress experienced by students, and improve teaching and learning. Diekelmann (1990) believes that conversations with students "need to be dialogues in which we hold mirrors up which reflect and call one another forth. Dialogue is engaged listening, seeking to understand, and being open to all possibilities" (p. 301).

An important element in developing positive relationships with students is the teacher's commitment to conduct teaching in caring ways. Faculty attitudes toward learners are characterized by a "deep respect for them as human beings and a concerted effort to deal with them at their level of understanding" (Hedin, 1989, p. 76). In establishing interpersonal relationships with students, the teacher is warm and open, highly student-centered, and predictable (Lowman, 1985).

Lowman (1985) believes the quality of instruction results from the teacher's skill at creating intellectual excitement and positive rapport with learners. "A teacher who is accomplished at both is most likely to be outstanding for all students and in any setting" (Lowman, 1985, p. 10). These dimensions combine to encourage and foster motivation of students to do their best work. Skill at creating the intellectual dimension relates to the teacher's knowledge and ability to present it to learners. The teacher's interpersonal rapport with students is critical in motivating them to learn. This dimension of teaching deals with the faculty's awareness of the interpersonal processes within the teaching situation and their skill in communicating with students in ways that foster motivation, enjoyment, excitement about learning, and independence in learning. The teacher "respects the students as individuals and sees them as capable of performing well" (Lowman, 1985, p. 16). While important for all teaching, this interpersonal dimension is critical in instructional situations which are one-to-one such as those encountered in the learning laboratory and clinical setting.

Personal Characteristics

Other characteristics of effective teaching relate to personal attributes of the teacher, which in many ways are associated with the dynamism of the faculty and enthusiasm for teaching in the clinical setting. This flair and enthusiasm for teaching come with enjoyment in working with students and confidence in one's own teaching ability and clinical skills. One of the benefits of self-confidence is that it enables the teacher to be genuinely enthusiastic about teaching. Eble (1988) emphasizes the strong force of the teacher's personality. "Denying the place of personality in teaching exposes us to a contrary danger of forgetting that *human* learning is the aim of teaching" (Eble, 1988, p. 16).

In an early study of teacher behaviors which facilitate or interfere with learning in the clinical setting, O'Shea and Parsons (1979) found that friendly, supportive, understanding, and enthusiastic behavior of the teacher promoted learning. In more recent studies characteristics of the teacher perceived as important in clinical teaching include demonstrating self-confidence, being enthusiastic, being open-minded and nonjudgmental, displaying a sense of humor, admitting mistakes and limitations, being cooperative and patient, and being flexible when the occasion calls for it (Bergman & Gaitskill, 1990; Knox & Mogan, 1987; Nehring, 1989).

Teaching requires a great deal of caring for others and giving of self. Cross (1986) believes that good teachers have certain characteristics in common—knowledge of their subject and enthusiasm for teaching. The personal qualities of the teacher are important in engaging the student in the learning process and motivating them to learn. Teaching is a dynamic endeavor that "builds bridges between the teacher's understanding and the student's learning" (Boyer, 1990, p.23). Table 5-1 summarizes characteristics of an effective clinical teacher in nursing.

Effective clinical teaching places many demands on faculty—demands for knowledge and clinical expertise, skill in interacting with students and others in the setting, and personal characteristics which promote learning. "Effective teaching in nursing requires knowledge about nursing and *how* to teach" (Oermann, 1990, p. 25). A teacher with knowledge and expertise in clinical practice is not a teacher if unable to communicate effectively with students and facilitate their learning in the practice setting.

TEACHER-STUDENT RELATIONSHIP

A humanistic climate that supports the process of learning is dependent on a caring relationship between teacher and student. The success of any clinical learning experience rests heavily on this relationship as learners pursue educational goals leading toward their development as professional practitioners.

The need for caring behaviors demonstrated within the teacher-student relationship is one of the themes of the curriculum revolution literature. Diekelmann (1989) has described the normal experience in nursing education between faculty and students as adversarial. Caring, however, requires "cooperation and collaboration" (Zerwekh, 1991,

Table 5-1
Characteristics of Effective Clinical Teacher in Nursing

Knowledge and Clinical Competence	Teaching Skills	Relationships with Students	Personal Characteristics
• Has extensive knowledge and clinical competence in area in which teaching	• Diagnoses learning needs, plans instruction, supervises students in clinical setting, and evaluates learning	• Develops interpersonal relationships with students characterized by —warmth —mutual respect —caring behaviors —concern for students —openness	• Is dynamic and enthusiastic
• Maintains up-to-date knowledge and clinical skills	• Presents information in organized way		• Enjoys clinical nursing practice and teaching in clinical setting
• Analyzes theories, synthesizes from multiple sources, and emphasizes conceptual understanding among students	• Emphasizes important points		• Is friendly, supportive, and understanding
	• Gives clear explanations and directions	• Is approachable	• Demonstrates self-confidence
• Assists learner in relating underlying theory to nursing practice	• Asks questions which facilitate learning and answers them clearly	• Provides support and encouragement	• Is fair in teaching and evaluation
• Is well-informed	• Demonstrates procedures/care practices effectively	• Listens attentively	• Displays a sense of humor
• Is able to communicate knowledge to learners	• Suggests multiple resources for student learning	• Respects rights of student to challenge, question, and express own views	• Admits mistakes and limitations
• Demonstrates clinical competence, expert clinical skills and judgment, and attitudes and values to be developed by student	• Is well prepared for clinical teaching	• Encourages students in self pursuit of knowledge	• Is cooperative and patient
	• Gives encouragement and praise as significant dimension of teaching	• Accepts differences among students	• Demonstrates flexibility
	• Communicates clear expectations to learners		• Is responsible and dependable
• Is good role model	• Employs teaching and evaluative practices that promote student independence		• Is committed to nursing and teaching in the clinical setting
	• Gives immediate and positive feedback on student progress		• Believes in learners and expresses this belief through teaching practices

p. 265). The interactions between teacher and student need to reflect a mutual process in which both parties contribute. The role of nursing student has always been challenging and sometimes frustrating; the pressures on students today are even greater as more and more students assume additional responsibilities outside of school, ones involving work and family. Hegyvary (1990) urges faculty to support and care for nursing students. This support and caring is demonstrated through the relationship established between faculty and student.

Just as the nurse-patient relationship is a helping one, so is the teacher-student relationship. Carl Rogers (1983) identified certain qualities of this relationship that facilitate learning. These qualities, similar to those necessary for any therapeutic encounter, include realness or genuineness, trust and respect for the learner, and empathetic understanding.

The teacher who exhibits realness or genuineness in a relationship is honest and open with students and willing to express his or her own feelings. Genuineness implies an ability to admit mistakes and acknowledge limitations.

Other qualities of this relationship include trust (important in promoting risk-taking behaviors in the clinical setting), and respect, i.e., accepting learners as they are. Trust communicates confidence in student ability to achieve in clinical practice; and in a trusting relationship with faculty, learners are more inclined to discover and seek out new experiences. Judgment of performance occurs, but feedback from faculty is viewed as a means of helping students learn and further develop their skills, not as a punitive process addressing negative aspects of performance as an end in itself.

Empathetic understanding is also a significant attribute of a strong teacher-student relationship. Empathy means the teacher can view a situation from the learner's perspective. The development of a helping relationship requires teacher responsiveness to the feelings of students and an ability to communicate that understanding to them. Carl Rogers (1983) writes, "When the teacher has the ability to understand the student's reactions from the inside, has a sensitive awareness of the way the process of education and learning seems *to the student*, then again the likelihood of significant learning is increased" (p. 125).

Studies by Aspy and Roebuck (1974) have demonstrated that the interpersonal skills of the teacher influence student learning. These researchers found that empathy, congruence (genuineness), and positive regard (respect), which Rogers identified as critical dimensions of any interpersonal relationship, were significantly related to cognitive learning. High levels of empathy, congruence, and positive regard provided by the teacher tend to enhance learning, and conversely, low levels of these conditions may impede it. Although these studies were conducted with elementary school students and teachers in a classroom setting, they have implications for nursing faculty in that Aspy and Roebuck have been able to demonstrate a relationship between teachers' interpersonal skills and student learning.

Using Aspy's scales for evaluating the interpersonal skills of the teacher, Karns and Schwab (1982) examined nursing students' perceptions of teaching behaviors that promote a positive relationship between the teacher and student. Although the sample was small, most of the behaviors identified by students were ones relating to the conditions of empathy, congruence, and positive regard.

Clinical practice is inherently stressful for students. The environment cannot be fully controlled, and the student is faced with unexpected occurrences and uncertainties. Results of research by Beck and Srivastava (1991) indicated that nursing students experienced high stress levels. Kleehammer, Hart, and Keck (1990) examined anxiety-producing situations in the clinical setting. Students expressed the highest anxiety during the initial clinical experience on the unit and the fear of making mistakes. In addition, students' anxiety increased in the clinical setting with nonsupportive faculty. Often, the clinical setting, client population, teacher, and even peers are unfamiliar to the learner. Clinical practice places the student in a vulnerable position in that learning occurs as a public event, in front of others—the teacher, clients, peers, agency staff, and sometimes even individuals from other disciplines. Perception of faculty as a threat forces students into "playing games" in an effort to survive in the system. Survival, rather than learning, becomes the emphasis. A trusting relationship between teacher and student is a prerequisite to reducing some of this stress and to the students' use of faculty as a resource for learning.

Teaching in the clinical setting requires a supportive learning environment, development of caring relationships with learners, and use of effective teaching behaviors. The teacher has responsibility for selecting learning experiences for students that reflect the objectives and take into consideration the goals and priorities of the clinical setting.

SELECTION OF LEARNING EXPERIENCES

Selection of learning experiences in the clinical setting requires collaboration of faculty, students, and agency staff but remains the responsibility of faculty. Retention of this responsibility by the teacher is important to fulfill the educational purposes of clinical practice. With some experiences, students are responsible for choosing the learning activities in which they will engage, and planning for those experiences then occurs between students and staff.

Criteria for the selection of learning experiences in the clinical setting include:

1. Appropriateness for the objectives of the experience
2. Availability of faculty
3. Appropriateness for learner's level of knowledge and skill, learning needs, and individual characteristics of learner
4. Provision for progressive development and continued growth of the learner
5. Compatibility with the philosophy and conceptual framework of the nursing program
6. Provision for variety

Learning experiences in the clinical setting are selected for the purpose of achieving the objectives for clinical practice. These experiences might involve interviewing a client or family, health teaching, providing care, conducting a conference, completing written assignments, and participating in other types of activities. The learning experiences vary according to the objectives regardless of whether these objectives are established by faculty or reflect personal learning goals of students.

Availability of faculty, or preceptors in the setting, with expertise in the area of practice and in sufficient number for student supervision represents another criterion in selecting experiences. The student-faculty ratio is dependent upon the objectives and level of the learner. Preceptorships, for example, allow for larger student-faculty ratios than do others requiring direct faculty supervision. Beginning students and those entering a new clinical area need closer supervision by the teacher than do learners who have experience in the practice specialty. An early study on teacher effectiveness revealed that the availability of faculty in the clinical setting facilitated student learning while being unavailable interfered with it (O'Shea & Parsons, 1979). Availability to work with students as the situation arises in the clinical setting has been identified as a characteristic of clinical teaching effectiveness (Bergman & Gaitskill, 1990). As such, the teacher's availability to supervise students needs to be considered in selecting clinical experiences for learners.

Selection of experiences in clinical practice depends on the learner's present level of knowledge and skills and individual learning needs. Not all students will have similar learning needs, and, therefore, it is unreasonable to expect them to complete the same learning activities.

Individual differences of students also must be considered in the selection of clinical experiences. One important difference relates to the student's aptitude or time required for mastery of a particular learning task. The time available for learning should reflect that required by the learner. Research has clearly demonstrated that students learn at different rates. Not only are there rate variations among students, but the rate at which a person learns is not constant over different learning tasks. The amount of time needed to learn is a function of the prerequisite knowledge and skills possessed by the student. If the learning experience assumes certain prerequisites that the student lacks, additional time is necessary in order to acquire these entry behaviors. This means that the learning experience initially should assist the student in acquiring entry behaviors in which he or she is deficient and then should provide for individual differences in rates of learning. It is recognized that with perseverance and time allowed for learning, students with varying aptitudes can achieve the objectives; but in most nursing programs, some time frames within which clinical objectives must be met to progress in the program are established.

Collaboration with learners in the selection of experiences provides for individual styles of learning, interests, and preferences. Merritt (1991) believes that planning instruction based on learning styles preferences, such as differences between field dependent-independent learning styles, has the potential for increasing motivation and learning (p. 241). It is important for students to participate actively in choosing experiences meaningful to them. Student participation in determining clinical learning activities is based on the objectives; student needs, interests, and aptitude; and the past experience of the learner (Infante, Forbes, Houldin, & Naylor, 1989). Russell (1990) suggests that student involvement in the instructional process may be a significant element of a successful learning experience.

Learning experiences in the clinical setting provide for progressive development of knowledge, skills, and values and for continued growth of the learner. Experiences build on preceding ones and modify those that follow. The nature of and way in which the experiences are organized are important in promoting continued growth of the learner.

The philosophy of the nursing program, with respect to statements about learning and teaching, influences the selection of clinical experiences. A philosophic statement that the learner is self-directed and actively involved in the learning process may be reflected in clinical practice in provisions for the student to participate in selecting experiences and to direct his or her own learning in accord with the stated goals of the experience. In the clinical setting, students learn the practice of nursing as described in the conceptual framework of the nursing program. The experiences selected should be congruent with this description of the nature of nursing practice. For instance, if the nursing program is based on an adaptation framework, experiences in clinical practice should assist learners in using this framework with clients.

Learning experiences in the clinical setting should provide for variety. The very nature of nursing itself, with its multiple activities and skills required, demands variation in clinical experiences. Variety in learning experiences can be a factor in maintaining student interest and promoting independent inquiry in the clinical setting.

INSTRUCTIONAL PROCESS

The instructional process may be viewed in terms of five interrelated components: clinical objectives, assessment of learner, instruction, formative evaluation, and summative evaluation. These follow a sequence of events as depicted in Figure 5-1.

Clinical Objectives

The first component relates to the clinical objectives established for the practice experience. These objectives provide the basis for teaching in the clinical setting because they specify the outcomes to be attained there. The clinical objectives are part of the overall course objectives and represent those behaviors to be attained in practice. While the clinical objectives are developed by the teacher, students set individual goals for learning in clinical practice which are also representative, then, of this first component.

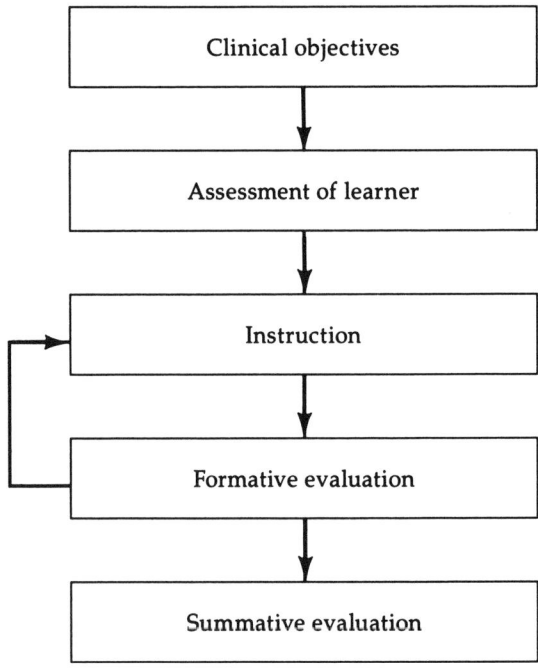

Figure 5-1
Instructional Process in the Clinical Field

Assessment of Learner

Instruction begins at the level of the learner, so the second component necessarily deals with assessment in terms of (1) entry behaviors, the prerequisite knowledge and skills for learning a particular task, and (2) relevant characteristics of the learner. These prerequisites constitute the necessary link between the students and attaining the objectives. Given this view, the learner must possess or acquire the necessary entry behaviors to achieve the clinical objectives established for the practice experience.

Assessment determines if learners possess the necessary prerequisites for accomplishing the objectives. This is an important step in the instructional process for if students lack the entry behaviors for a given learning situation, even high-quality instruction will not overcome the effect of this lack unless that teaching is directed toward remedying these deficiencies (Bloom, 1976). Assessment reveals to the teacher whether or not the instruction needs to assist the learner in acquiring the prerequisite behaviors. Assessment might also reveal that some students have already achieved certain objectives and are able to move on to other learning tasks.

Assessment also includes determining the affective characteristics of the learner, "a complex compound of interests, attitudes, and self-views" (Bloom, 1976, p. 75) which vary greatly among students. Learning is facilitated when students are interested in the practice experience and have a desire to learn. Bloom believes that individuals tend to like activities which they perceive they have done or can do successfully. This perception is determined by previous experiences with similar learning tasks. If students perceive they have completed prior related tasks successfully, they are likely to approach the next similar learning situation with a positive affect. This raises the question as to the influence of student perception of the relationship with the teacher and success with learning in the clinical setting on subsequent related clinical experiences. Students who believe they have performed unsuccessfully in the past with interviewing, for instance, may approach subsequent learning experiences involving interactions with clients with some degree of negative affect.

Another related matter is whether students view the clinical experience as relevant to their individual goals. The learner who perceives some relationship between the present learning situation and experiences and future goals is more likely to be motivated to learn. Student establishment of own goals for learning provides a strategy for maintaining interest and motivation.

Assessment also reveals differences in rates of learning, cognitive styles, and cultural patterns among students relevant to planning the instruction. These differences influence teaching methods, types of learning experiences, time allowed for learning, and teacher behavior.

Learner assessment may be carried out by: (1) questioning, (2) observation of performance, (3) written tests, and (4) student self-evaluation.

Instruction

Instruction, the third component, pertains to the actual teaching process. This phase involves the selection of teaching methods and learning experiences for facilitating attainment of the objectives or initially assisting the student in acquiring any lacking prerequisite behaviors, development of the learning environment, and interaction with students and staff in the process of carrying out the instruction. Research continually reminds faculty of the wide range of differences among students and need for these to be taken into account in the instruction.

Regardless of the specific experiences in which students engage, the instruction should provide for clear directions and explanations to learners, active involvement of the student in the experience, practice of behaviors to be learned, immediate feedback, and reinforcement for learning. The teacher adapts the extent of the directions, amount of participation and practice, and use of reinforcement to the individual's needs.

Formative Evaluation

The remaining two components of the instructional process refer to evaluation of the learner. Formative evaluation provides feedback to students as to their progress in achieving the objectives and is continuous throughout the practice experience. Evaluation which is formative in nature serves a diagnostic purpose because it informs students as to areas where further learning is necessary. This information is then used to plan additional instruction. For this reason, formative evaluation is depicted in Figure 5-1 with a connecting line to the instructional component. Formative evaluation alone only improves learning to a small degree and therefore needs to be accompanied by supplemental instruction whereby students can correct their learning difficulties. Since formative evaluation is an integral part of the instruction, the resulting data are not subjected to the grading process.

Summative Evaluation

Summative evaluation, in contrast, is conducted at the conclusion of certain clinical experiences or the course to determine if the objectives have been achieved. This type of evaluation provides data for arriving at grades in clinical practice. In summative evaluation there is a concept of finality, stating "what is rather than what is and what can be" (Reilly & Oermann, 1990, p. 128). Summative evaluation is concerned with how students have achieved the objectives of the learning experience.

The instructional process is depicted here in terms of five components beginning with the identification of clinical objectives and proceeding through assessment of the learner, planning and carrying out the instruction, and evaluating student learning in relation to the objectives. For the instruction to be effective, individual differences of learners must be taken into account in each phase of the process.

SUMMARY

Development of a climate for learning is concerned with the setting in which clinical practice takes place, interpersonal relationship established between the teacher and student, and the way in which the teaching process is carried out in the clinical setting. Teaching is an interactional process; it is facilitating rather than controlling. Teaching occurs most effectively in a climate of trust, authenticity, and caring where learners are supported as they enter into learning experiences in the clinical setting. Teaching, like nursing, is humanistic and caring, involving diagnosis of learning needs and interventions geared to developing the learner's knowledge and skills further. It reflects concern for the individual learner and learner's own goals.

In teaching in the clinical setting, there are many faculty behaviors and characteristics which promote learning—knowledge of nursing, clinical competence, interpersonal relations with students both on a one-to-one basis and as a group, teaching practices and skill in the instructional process, availability to students, and personal characteristics such as enthusiasm. The teacher respects the learner as an individual and recognizes and builds upon the wealth and diversity of experiences learners bring to the clinical setting.

In clinical practice, the teacher through interaction with the learner facilitates student attainment of the objectives and individual learning goals, providing the supportive environment required for learning to take place. The process of instruction may be viewed in terms of five components: development of clinical objectives, assessment of the learner, instruction, incorporation of formative evaluation, and provision for summative evaluation. Through the instructional process and within a climate for learning which accepts individual differences, respects learners, and values their input into the learning process, students in the clinical setting are encouraged to learn and develop knowledge and skills further.

REFERENCES

Aspy, D. N., & Roebuck, F. N. (1974). From humane ideas to human technology and back again many times. *Education, 95*, 163–171.

Beck, D. L., & Srivastava, R. (1991). Perceived level and sources of stress in baccalaureate nursing students. *Journal of Nursing Education, 30*(3), 127–133.

Bergman, K., & Gaitskill, T. (1990). Faculty and student perceptions of effective clinical teachers: An extension study. *Journal of Professional Nursing, 6*(1), 33–44.

Bloom, B. S. (1976). *Human characteristics and school learning.* New York: McGraw-Hill.

Boyer, E. L. (1990). *Scholarship reconsidered: Priorities for the professoriate.* Princeton, NJ: Carnegie Foundation for the Advancement of Teaching.

Brown, S. T. (1981). Faculty and student perceptions of effective clinical teachers. *Journal of Nursing Education, 20*(9), 4-15.
Clayton, G. M., & Murray, J. P. (1989). Faculty-student relationships: Catalytic connections. *Curriculum revolution: Reconceptualizing nursing education* (pp. 43-53). New York: National League for Nursing.
Cross, K. P. (1986). A proposal to improve teaching. *AAHE Bulletin, 39*(1), 9-15.
Diekelmann, N. (1989). The nursing curriculum: Lived experiences of students. *Curriculum revolution: Reconceptualizing nursing education* (pp. 25-41). New York: National League for Nursing.
Diekelmann, N. (1990). Nursing education: Caring, dialogue, and practice. *Journal of Nursing Education, 29*(7), 300-305.
Eble, K. E. (1988). *The craft of teaching* (2nd ed.). San Francisco: Jossey-Bass.
Edwards, E. J. (1991). Use of listening skills when advising nursing students in clinical experiences. *Journal of Nursing Education, 30*(7), 328-329.
Flagler, S., Loper-Powers, S., & Spitzer, A. (1988). Clinical teaching is more than evaluation alone! *Journal of Nursing Education, 27*(8), 342-348.
Greer, P. S. (1990). The one minute clinical instructor: An application of the principles of the one minute manager. *Journal of Nursing Education, 29*(1), 37-38.
Hedin, B. A. (1989). Expert clinical teaching. *Curriculum revolution: Reconceptualizing nursing education* (pp. 71-89). New York: National League for Nursing.
Hegyvary, S. T. (1990). The need for care of nursing students. *Journal of Professional Nursing, 6*(4), 190.
Infante, M. S., Forbes, E. J., Houldin, A. D., & Naylor, M. D. (1989). A clinical teaching project: Examination of a clinical teaching model. *Journal of Professional Nursing, 5*(3), 132-139.
Karns, P. J., & Schwab, T. A. (1982). Therapeutic communication and clinical instruction. *Nursing Outlook, 30*, 39-43.
Kleehammer, K., Hart, A. L., & Keck, J. F. (1990). Nursing students' perceptions of anxiety-producing situations in the clinical setting. *Journal of Nursing Education, 29*(4), 183-187.
Knox, J. E., & Mogan, J. (1987). Characteristics of 'best' and 'worst' clinical teachers as perceived by university nursing faculty and students. *Journal of Advanced Nursing, 12*, 331-337.
Lowman, J. (1985). *Mastering the techniques of teaching*. San Francisco: Jossey-Bass.
Merritt, S. L. (1991). The abilities and aptitudes of students must be considered in program design. *Nursing & Health Care, 12*(5), 240-242.
Nehring, V. (1990). Nursing clinical teacher effectiveness inventory: A replication study of the characteristics of 'best' and 'worst' clinical teachers as

perceived by nursing faculty and students. *Journal of Advanced Nursing, 15*(8), 934-940.

O'Shea, H. S., & Parsons, M. K. (1979). Clinical instruction: Effective/and ineffective teacher behaviors. *Nursing Outlook, 27,* 411-415.

Oermann, M. H. (1990). Research on teaching methods. In G. M. Clayton & P. A. Baj (Eds.). *Research in Nursing Education* (Vol. III, pp. 1-31). New York: National League for Nursing.

Pugh, E. J. (1988). Soliciting student input to improve clinical teaching. *Nurse Educator, 13*(5), 28-33.

Rauen, K. C. (1974). The clinical instructor as role model. *Nurse Educator, 13*(8), 33-40.

Reilly, D. E., & Oermann, M. H. (1990). *Behavioral objectives: Evaluation in nursing* (3rd ed.). New York: National League for Nursing.

Rogers, C. R. (1983). *Freedom to learn for the 80s.* Columbus, OH: Chas. E. Merrill.

Russell, J. M. (1990). Relationships among preference for educational structure, self-directed learning, instructional methods, and achievement. *Journal of Professional Nursing, 6*(2), 86-93.

Windsor, A. (1987). Nursing students' perceptions of clinical experience. *Journal of Nursing Education, 26,* 150-154.

Zerwekh, J. (1991). Undoing the habit of hostility. *Journal of Professional Nursing, 7*(5), 265.

BIBLIOGRAPHY

Anderson, C. A. (1989). Type and expectations of faculty. *Journal of Professional Nursing, 5*(5), 250-255.

Bevis, E. O., & Murray, J. P. (1990). The essence of the curriculum revolution: Emancipatory teaching. *Journal of Nursing Education, 29*(7), 326-331.

Boland, D. L., & Sims, S. L. (1988). A comprehensive approach to faculty evaluation. *Journal of Nursing Education, 27*(8), 354-358.

Carlson, D. S., Lubiejewski, M. A., & Polaski, A. L. (1987). Communicating leveled clinical expectations to nursing students. *Journal of Nursing Education, 26*(5), 194-196.

Dawson, N. (1986). Hours of contact and their relationship to students' evaluations of teaching effectiveness. *Journal of Nursing Education, 25*(6), 236-239.

DeBack, V. (1991). The National Commission on Nursing Implementation Project. *Nursing Outlook, 39*(3), 124-127.

del Bueno, D. J., Griffin, L. R., Burke, S. M., & Foley, M. A. (1990). The clinical teacher: A critical link in competence development. *Journal of Nursing Staff Development, 6*(3), 135-138.

Donovan, M. S. (1989). The 'high-risk' student: An ethical challenge for faculty. *Journal of Professional Nursing, 5*(3), 120.

Gien, L. T. (1991). Evaluation of faculty teaching effectiveness—Toward accountability in education. *Journal of Nursing Education, 30*(2), 92-94.

Karuhije, H. F. (1986). Educational preparation for clinical teaching: Perceptions of the nurse educator. *Journal of Nursing Education, 25*(4), 137-143.

Klaassens, E. L. (1988). Improving teaching for thinking. *Nurse Educator, 13*(6), 15-19.

Lee, E. J. (1987). Analysis of stressful clinical and didactic incidents reported by returning registered nurses. *Journal of Nursing Education, 26*(9), 372-379.

Lindeman, C. A. (1989). Clinical teaching: Paradoxes and paradigms. *Curriculum revolution: Reconceptualizing nursing education* (pp. 55-69). New York: National League for Nursing.

Lindeman, C. A. (1989). Curriculum revolution: Reconceptualizing clinical nursing education. *Nursing & Health Care, 10*(1), 23-28.

McCabe, B. H. (1985). The improvement of instruction in the clinical area: A challenge waiting to be met. *Journal of Nursing Education, 24*(6), 255-257.

Monahan, R. S. (1991). Potential outcomes of clinical experience. *Journal of Nursing Education, 30*(4), 176-181.

Myrick, F. (1991). The plight of clinical teaching in baccalaureate nursing education. *Journal of Nursing Education, 30*(1), 44-46.

Pagana, K. D. (1990). The relationship of hardiness and social support to student appraisal of stress in an initial clinical nursing situation. *Journal of Nursing Education, 29,* 255-261.

Pugh, B. J. (1991). Becoming an intentional teacher. *Nurse Educator, 16*(3), 5-6.

Sorcinelli, M. D., & Cunningham, H. (1991). Developing teaching skills through individual consultation. *Nurse Educator, 16*(3), 7-11.

Talarczyk, G. (1989). Aptitude, previous education: Students' perceptions of roles, effort, and performance. *Journal of Nursing Education, 26,* 380-383.

Theis, E. C. (1988). Nursing students' perspectives of unethical teaching behaviors. *Journal of Nursing Education, 27,* 102-106.

Thurston, H. I., Flood, M. A., Shupe, I. S., & Gerald, K. B. (1989). Values held by nursing faculty and students in a university setting. *Journal of Professional Nursing, 5*(4), 199-207.

Van Ort, S., Noyes, A., & Longman, A. (1986). Developing and implementing a model for evaluating teaching effectiveness. *Image: Journal of Nursing Scholarship, 18*(3), 114-117.

Williams, C. A. (1988). Faculty practice and knowledge development: Will there be a linkage? *Journal of Professional Nursing, 4*(5), 317.

Williams, R. A. (1988). The relationship of cognitive styles and stress in nursing students. *Western Journal of Nursing Research, 10,* 449–462.

Wang, A. M., & Blumberg, P. (1983). A study of interaction techniques of nursing faculty in the clinical area. *Journal of Nursing Education, 22*(4), 144–150.

Wong, J., & Wong, S. (1987). Towards effective clinical teaching in nursing. *Journal of Advanced Nursing, 12,* 505–513.

Zimmerman, L., & Waltman, N. (1986). Effective clinical behavior of faculty: A review of the literature. *Nurse Educator, 11,* 31–34.

6

Teaching Methods

The multipurpose nature of the clinical field, types of learning outcomes, diversity of nursing competencies, and differences among learners and teachers require various methods for teaching in the practice setting. Teaching method refers to a way of organizing and presenting the instruction reflective of a theoretical perspective of teaching and learning and directed toward achieving specific learning outcomes. No one method is sufficient for teaching nursing in the clinical setting. The teacher, therefore, chooses from a repertoire of methods depending on the objectives, individual characteristics of the learner, his or her own teaching abilities and conceptual framework of the teaching-learning process. Methods particularly relevant to teaching in the clinical setting are the focus of this chapter.

The chapter is organized according to seven classifications of teaching methods. Each category is presented as follows: first, a discussion of the theoretical base for the classification and second, a description of the teaching methods included in it and guidelines for use of the methods.

CRITERIA FOR SELECTION OF TEACHING METHODS

Planning for the clinical practice experience includes the decision as to methods to use for promoting achievement of the objectives. In making this decision, the teacher considers the nature of the objectives, entry behaviors and characteristics of the learner, qualities and skills of the teacher as well as availability in relation to the teacher-student ratio, characteristics of the clinical setting, and particular attributes and limitations of the teaching method itself. Criteria for the selection of clinical teaching methods include:

1. Appropriateness for the objectives of the practice experience in relation to the particular attributes of the method.
2. Appropriateness for learners in terms of abilities, experience, and other characteristics.
3. Compatibility with the teacher's skill and conceptual framework of the teaching-learning process.
4. Suitability in terms of availability of resources and constraints of the clinical setting.
5. Congruence with the philosophy of the nursing program in relation to faculty beliefs about teaching and learning.
6. Provision for variety, in accord with the various competencies to be achieved.

The particular attributes of each method make some strategies more appropriate than others for fostering certain types of learning. The question for faculty is which methods are the best ones for achieving the clinical objectives. For many objectives, several methods might be used, thereby allowing for individual differences among learners and teacher preference. For example, assisting students to apply concepts of teaching and learning to patient education may be accomplished through experiential methods such as a simulation or a patient assignment in which the student carries out instruction with a client, through use of media, or by observation of patient teaching combined with discussion. Other objectives, however, such as those relating to psychomotor skill development, are more limited as to methods that are appropriate.

Knowledge of the learner provides another source of data for making the decision as to teaching strategies. Methods should be appropriate for the learners who will participate in them in terms of abilities, experience, cognitive styles and other relevant characteristics. Role play may not be suitable if students lack the necessary concepts for analyzing the outcomes of the role play situation and are unfamiliar with the other participants. Use of experiential methods, for instance, patient assignment, depends on the learner's present level of knowledge and skill and on the kinds of related experiences the student has had in field practice. Teaching methods also need to reflect individual differences among learners. Field-dependent learners, for instance, prefer methods that involve interactions with others more so than do learners who are field-independent.

Choice of methods is made ordinarily by the teacher but might also be made cooperatively by teacher and learner or even, in some situations, by the learner. Student input into selection of methods provides a means and evidence of attending to the interests of the learner and preferences for a teaching method if more than one is appropriate for the objectives.

Methods should capitalize on faculty strengths and should be compatible with teaching abilities. This is not to say that faculty should avoid trying out new strategies, but with some methods, the teacher may need further development of his or her own skills before using a method in the clinical setting. The selection of methods also reflects the faculty's own style of teaching, preference for particular strategies, and one's own beliefs about clinical teaching and ways of promoting learning in the practice setting. One component of the faculty's conceptual framework of teaching and learning is the relationship between various teaching methods and the learning process.

Teaching methods for clinical practice reflect the resources available and constraints of the setting and clinical teaching situation. Knowledge of the requirements of the methods for effective implementation, therefore, is important in the selection of strategies. Considerations in relation to this criterion include: (1) the time required for use of the teaching method and faculty time in preparing for it; (2) requirements of the method, such as space within the clinical setting and related equipment and supplies; (3) costs entailed with purchase, continued use, and administration; and (4) number of participants that permit effective implementation. Faculty might also consider the context of the teaching situation in terms of the time when the method will be used. Late afternoon of a day in which students engaged in field practice may not be an appropriate time for a teacher-centered method; one where learners participate actively in the instruction may be better suited.

The philosophy of the nursing program influences the selection of clinical teaching methods. Strategies should be congruent with the beliefs expressed in the philosophy regarding teaching and learning.

Variety in teaching methods, as long as it is in accord with the competencies to be achieved, may be advantageous in maintaining student interest. In many instances different teaching methods are appropriate which enable the teacher to vary the instructional strategies being used in the clinical setting.

CLINICAL TEACHING METHODS

Clinical teaching methods available to faculty are classified in relation to the primary purposes served by each strategy. These categories are:

1. Experiential
2. Problem solving
3. Conference
4. Observation
5. Multimedia
6. Self-directed
7. Preceptorship and other models of concentrated practice

Some teaching methods can serve several purposes and are not confined by the basic categorization. For example, patient assignment, while classified as an experiential method because it provides for actual participation in the events to be learned, also promotes problem-solving learning with real clients and problems.

Experiential

Experiential teaching methods provide for direct experiencing of events, either through clinical practice involving interaction with real clients and others in the field or through contrived experiences of reality such as with simulations and role play. Learning results from actual participation in the events to be learned.

Experiential methods are based on a phenomenologic concept of learning. They provide for interaction of learners with the environment from which the learners derive personal meaning. Learners differ in their perception of events in the environment and the meanings given to phenomena, and thus, the learning outcomes evolving from the experience vary with the learner. Experiential methods recognize the importance of perception and insight in learning. They involve the whole learner in cognitive, psychomotor and affective aspects of the learning event. Because of this involvement, there is an important affective dimension to the learning, regardless of whether the experience is directed toward cognitive or psychomotor outcomes. Experiential methods provide for actual participation of the learner in the events to be learned and recognize the ability of the individual to derive personal meaning from the experience.

Experiential clinical teaching methods include:

1. Clinical assignment
2. Written assignments, which often accompany experiences in the practice setting
3. Simulation and game

Clinical Assignment. Clinical assignment involves patient care; other kinds of experiences with clients; and practice experiences with peers, nursing staff, and members of other disciplines. Clinical assignment is essential in assisting students to use concepts and theories in practice, learn how to learn, develop skill in handling ambiguity, and become socialized into the profession. Experiences in care of clients and with others in the clinical setting facilitate the development of problem-solving, decision-making, and critical thinking skills; provide opportunity for moral and ethical decision making relative to client, setting, and self; and enable learners to develop and refine psychomotor skills. Nursing is people oriented, and experiences in practice enable students to learn to work with others.

Clinical practice provides experiences for developing the thinking *processes* used by students to solve client and other problems. In developing critical thinking skills, students need experience in collecting data, differentiating relevant from irrelevant data, drawing inferences from the data and evaluating them, and making decisions about the problems as well as nursing interventions. A patient assignment provides the opportunity to carry out this thinking process with clients and exposure to different types of problems and solutions. In this context the teacher also has the opportunity to examine with the student and reinforce the process of thinking as well as the outcome.

Miller and Malcolm (1990) call upon faculty to encourage and reinforce the spirit of inquiry and independent thought as a means of fostering critical thinking (p. 73). Clinical assignments and related discussions provide an important strategy for meeting this goal.

In the clinical setting, students experience unfamiliar situations where the problem is unclear and encounter problems without well defined solutions. These types of experiences are important in learning to "think like a professional." In practice with clients, students learn forms of inquiry used by practitioners in applying knowledge to particular cases. They also learn to make "new sense of uncertain, unique or conflicted situations of practice," thereby learning that existing professional knowledge does not fit every client case and every problem encountered in practice does not have a right answer (Schön, 1990, p. 39). Through the clinical experience students learn a reflection-in-action that is beyond the rules of inquiry. They develop new methods of thinking, reasoning, and understanding and have an opportunity to test new strategies for action and ways of framing problems (Schön, 1990, p. 39).

The nature of the clinical assignment is dependent upon the objectives, individual learning needs, and knowledge base of the learner. In some instances, the assignment may be care of a client or group of clients. In other instances, students may be assigned or select specific types of learning experiences with clients or others in the setting. This is particularly true in early stages of clinical experience. For example, when the goal is the development of communication skills, the clinical assignment emphasizes interacting with clients rather than their care per se. The teacher decides whether an assignment involving complete care of the client is the most appropriate strategy for the given practice experience.

Clinical assignments provide for progressive development of the learner. They build upon preceding experiences and reflect the learner's needs and abilities. In developing clinical assignments for a group of learners, faculty also takes into account the time needed for supervision. Assignments are best developed when faculty and agency personnel concur on goals, types of experiences, specific responsibilities of students, and the time learners are in the setting. Student preparation for a clinical assignment may involve library research, laboratory practice, and visitation in the clinical setting. At the conclusion of clinical assignments, conferences and other types of discussions are important to assist learners in examining the experiences and setting directions for future learning.

Written Assignments. Written assignments are used to promote problem-solving learning in relation to clients and other problems encountered in the practice setting. They help learners to identify and reflect upon their values and beliefs, improve understanding of a particular aspect of clinical practice, and develop written communication skills.

Written assignments which accompany the clinical experience are effective strategies for promoting the development of critical thinking skills. For this purpose assignments allow the student to puzzle over an issue or idea and arrive at relevant conclusions. Written assignments such as these provide opportunity for students to focus on real problems they have encountered in the clinical area, ones which they have experienced personally. Meyers (1986) believes that students must "feel that they are struggling with real problems and issues" for the assignment to promote critical thinking (p. 73). Meyers also recommends more and shorter assignments rather than fewer and longer ones. A series of short papers requiring an analysis of a clinical problem, a situation experienced in clinical, or an issue encountered involving either a client or staff provide for repetition and practice in critical thinking over time. Another advantage of shorter and more frequent assignments is that the teacher may give immediate feedback to learners. Written assignments enhance understanding of content and ability to make decisions in clinical practice (Allen, Bowers, & Diekelmann, 1989, p. 9).

They also foster development of skill in writing. Written assignments may be completed prior to clinical practice, concurrent with practice, or subsequent to it. Types of written assignments relevant to clinical practice include nursing care plans, case studies, teaching plans, process recordings, experiential diaries, learning logs, reports, and other forms of written work.

Nursing Care Plans. Nursing care plans enable the learner to analyze the client's health care problems and develop a plan which incorporates goal setting and a selection of care activities and provides direction for evaluation. The format of the care plan may be that of a specific clinical agency in which the student is involved in practice or one developed by faculty for use as a learning strategy, in a particular course or throughout the program. The intent of the learning care plan, which tends to be more detailed and comprehensive than the practice plan, is to assist in the development of the knowledge base for practice. The number of learning care plans is dependent upon the student's learning needs, for the ultimate goal of teaching should be to move the student to the practice model as soon as possible.

In some settings students may develop computerized care plans. Some hospital information systems provide a directory of standardized care plans which may be generated from the system and then adapted for the specific patient (Brown, 1991, p. 206). Regardless of the way in which it is developed, a care plan may be stored in the computer and then updated as needed. Strength and Keen-Payne (1991) describe a system for computerized patient care documentation at the bedside which in the future will allow for the development of computerized care plans according to NANDA diagnosis. Integration of computer documentation in the clinical setting and need for students to develop skill in its use will continue to be an important outcome of clinical practice.

Whether the care plan is developed in print form or generated from a computer system, faculty need to be clear as to the purpose of this assignment. A written care plan may not necessarily represent critical thinking on the part of the learner nor promote its development. In relation to this, Tanner (1986) writes, "we have no empiric evidence to support continued reliance on the written nursing care plan as the predominant instructional method, nor is there evidence to eliminate it entirely" (p. 9). The care plan may or may not reflect the complexity of thought and judgment needed to arrive at decisions regarding client problems and care. Care plans when accompanied by discussion with the teacher can more readily focus on the critical thinking process underlying the resulting care plan.

Case Study. Case study represents a holistic picture of a client's health care problems and requires more in-depth analysis of these problems than a care plan. At best, it requires from the learner an explanation of relevant theories and principles. When used as a clinical teaching strategy, the case study is based on a client for whom the student is responsible for care or is derived from a clinical situation in which the student has been previously involved. The case study might be presented in conference for peer review.

Analysis of a case provides opportunity for the students to: (1) examine the interrelationships of multiple phenomena in the clinical situation; (2) enlarge own knowledge base; (3) develop skill in problem solving and critical thinking; (4) examine multiple approaches to problems, compare them, and decide upon approaches to be used in this situation; (5) provide a supporting rationale for decisions made; and (6) organize ideas logically in written form. Case studies may also be used to teach ethics (Waite, Duckett, Schmitz, Crisham, & Ryden, 1989) and moral judgment in the clinical setting. When using case studies, it is important that students possess sufficient depth of understanding and the theoretical background necessary for analyzing the clinical situation under review.

Teaching Plan. A written teaching plan enables learners to apply concepts of learning and teaching in meeting the educational needs of patients, families and staff. In terms of clients, the teaching plan is part of the total plan of care which addresses teaching as an intervention strategy. There are many formats with which teaching plans may be developed; in general, there are five major parts: objectives, content, teaching methods, learning activities, and evaluation. Plans are most effective when developed in settings where teaching is an on-going activity.

Process Recording. For objectives relating to the development of skill in interacting with others, the process recording provides a means for learners to record and then analyze their communications. A process recording consists of a written record of the communication that occurred between the learner and client, peer or another member of the health care team (Reilly & Oermann, 1990) and an analysis of that interaction. With this method, the learner is able to examine the client's and his or her own verbal and nonverbal behaviors, thereby increasing understanding of the client and improving learner's interaction skills.

The focus of the process recording depends on the purposes to be accomplished. If the objectives relate to nonverbal communication, for instance, then the written report and subsequent analysis of the interaction may emphasize nonverbal behaviors of the participants. Because this assignment is time consuming for students and for faculty who review it and provide feedback, the number of recordings should be determined by the needs of the student. Continuance of the assignment beyond its value for learning results in boredom for students which, in turn, may precipitate careless or less-than-honest completion of the process recording. Learners must also have time immediately following the interaction for writing the report. One format for a process recording is presented in Table 6-1.

Experiential Diary and Learning Log. Similar to a process recording, experiential diaries and learning logs also provide a means of recording experiences related to clinical practice. Diary writing is a dialogue with self, representing a record of the student's feelings, reactions, attitudes, perceptions, and activities regarding experiences in the clinical setting. Diary writing prepares learners for working with clients and families and enables them to reflect on their experiences and derive personal meaning from them. Spontaneous responses result when there are no instructions as to the format of the presentation. The message, "write as though you were writing your own diary," suffices.

Early on, Reilly (1958) demonstrated the use of diaries in determining the nature of learning experiences in the clinical setting. Students wrote a diary after their first experience in the clinical setting, one month later, and at the time they entered a new setting. A content analysis of the diaries provided faculty with cues for planning subsequent learning experiences.

Learning log, a form of diary, is a sequential record of learning experiences usually documented in relation to specific clinical objectives. Students may be directed by faculty as to notations to be made in the log, depending on the objectives associated with the experience, or may be encouraged to formulate their own notations relevant to the objectives.

Table 6-1
Guidelines for Nurse-Patient Process Recording[a]

Milieu	Patient	Nurse	Feelings	Analysis
Describe environment in which patient and nurse are interacting. Include physical and social aspects and feeling tone of environment. Indicate changes in the milieu that occur throughout the interaction. Identify effects of milieu on the interaction. Identify modifications in milieu planned by nurse.	Describe patient's appearance. Describe patients's nonverbal communication. Record patient's verbal communication, using direct quotes whenever possible.	Describe nurse's nonverbal communication. Record nurse's verbal communication, using direct quotes whenever possible.	Describe nurse's *feelings*, e.g., anger, fear, relief, comfort, pleasure. Identify changes in feelings as interaction progresses.	1. Analyze nonverbal and verbal meanings of patient's communication. 2. Analyze nurse's responses to client's behavior, both verbal and nonverbal. 3. Identify specific communication skills used by nurse (e.g., open-ended questions, reflection, etc.). 4. Identify use or nonuse of empathetic responses by nurse. 5. Identify blocks nurse may have used and why such blocks may have occurred. 6. Describe effects of nurse's feelings, needs, attitudes, values and beliefs on nurse's behavior and on the interaction. 7. Identify physical, environmental, and cultural variables that may have affected the interaction. 8. Describe effect of client's behavior on nurse and on the interaction. 9. Describe implications for nursing actions.

[a] Adapted from Wayne State University College of Nursing.

Other Assignments. Other written assignments appropriate for clinical practice include reports, such as those of field trips; papers; and written work students complete about observations made in the field and of practice experiences in which they have engaged.

Simulation and Game. Another category of experiential teaching methods includes simulations and games. While not replacing direct involvement with clients, simulations and games prepare learners for clinical practice by providing opportunity to develop and test cognitive skills in a relatively risk-free environment where the consequences of any mistakes are less costly than they would be with real clients, to apply theories of action before required to use those theories in practice, to learn complex skills in a more controlled setting than the field, to practice psychomotor skills, and to gain a perspective of what a clinical situation might be like for others. Experiencing an event in a simulated situation or through a game before encountering it in the field promotes learning in that the student is more confident as to possible ways of handling the situation and is more sensitive to the client's perspective.

Simulation. A simulation creates an experience that represents reality; in essence, it mimics a real-life situation. Simulations provide "a realistic experience for students without the constraints and distractions usually found within the real-life situation" (Hanna, 1991, p. 28). Simulations may or may not use accompanying media such as videotapes, computers, print materials, and others to portray the real clinical situation. With a simulation, the teacher can control the learning situation more easily than in the clinical setting, for instance, in terms of time, distractions, patient variables, and interruptions. Evans (1989) discusses advantages of using simulations for reviewing clinical skills such as cardiopulmonary resuscitation, suctioning, and inserting intravenous lines (p. 65). Hanna (1991) also suggests that a simulation facilitates affective learning in that students can critique their own behaviors, responses, and feelings before encountering similar situations in the clinical field.

There are different types of simulations appropriate for use in teaching in the clinical setting. In the case study method, information relative to a clinical situation is presented to the learner and usually requires that some decision be made. Information is gradually added to the case, often reflecting the consequences of the learner's decision, thereby simulating the progression of events in the real clinical situation. In this way, students learn how to solve clinical problems in a contrived setting and receive immediate feedback on the consequences of their decisions. The simulation may also provide opportunity for practice of psychomotor skills relevant to the clinical situation and client problems being simulated.

Plunkett and Olivieri (1989) describe the use of a simulation combined with videotaping intended to assist the student in developing skills in diagnostic reasoning. Emphasis is placed on generating multiple hypotheses from the data and exploring each one instead of arriving at one correct hypothesis or nursing diagnosis. Baldwin and Schaffer (1990) describe the use of a continuing case study in which the people and health status change over time. The continuing case study incorporates multiple scenarios and allows the students to act out different roles.

The simulation may be presented in paper and pencil format, through audiovisual media (frequently involving videotaping), and by computer. In a computer simulation of a clinical problem, the student responds to data presented by the computer, makes a decision, and receives feedback on the consequences of that decision. With some computer programs, the patient's status is altered by the decisions made which vividly communicates to the learner the outcomes of the decision-making process.

Interactive video (IAV) instruction combines the computer simulation with videotape in such a way that video segments are shown as the learner responds to the material presented in the computer simulation. The student is thus able to view the client's progress in this simulated situation and respond to visual and auditory scenarios, creating an experience that more closely mimics a real-life dilemma than would use of either a computer simulation or videotape alone.

Another type of simulation common in nursing education involves the use of models of the human body for teaching clinical skills, such as in the form of manikins, like "Mrs. Chase," for practicing basic nursing procedures. Many other models are available for teaching specific skills—breast examination, intramuscular and intravenous injections, and urinary catheterization, to name a few. Models enable students to practice skills in a safe environment and increase their confidence in performing them before having to use and often adapt those skills with clients.

Another form of simulation involves the use of peers and other persons who act in the role of client and behave as a patient would in that situation. Simulated patients may be used for the practice of psychomotor skills, taking a health history, physical assessment, and other experiences where a live patient is needed to represent effectively the real-life situation. The simulation may be videotaped so that participants are able to analyze their own behaviors or to permit evaluation by others.

Role Play. In role play, the learner portrays a specific individual and is generally given much freedom to act out that role spontaneously. Role play is particularly appropriate for objectives related to developing interpersonal relationships with clients, peers, and other health care providers. In general, two students act out the roles and the rest of the students in the clinical group observe, analyze, and provide feedback to the role players. Role play may be combined with videotaping to allow for learner analysis at the completion of the activity.

In planning for the role play, the clinical situation and roles are described briefly, allowing for creativity in portraying the roles. The time for the role play is typically 10 to 15 minutes, followed by a debriefing session in which students' observations and analysis of the role play are discussed. In the debriefing, the outcomes of the role play are considered in relation to the objectives and clinical practice. Discussion is limited to the role play experience rather than the acting ability or individual characteristics of the players.

Game. In comparison to a simulation, a game is a contest with rules, goals, and activities to perform. Games use competition or collaboration that leads to winning (Hanna, 1991). They may be played in groups or individually. Games for clinical teaching include crossword puzzles to teach medical terminology and other information about client care, question and answer games on clinical problems and interventions, trivia questions, and board games on clinical topics and nursing management.

Simulation Games. A simulation game combines properties of simulations and games, allowing learners to experience aspects of the real world but in the form of a game. Hanna (1991) describes simulation games as a variation of a simulation that adds the element of competition and collaboration, with the goal of winning, to the real-life role play (p. 28). Some illustrations of simulation games include: *Starpower* (Simile II) in which participants learn about power and the distribution of wealth through the trading of chips, simulating a society of have and have nots; *Into Aging* (Slack), for demonstrating how an older person is influenced by health professionals and other persons with negative attitudes and information about aging; *Blood Money* (Games/Simulations Inc.) which teaches about some of the problems faced by hemophiliacs within the health care system; *In Pursuit of Accreditation*, developed in the format of *Trivial Pursuit*, which prepares faculty for a National League for Nursing accreditation (Fitzgerald & McCurren, 1988); and *Researcher for a Day*, a simulated research experience appropriate for clinical problems (Blenner, 1991).

Simulations and games provide for experiential learning with an experience that represents a real-life situation in various ways. They have potential for raising motivation and interest in an area of clinical nursing, sensitizing students to what a situation might be like for others, assisting learners in developing decision-making skills, and enabling them to practice in a relatively safe environment.

Discussion, referred to as debriefing, following a simulation and game is important for students to (1) identify the concepts learned, (2) relate their learning to the objectives, (3) discuss application to clinical practice, and (4) evaluate the experience. The format of and questions for the debriefing session should be identified by the teacher prior to the activity. With some types of simulations and games, debriefing is in written form for completion independently by the learner or is part of the computer program.

In using a simulation/game, consideration is given to its requirements, for example, number of participants, time needed to prepare for and engage in the simulation/game, equipment, props, cost, space, and constraints of the teaching situation. Pretesting the simulation/game with a group of students familiarizes faculty with it, how it is played, equipment and materials needed, directions to be given to students, and the teacher's own role, which facilitates implementation and provides a means of evaluating its usefulness. Considerations by faculty in planning for use of simulation/game are included in Table 6-2.

Table 6-2
Planning Considerations for Use of Simulation/Game

Objectives:
Does the simulation/game relate to the objectives to be attained by learners?
What other goals might be met through the simulation/game?

Cost:
Is the cost of the simulation/game, for purchase (if commercially available), development (if to be developed by faculty), and continued use within the budgetary constraints of the nursing program?

Participants:
What is the minimum and maximum number of learners to participate in the simulation/game?
Is this number within the constraints of the teaching situation in which the simulation/game will be used?
What roles might other students assume if unable to engage in the simulation/game?
Do the intended learners have the necessary theoretical background and skill level for engaging in and learning from the simulation/game?
What preparation will be needed on the part of students to participate in the simulation/game?

Time:
What are time requirements for use of the simulation/game: preparation time for faculty? time for the simulation/game? time for debriefing after it is completed?
Are these within the constraints of the teaching situation?

Setting:
How much space is required for the simulation/game?
Is the required space available in the setting in which students will be?

Materials:
What equipment, supplies, props, and other materials are required by the simulation/game?
Are these available in the setting, or may they be easily transported there?

Debriefing:
Does the simulation/game have guidelines for debriefing?
What are important questions to be explored in the debriefing session?

Problem Solving

Problem-solving methods assist learners in analyzing a clinical situation with the intent of defining problems to be solved, deciding on actions to be taken, applying knowledge to a clinical problem, and clarifying one's own beliefs and values. They encourage divergent thinking, the derivation of more than one solution to a problem, which is essential for effective problem solving in practice and transfer of learning, stressing the connection between previous experiences and learning with new problems.

Problem-solving methods derive much of their theoretical base from cognitive-field theory. They also draw upon information processing theory and decision theory.

Problem-solving teaching methods appropriate for clinical practice include:

1. Problem-solving situation
2. Decision-making situation
3. Critical incident

Problem-solving Situation. A problem-solving situation represents a description of a clinical event for the purposes of defining problems to be solved as indicated in the situation, identifying relevant data significant to understanding the nature of the problem, proposing hypotheses, identifying appropriate nursing actions to be taken in the situation and underlying theoretical bases for such actions, and applying theory to practice. This method serves as one means of assisting students in applying the conceptual model of nursing upon which the curriculum is based to issues and problems in clinical practice.

If sufficient assessment data are presented in the case, questions can be directed toward critical thinking and leading the student through the clinical judgment process. Students can be asked to identify and cluster cues in the assessment data; differentiate relevant from irrelevant data; generate tentative hypotheses as to nursing diagnoses, with supporting data; evaluate those hypotheses; and arrive at a decision considering alternatives proposed. In addition, students can be asked to consider multiple interventions, weigh the consequences of each, and decide upon nursing management.

Problem-solving situations also can be used to address complex clinical practice problems and provide reflection-in-action experience in which new problem statements, methods of reasoning, and strategies of action are developed. Situations such as these assist students in dealing with the reality of practice concerns and realizing that not all problems have one single answer nor are they all readily solved empirically. The ambiguous nature of many problems faced clinically and multiple solutions possible may be presented and taught through problem-solving situations.

Problem-solving situations may be client, staff, or setting oriented or may represent issues affecting nursing practice and care delivery. They may be written, presented through multimedia, or generated from the student's clinical experience. Questions directed toward the problem situation may be in a written form or raised by the teacher or students in discussion of the situation. The types of questions asked, however, are important if the intent of the teaching strategy is to promote critical thinking skills. Questions need to ask the learner to consider other possibilities, alternate approaches, and different perspectives to the situation. The following example illustrates a problem-solving situation.

Problem-Solving Situation

Objectives
   Identifies universal, developmental, and health deviation self-care requisites.
   Relates concepts of self-care theory to client situation.
   Identifies nursing measures for meeting client's self-care needs.

Situation
Mr. A. is a 60-year-old patient who recently had a laryngectomy. His incision is healing and only requires a dressing change once daily. He has been unable to sleep for the last two evenings because of pain in his neck radiating to his shoulder. Mr. A. admits to being a problem drinker and to having a long history of smoking. Over the past two years, he has lost a significant amount of weight. He lives alone and is presently unemployed.

   Mr. A. rings the call bell for the nurse and writes on his memo pad, "I can't stand it anymore—the pain is too much for me."

1. What are Mr. A.'s universal, developmental, and health deviation self-care requisites?
2. On the basis of this information, what are the probable self-care demands?
3. What questions would you ask Mr. A. and what observations would you make to determine Mr. A.'s potential capability for self-care?
4. What actions should the nurse take in regard to Mr. A.'s statement?

Decision-Making Situation. A decision-making situation is a form of problem solving in which a decision is required. Learners examine the data presented, identify alternatives for action and consequences of each, establish priorities, and then make a decision. Reilly and Oermann (1990) describe another type of decision-making situation in which the decision is stated and learners indicate agreement or disagreement with a supporting rationale for the position chosen.

Decision-making situations may involve decisions relative to clients, staff, and communication with other disciplines. Like problem solving, the questions for discussion may be in written form or may be raised by the teacher during conference. Students may complete the decision-making situation individually or in small groups, but it is important that they have an opportunity for discussion to capture the thought underlying process used in responding to the situation.

The following example illustrates a decision-making situation.

Decision-Making Situation

Objectives
Uses the decision-making process in identifying nursing actions.

Situation
In reviewing a patient's chart, Ms. C., a registered nurse, finds that the order for Digoxin is considerably larger than the usual dose. She confirms this in a reference book and explains the situation to the head nurse. After reviewing the order on the patient's chart, the head nurse tells Ms. C., "Give the medication. I'm sure Dr. Smith had a reason for ordering this dose."

1. What is your assessment of the situation?
2. Identify three possible courses of action that might be taken.
3. Describe the possible consequences of each course of action.
4. Which course of action would you choose?
5. Why did you select the course of action you did?

Critical Incident. The incident process, also designed to assist students in developing skill in reflective thinking, is built around a single incident or clinical event. Through group discussion, learners seek information about the incident, identify the problem, describe their approach and supporting rationale, and then generalize from the incident to other clinical experiences.

Generally, the incident is described briefly in written form, although it might be presented verbally by the teacher or by a student. The incident should be generated from a practice experience in which the learner or faculty has recently been involved. Incidents may be client, staff, or setting oriented. The person directing the discussion, the teacher or one of the students, should have knowledge of the incident.

Cooper (1981) describes five phases of the incident process:

1. Studying the incident and formulating questions to gather more information about it.
2. Asking questions in an effort to acquire sufficient information to identify the problem. In this phase, the discussion leader provides only facts relative to the incident under study.
3. Identifying the problem.
4. Exploring possible alternative actions and making a decision individually as to which alternative to select, including a rationale for the choice. After learners defend their individual choices to the group, the group, in turn, comes to agreement as to the most appropriate action to be taken, followed by a report by the discussion leader as to what actually occurred.
5. Generalizing from the incident to other clinical experiences, considering ways in which the concepts learned are applicable to other situations, and reflecting on the case as a whole.

There are many incidents associated with clinical practice that could be used. A few illustrations are included.

Incidents

Mr. B., 75 years old, was diagnosed recently with inoperable metastatic lung cancer. In a home visit, the nurse notices that Mr. B. has continued smoking.

John, a 17-year-old diabetic, comes to the clinic with a blood sugar of 360. He tells the nurse, "I was partying and maybe had too much to drink. My doctor said I could eat whatever I wanted since I'm still growing."

Conference

The clinical conference is a form of group discussion about some aspect of clinical practice. Conferences promote problem-solving learning in that the group undertakes critical analysis of a problem and explores alternate and creative approaches. With this method, students are able to talk through the problem-solving process and receive immediate feedback from peers and the teacher. In a conference, the group of learners gains exposure to varied clinical situations, many of which students may not encounter themselves. Conferences also provide opportunity for peer review, discussion of concerns and analysis of issues relative to clinical practice, and problem solving by different disciplines.

In addition to these outcomes, group discussions have other benefits. In a conference, students have a chance to interact with one another and with the teacher, using each other as resources for learning. Discussion enhances the ability to formulate ideas and express them clearly; gives learners an opportunity to be recognized for their contributions; increases confidence in interacting in a group format; and provides a place for them to explore feelings, attitudes, and values affecting practice. In a discussion, students can develop skills in group process.

The relationships between the teacher and learner and within the group are significant in promoting discussion, for learners need to be comfortable with peers and other participants and particularly with the teacher to express their views and feelings and take risks in responding to questions. The teacher's behavior often influences whether or not students will participate in a conference and their willingness to be honest and open. The faculty's general stance can invite or discourage student participation.

Types of conferences relevant for teaching in the clinical setting include:

1. Preconference, postconference, and other types of clinical conferences
2. Nursing and multidisciplinary conferences

Pre- and postconferences relate directly to the clinical practice experience. Preconferences prepare students for their experiences in the practice setting; assist them in identifying client problems, planning care, and evaluating outcomes; and provide a means for students to discuss with faculty (and with peers if in a group format) questions about their clients. These conferences enable the teacher to identify concerns and feelings of students regarding the practice experience. Preconferences may be one-to-one or in a group depending on learner needs, teacher preference, and context within which the clinical experience takes place.

Postconferences take place following clinical practice, such as the end of an experience in which students have been in the field or after a specific learning experience completed by an individual or group of learners, for instance, an observational experience. These postclinical discussions provide an opportunity for group problem solving, in relation to problems in which students are involved in practice, and for sharing of clinical experiences among the group. Postconferences provide an effective strategy for critical thinking. The decisions made by students and other alternatives possible, which were generated in the discussion, can be examined by the group. The teacher and students can focus on the thinking process used in clinical and propose other strategies.

Clinical conferences may also be used for reviewing and critiquing each other's work. Peer review enables learners to gain experience and skill in the process of evaluating another's practice, similar to what takes place in the work setting. In a conference intended for peer review, the criteria for critique of another's work should be explicit and understood by learners. In addition, students must be comfortable with one another and value feedback from peers for such a review to be effective. Experience in peer review within the educational process prepares learners for carrying this out in their own practice.

Conferences also provide an opportunity for discussion of issues affecting nursing practice not necessarily generated from the clinical experience but relevant to it (Oermann & Gignac, 1991). In a conference learners can explore economic, political, social and ethical issues and their implication for nursing practice in general and in the particular clinical setting in which they are having experience. Teleconferences may also be used.

Nursing and multidisciplinary conferences emphasize the process of collaborative decision-making in which plans for client care are developed, evaluated, and revised; implementation of the plan may also be examined. Participants in these conferences range from a group of nurses in one particular setting to a multidisciplinary team. Regardless of the composition, the intent is to engage in group problem-solving.

As early as 1958, Reilly described the value for student learning of multidisciplinary conferences in her study of clinical conferences attended by nursing and medical students. Students reported that these conferences "contributed to improved patient care by furthering mutual understanding" among disciplines (Reilly, 1958, p. 24). Multidisciplinary conferences also enable learners and practitioners to explore different perspectives of issues affecting care and the delivery of that care. In the health care field, collaboration among professionals is needed to provide effective care (Oermann, 1991b, p. 9).

Observation

Observation of an actual experience in the field or of a demonstration provides for learning through modeling. According to social learning theory (Bandura, 1977), modeling promotes learning by informing the learner of what the behavior to be developed is like. From observation of others, the learner forms an image of how new behaviors are performed which serves as a guide for future learning.

Observational teaching methods include:

1. Observation in the clinical setting
2. Field trip
3. Nursing rounds
4. Demonstration

Observation in the Clinical Setting. Observation in the clinical setting (1) prepares learners for future experiences with clients, giving them a perspective of what the care or specific intervention is like; (2) enables them to view others in practice, which serves as a guide for development of their own behaviors; (3) makes it possible for students to observe a clinical situation with which they may not have an opportunity to be involved themselves; and (4) provides a means for improving their own observation skills. Participatory observation, in which learners participate in activities as they are observing, minimizes the effects of their presence by making them less noticeable and setting clients and others at ease. A balance needs to be established between such participation and attending to the observations so the participation does not interfere with making skillful observations.

Observation may be done individually or in small groups, depending on the situation being observed. With group observation, it is particularly important that careful consideration be given to the effect on those observed.

Field Trip. The field trip provides an opportunity for observations outside of the clinical setting in which students are presently involved in practice. Students gain experiences that are generally not available in their own setting to augment current knowledge and acquire a broader perspective of the health care problem or issue under discussion.

A field trip may be taken to any site pertinent to the clinical objectives, for instance, rehabilitation and long term care facilities, clinics, day care centers, group meetings within the community, shelters, hospices, and other settings which would facilitate students' understanding of different dimensions of the client's care. Blainey (1991) recommends using clinical focus guidelines for experiences where the teacher is not present. These guidelines are derived from the course objectives and state how students prepare for the experience, what observations should be completed, and what evaluation should be conducted by the student. Arrangements must be made by faculty with the clinical agency to clarify the purpose of the field trip, kinds of observational experiences desired, level and number of students, length of time in the agency, and other specifics of the experience. Evaluation by faculty, students, and clinical agency personnel of the observational experience is critical in planning for subsequent field trips to the particular setting.

For some experiences, a written guide is valuable to assist learners in focusing their observations. When the observation is of clients or families, permission should be obtained from them and/or the practitioner responsible for care. Discussion of the observations provides an opportunity for sharing among learners, having questions answered, relating the experience to practice, evaluating the experience, and proposing recommendations regarding future observations of a similar nature.

Nursing Rounds. Nursing rounds involve the observation and often interview of a client or several clients in the setting, generally followed by group discussion. Through an actual visit to the client, students are able to observe the client's condition, review the care provided, and collect information from the patient. Rounds also provide an opportunity for demonstrating a particular nursing intervention or the result of an intervention and for learners to observe interaction of the teacher, peer, or nursing staff (if participating in the rounds) with the client. Observing the client in the client's own environment contributes to discussion about that individual's care.

Rounds may be conducted by the teacher, by students (of their own clients), or by nursing staff. After arrangements have been completed for the nursing rounds, Cooper (1982b) recommends that the rounds begin with an introduction of the patient to the students, emphasizing the client's contribution to their learning, followed by discussion with the client, observations, and any demonstrations. Discussion of the observations made should take place following the nursing rounds and out of the client's presence. In the discussion, students are able to reflect on their observations; review the patient's problems and care, considering additional data obtained in the rounds; propose alternate interventions if appropriate; apply knowledge to the particular client situation; and relate their observations to other patients and to future learning.

Major difficulties in use of nursing rounds concern respecting the client's privacy during the observation and interview and assuring that the client desires to participate. Permission from the client should always be obtained in advance, and clients should understand their right to refuse participation. Clients should be encouraged to indicate when they no longer desire to continue with the nursing rounds.

Demonstration. Demonstration involves a presentation of how to perform a procedure or technique, how to use equipment, and how to interact with others (Cooper, 1982a). It provides for learning through visual and auditory modes and thus enables students to observe a procedure and its component steps while having those steps and underlying principles explained. Oermann (1990a) emphasizes that in beginning skill learning, demonstration of the procedure is important, for at this point learners observe the skill, develop a mental image of the way in which it should be performed, and then practice it until their own performance reflects their mental image (p. 204).

A demonstration may be performed in the learning laboratory or clinical field. In the laboratory, the teacher has greater control over the demonstration, there are fewer distractions, and students are able to practice the procedure more easily than usually possible in the clinical setting. Some demonstrations are best taught with patients, real or simulated. For those carried out with real clients, it is important that they be selected and prepared for the experience similarly as in the instance of nursing rounds. Regardless of the setting, the presentation may be in small groups or with an individual learner. The demonstrator may be the teacher, a staff nurse, or others with expertise in the procedure; or the demonstration may be presented in media, such as, interactive video, a videotape, or a film.

As with other observational teaching methods, students need information as to the purpose of the demonstration and important points on which to focus attention. Verbal directions of the teacher during the presentation serve as a means of emphasizing these relevant aspects. Explanations of the underlying principles, while important to the demonstration, need to take place before the demonstration begins and following it, not during the actual presentation when the focus should be on the procedure itself.

For some procedures, particularly if they are complex or require advanced skill, the demonstration in its entirety or selected segments may need to be repeated. de Tornyay and Thompson (1987) recommend using a video camera during a demonstration involving intricate hand movements so all learners are able to visualize the movements on a television screen (p. 64). Practice is essential to allow learners to try out the procedure observed, receive feedback and additional instruction from the teacher, and develop confidence in performance. In a study by Baldwin, Hill, and Hanson (1991), faculty assistance in terms of demonstrating a skill and supervising practice was found to be an important factor in learning the skill. Because learning occurs at different rates, the amount of practice needed will differ among students. Practice may be completed independently once the procedure has been performed satisfactorily. Additional guidelines for carrying out the demonstration are presented in Table 6-3.

Multimedia

Media provide for multisensory learning. Depending on the form, they communicate a message to the learner through varied sensory modes: visual, such as with slides and filmstrips; auditory, as with audiotapes; tactile with use of models and other objects to be manipulated; and often through a combination of these, such as videotape recordings and interactive video. In general, the more senses involved the easier it is for learners to conceptualize the message communicated. Auditory learning requires students to visualize internally what is heard. Combining auditory and visual modes enables learners to hear and see the message simultaneously, which permits visualization of the concept or activity to be learned and provides an accompanying description of it. Media create a vicarious experience for learners. They give learners an idea of what a situation is like, which is important in preparing them for clinical practice and for their own experiencing of that situation.

In a review by Oermann (1990b) of research on teaching methods in nursing from 1965 to 1988, 28 studies involved multimedia. In these studies, a range of multimedia was examined: videotapes, slides, films, audiotapes, programmed instruction, and other print and nonprint media. Findings indicated that media are effective in promoting cognitive

Table 6-3
Guidelines for Presenting a Demonstration

Preparation:
1. Identify relevant readings and other activities to prepare learners for demonstration.
2. For complex procedures, develop written guidelines for focusing observations during demonstration.
3. Practice demonstration beforehand so skilled in performing procedure and manipulating any related equipment.
4. Time demonstration beforehand including time for:
    Preparation
    Introduction to demonstration
    Actual demonstration
    Discussion following demonstration
    Practice by learners
    Clean up

Before Demonstration:
1. Prepare materials and equipment before learners arrive and test equipment to assure working order.
2. Arrange materials and equipment so they can be visualized by all learners.
3. Introduce purpose of demonstration and provide overview of procedure to be demonstrated.
4. Review materials and equipment used in procedure.
5. Discuss underlying principles prior to beginning demonstration.
6. Identify important features to be observed in demonstration.
7. Check that all learners can see demonstration and hear related explanation.

Demonstration:
1. Demonstrate steps of procedure in same sequence as would be followed in practice.
2. Describe procedure as demonstrating it with emphasis on procedure itself and important points in performing it.
3. Avoid details that are not essential to proper performance.
4. Emphasize how procedure is performed rather than how not to perform it.
5. Monitor pace of demonstration.

After Demonstration:
1. Repeat demonstration or segments of it if students need further observation of procedure.
2. Discuss procedure immediately following demonstration and review again important points in performing it.
3. Provide opportunity for supervised practice considering individual differences of learners as to amount of practice, feedback, and reinforcement needed.
4. Take into consideration left-handed learners if relevant to performance of procedure.
5. Evaluate demonstration and identify areas for modification with subsequent ones.

learning, retention of knowledge, and performance. There also appear to be benefits of using media for affective learning although further research is indicated in this area.

Media have an advantage of being able to show remote and inaccessible processes and events, close-up pictures, and procedures in which learners may not have an opportunity to observe or participate in themselves. With psychomotor skills, media provide a means of demonstrating the skill and emphasizing the critical elements in performing it. Media also promote affective learning by introducing learners to clinical situations that can be examined for value connotations. Situations depicted through media lend themselves to critical analysis by learners, individually or in small groups, from an affective perspective.

Videotape recordings and interactive video (IAV) represent important teaching methods for promoting problem-solving, decision-making and critical thinking skills among learners. Videotapes can create a vicarious experience for students; they can present a simulated situation in which students analyze and discuss the underlying thought process used in arriving at their decisions. Learners may be asked to role play and perform as they would in the clinical field. Matthews and Viens (1988) describe a teaching strategy involving videotaping in which students are presented data about a client, followed by their acting out the roles of patient, nurse, and evaluator.

Videotapes and IAV are particularly appropriate for assisting students in developing cognitive skills. The patient scenario presented in the videotape or IAV may be analyzed in terms of cues presented in the data, additional data needed for decision-making, tentative hypotheses and supporting data, and evaluation of each hypothesis to determine nursing diagnoses. Discussion can also be carried out to examine nursing management and alternative interventions. The videotape and IAV provide a real image of the patient situation not possible through print material alone.

There is a wide range of print and nonprint media available for clinical teaching, as indicated in Table 6-4. Oermann (1984a, 1984b) has developed an instrument for evaluating the quality of media prior to its use. It is important for learners to develop skill in evaluating the quality of care as seen in the media, judging the appropriateness of specific interventions and procedures for setting and practice, and adapting, if necessary,

Table 6-4
Types of Media

Print	Nonprint
Handout	Audiotape/record
Pamphlet	Computer
Programmed instruction (printed)	Film
Textbook	Filmloop
Workbook/study guide	Filmstrip
	Model
	Multimedia program
	Overhead transparency
	Photograph
	Real object
	Slide
	Television
	Videotape

what they have learned in the multimedia for use with clients and others in the clinical setting.

Computer-assisted Instruction. Computer-assisted instruction (CAI) provides for active involvement of the learner in responding to questions asked by the computer and making decisions regarding clinical situations presented. CAI also allows for differing rates of learning. CAI may be used to assist learners in acquiring knowledge needed for care of clients, analyzing data, deciding on clinical problems, selecting intervention strategies, and evaluating care.

There are several types of CAI: drill and practice, tutorial, simulation, and IAV.

In *drill and practice* questions are presented to learners seeking a response from them. The computer program then provides immediate feedback in terms of the response. Factual information, such as definitions of terms, laboratory values, and calculating dosages of medications, is particularly appropriate for drill and practice.

Tutorial provides for more feedback than with drill and practice. The computer presents information to the learner, then asks questions about the material, branching forward if the student responds correctly or backward if remediation is necessary (Hassett, 1984).

A *computer simulation* presents a real-life situation enabling the learner to make a series of clinical decisions similar to ones necessary in actual practice. The learner's decisions influence the information presented subsequently. Simulations are particularly appropriate for assisting students in analyzing client data, identifying nursing diagnoses from the data presented, proposing interventions, and evaluating the effectiveness of the approaches. One of the major advantages of computer simulations is in promoting critical thinking and problem-solving (de Tornyay & Thompson, 1987; Lowdermilk & Fishel, 1991). Students have expressed preference for computer applications on clinical practice rather than other topics (Van Dover & Boblin, 1991).

IAV combines the branching power of the computer with the reality of video (Rizzolo, 1990) to allow for visualization of the client situation and active involvement in the simulated data collection and analysis, planning care, intervening, and evaluating the results of decisions made. With IAV the system provides immediate feedback on the student's responses; the student also has the ability to access video segments to clarify those responses (Battista-Calderone, 1989). IAV has the potential to address multiple learning styles and needs of learners; allow students to experiment, explore alternatives, and see consequences without risk to the client; and evaluate client assessment, management, and decision-making, among other outcomes (Rizzolo, 1990). Difficulties with IAV relate to its cost and equipment needs.

In a study by Schare, Dunn, Clark, Soled, and Gilman (1991), IAV was found to be as effective as a traditional lecture in terms of cognitive achievement. Students, however, expressed a more positive attitude toward learning as a result of the IAV. These findings are similar to Oermann's (1990b) review of research on CAI in which CAI, regardless of its type, was found to be as effective as other instructional strategies for cognitive learning. Chang (1986) also concluded that CAI was time saving in comparison with traditional teaching methods.

IAV is used similarly to other resource materials for clinical learning. In many instances only parts of the IAV are assigned to reflect the particular outcomes of the clinical experience or learner needs. If only certain parts are to be completed, learners should receive explicit directions in terms of the menus and options.

Self-Directed

Self-directed teaching methods are based on a phenomenologic concept of learning that recognizes learning as an individual process requiring active involvement of the learner. This view acknowledges the uniqueness of the individual and his or her ability to make choices and decisions about learning. There is sufficient evidence to support the wide range of individual differences among learners. Students enter the learning situation with different levels of knowledge and skill, past experiences, cultural backgrounds, cognitive styles, teaching preferences, and rates of learning. Self-directed teaching methods attempt to reflect individual differences and needs among learners. With these methods, the responsibility for learning rests with the learner.

There are multiple strategies for self-directed learning. The degree of learner choice and control over the learning experience differs with the method. Learning contract and independent study, for example, are designed and controlled by the learner while other strategies, such as modules, multimedia programs, and computer-assisted instruction, are developed by the teacher or are available commercially. Even though the teacher may be responsible for the design or selection of the instructional materials, the learner can still choose alternate or additional learning activities, select the setting (home, work, library, or elsewhere) in which the learning will take place, and control the amount of time in learning and pace (Bell & Bell, 1983).

Three self-directed teaching methods are described:

1. Learning contract
2. Independent study
3. Self-paced module

Learning Contract. A learning contract represents a written agreement between the teacher and learner specifying their responsibilities in terms of outcomes to be achieved. The learner then fulfills the contract independently. Contracts enable learners to pursue individual objectives related to clinical practice, which are compatible with overall program and course goals, according to their preferred styles of learning and with learning activities and resources identified by them. They also provide for choice in evaluation methods and process. In discussing the use of contracts, Carl Rogers (1983) writes: "Contracts provide a sort of transitional experience between complete freedom to learn whatever is of interest and learning that is relatively free, but that is within the limits of some institutional demand and course requirement" (p. 149).

The contract, developed by the learner in collaboration with faculty or a preceptor, generally includes the following components:

1. Goals and objectives to be achieved in clinical practice upon completion of the contract.
2. Types of learning activities to be carried out within a designated time frame.
3. Expectations of the faculty/preceptor and student.
4. Evaluation methods and materials and other evidence to be submitted.
5. Credit allocation and grading, if applicable.
6. Date for completion of the contract.

A format for a learning contract is illustrated in Table 6-5.

Independent Study. In independent study the learner is given freedom to manage his or her own learning without the formalized procedure of negotiating a learning contract. The objectives to be achieved through independent study may be determined by the learner in collaboration with the teacher or by the teacher with the student then independently pursuing relevant experiences. Independent study is valuable in meeting individual learning needs of students relative to practice, assisting them in preparation for a clinical experience, and enabling them to investigate a particular clinical problem in depth. Learners may need an orientation to independent study and how to proceed with it.

Self-Paced Module. Self-paced modules represent another means of individualizing instruction and providing for self-directed learning. A module is a self-contained unit of instruction which is completed independently by the learner. Students progress through the module at their own rates of learning, taking as much time as necessary to achieve mastery. Depending on their learning needs, students may omit learning activities, repeat them, or participate in additional ones. The learning activities often represent various strategies, such as

Table 6-5
Learning Contract

Name _____   Course _____
Dates:
   Started _____   Clinical Agency _____
   Completed _____   Faculty _____
Credits _____   Preceptor _____
Grade _____
Nature of clinical practice experience: _____
_____
_____
_____
_____

Section I: Goals and Objectives

A. *Goals:* Write a statement of your goals for this clinical practice experience. Identify how these goals relate to your professional goals. _____

_____
_____
_____
_____

B. *Objectives:* Write the objectives for this experience that you expect to achieve.

_____
_____
_____
_____

Section II: Learning Activities

A. *Learning Activities:* Identify learning activities which you will carry out to achieve these objectives. _____

_____
_____
_____

Table 6-5 *(Continued)*

B. *Schedule of Activities:* Project a calendar of activities. (Consult with faculty/preceptor where relevant). _____

Section III: Evaluation

A. *Evaluation Methods:* Identify evaluation methods and materials to be submitted.

B. *Evaluation Report:* Prepare a written evaluation report of the clinical experience in terms of stated goals and objectives. _____

Student Signature _____ Date _____

Faculty Signature _____ Date _____

Preceptor Signature _____ Date _____

media and readings. Through pretests that enable them to identify objectives already attained, learners are able to determine the most appropriate point in the module at which to begin the instruction.

For clinical practice, a module may be used for acquisition of knowledge and development of skills as a prerequisite to practice, preparation for specific clinical experiences, review of content or skills, and for learning beyond any particular clinical requirement. Modules are appropriate for use in orientation of nurses to a clinical setting (Rufo, 1985) and for updating their knowledge and skills in practice.

A self-paced module generally contains the following components:

1. Purpose of module.
2. Pretest for determining objectives already met.
3. Objectives and any prerequisites.
4. Learning activities, allowing for choice and assisting in application of content to clinical practice, and resources for learning.
5. Posttest or other evaluation strategy for determining if students attained the objectives.

It also is important that a strategy such as use of questions be incorporated in the module to allow for periodic assessment of progress toward meeting the objectives and provide feedback to learners as they are completing the instruction.

Preceptorship and Other Models of Concentrated Practice

Clinical preceptors are staff nurses and other nursing practitioners in a clinical setting who serve as role model and teacher for students, new graduates, and other nurses through a one-to-one relationship. Preceptorships are based on the concept of modeling. Learners acquire or modify behaviors by observing vicariously a model who has the behaviors needed by the learner and having an opportunity to practice those behaviors. Andersen (1991) found that preceptors, when working with students, use a variety of teaching behaviors, an important one being role modeling.

In the role of teacher, the preceptor provides instruction for learners based on identified objectives and individual learner needs, provides feedback, assists learners in integrating education and work values, and is involved in their evaluation. The learner, in turn, has an opportunity to work with a competent role model involved in client and unit-based decisions.

Many of the experiences involving preceptors, whether for students or new graduates, are designed to facilitate the transition from the student role to that of staff nurse. By working on a one-to-one basis with a practitioner functioning in the role, students and new graduates are able to model behaviors of the practitioner and become socialized into the professional role. Preceptors provide an opportunity for the development of a mentor relationship with the learner, important in facilitating role transition.

The preceptor guides the student or orientee in gaining the knowledge and skills needed for care of clients and learning about the role and responsibilities of the nurse in that setting (Bizek & Oermann, 1990). This one-to-one relationship between the preceptor and learner provides for close supervision and immediate feedback on performance; learners develop competence in performing clinical skills and increase self-confidence in their new role. For the preceptor, the role presents a professional challenge and a source of stimulation. Bizek and Oermann (1990) believe that "participating in the growth and development of a beginning practitioner can be a source of satisfaction for the preceptor" (p. 440).

There are various ways in which preceptors may be incorporated within nursing education programs depending on the goals to be achieved. Clinical courses, particularly those offered in the student's final semester or during the summer preceding the last year of study, may be designed to include the use of preceptors who act as role model and teacher for the student to whom assigned.

The literature abounds with reports on preceptorships in nursing programs. Reports on the effectiveness of preceptorships cite benefits gained on the part of students themselves (Barker, 1985; Clayton, Broome, & Ellis, 1989; Hughes, Wade, & Peters, 1991; Jairath, Costello, Wallace, & Rudy, 1991; Kilcullen, 1985; Koehler, Broome, Clayton, & Morse, 1988; Myrick, 1988; Scheetz, 1989; Spears, 1986; Turkoski, 1987) and for the preceptors and settings in which they practice (Barker, 1985; Hsieh & Knowles, 1990; Koehler et al., 1988; Miner & Schueler, 1987; Swayne, 1986).

Clayton et al. (1989) studied the relationship between a preceptorship experience and role socialization of graduate nurses. Findings suggested that working with a preceptor enhanced transition to the staff nurse role. Scheetz (1989) found that students who participated in a preceptorship experience had significantly greater gains in clinical competence than students who worked as nursing assistants in noninstructional clinical settings. Further empirical study on preceptorship, however, is still needed particularly since it is becoming, in Myrick's terms, one of the "most acceptable alternate method[s] of clinical teaching" (Myrick, 1988, p. 591).

Experiences involving preceptors may also focus on the development of knowledge and clinical skills in a particular area of nursing practice. Often students select their own area of practice and clinical setting depending upon their objectives. The kinds of experiences in which students engage and the amount of time spent in the agency vary with the nursing program and objectives to be achieved.

Oermann (1991a) and Oermann and Provenzano (1992) have examined the outcomes of an undergraduate critical care course in which students select the type of critical care setting in which they want to practice and are then paired with a preceptor for their clinical experience. One of the benefits cited by students in working with preceptors in this setting is improved transition into practice (Oermann, 1991a; Oermann, Dunn, Munro, & Monahan, in press).

When preceptors are used for clinical teaching, faculty functions in a different role than with other clinical courses. In general, the teacher is responsible for: (1) planning the experience with agency personnel and with the preceptor; (2) orienting students to the course, use of preceptors for clinical instruction, and faculty role; (3) assisting preceptors with educational problems that arise; (4) monitoring the experience and student achievement of the objectives; and (5) participating in evaluation. Although preceptors provide the clinical instruction, faculty has overall responsibility for the experience and an important role in monitoring it so student and program objectives are attained.

In clinical agencies, preceptors as part of an orientation program facilitate role transition of the new graduate and entry into the work setting. Preceptors have also been used to assist experienced nurses in changing roles in the setting or moving into a new area of clinical practice.

Other models of concentrated clinical practice, such as externship, cooperative education, and internship, are also aimed at facilitating the transition from the student to staff nurse role, improving the learner's clinical and leadership skills, and increasing self-confidence in practice. Concentrated practice is developed within some kind of system or pattern that includes experience with the practitioner role. Such practice, by enabling learners to function in the role for which they are preparing, provides a means of bridging the gap between school and work. This intensive clinical experience provides for experiential learning and the development of problem-solving and decision-making skills and reflects concepts of modeling, particularly with those strategies in which the student or new graduate works with a preceptor.

Three modes of concentrated clinical practice include:

1. Externship
2. Cooperative education/Work study
3. Internship

Externship. An externship provides opportunity for students to gain experience in a practice setting and receive both academic credit from the college/university and a salary from the agency, frequently at the rate of ancillary personnel, for the experience. The externship serves to improve the student's knowledge and performance through a variety of experiences in direct patient care under the direction of a preceptor. Oermann and Navin (1992) found that new graduates who had an externship experience while enrolled in their basic nursing program rated their competency in performing psychomotor skills and their clinical competence overall at a significantly higher level than non-externs. The authors suggest that the externship may have increased the nurse's confidence in performing skills and providing care to patients. Often offered in the summer preceding the final year of study, externships vary as to the number of credit hours, extent of time in the clinical setting, kinds of experiences in which students engage, and supervision of the learner. Students are frequently supervised by preceptors with periodic contact with faculty who retain responsibility for planning, monitoring, and evaluating the experience.

Cooperative Education/Work Study. Cooperative education unites educational institutions, employers, and students in developing a career related work experience which is integrated within the curriculum (Siedenberg, 1989). Cusack, Joos, and Simenc (1990) identify two types of cooperative programs: part-time or parallel plan and full-time alternating plan. In the part-time parallel plan, the student carries a full-time course load during a semester and also works part-time in a clinical setting. In this design students work in the clinical agency as they progress through the nursing program.

The full-time alternating plan allows a student to alternate one semester of study with one semester of full-time paid work. This model of work-study provides flexibility for the student to leave the educational setting for a period of time to engage in concentrated clinical practice, although usually in an ancillary position, and obtain experience with other systems of care. In this type of experience, employment is arranged by the nursing program or student and is limited to a specified length of time, for instance, a semester, generally coinciding with the student's academic schedule (Waters, Limon, & Spencer, 1983). Faculty has a role in counseling students in the selection of clinical settings and type of experience so that the work-study is an integral part of the total nursing program.

Internship. An internship refers to a work period immediately following the educational program. With this model, the practice experience takes place after completion of the program rather than during it, as with externship and cooperative education, and thus is arranged by the clinical setting in which the new graduate is employed. An internship represents a supervised orientation program aimed at facilitating the transition from student to staff nurse (Roell, 1981).

SUMMARY

Planning for the clinical practice experience includes deciding on the teaching methods for promoting achievement of the objectives. No one teaching method is inclusive because of the multipurpose nature of the setting, multiple activities inherent in nursing, variation in purpose and objectives for a specific clinical experience, and differences among learners and teachers. Teaching methods are classified as experiential, problem-solving, conference, observation, media, self-directed, and preceptorships.

Experiential methods provide for direct experiencing of events either through clinical practice involving interaction with real clients and others in the field or through contrived experiences of reality, such as with simulations and role play. These methods include clinical assignment, various written assignments, and simulation/game.

Problem-solving methods assist learners in analyzing a clinical situation to identify problems to be solved and relevant actions to be taken and in applying knowledge to a clinical problem. There are three types of problem-solving methods appropriate for teaching in clinical: problem-solving situation, decision-making situation, and critical incident.

Clinical conferences are group discussions about some aspect of clinical practice. Pre- and postconferences and other types of conferences promote problem-solving about client care and other aspects of practice in the clinical setting. These discussions also provide a means of assisting students in their critical thinking and examining affective dimensions of client care.

Observational teaching methods include observation in the clinical setting, field trip, nursing rounds, and demonstration. A wide range of multimedia is also appropriate for clinical teaching.

Self-directed methods recognize learning as an individual process requiring active involvement of the learner. Strategies classified as self-directed include learning contract, independent study, and self-paced module.

Preceptorships and other models of concentrated practice, such as externships, facilitate transition from the student to staff nurse role. These methods also promote the development of the learner's clinical skills and confidence in his or her own ability in practice.

Criteria assist faculty in relating teaching methods to the demands of the learning situation. The teacher's task is to choose from these classifications methods that fit with the objectives, learners, teacher, and clinical setting in which the practice takes place.

REFERENCES

Allen, D. G., Bowers, B., & Diekelmann, N. (1989). Writing to learn: A reconceptualization of thinking and writing in the nursing curriculum. *Journal of Nursing Education, 28*(1), 6-11.

Andersen, S. L. (1991). Preceptor teaching strategies: Behaviors that facilitate role transition in senior nursing students. *Journal of Nursing Staff Development, 7*(4), 171-175.

Baldwin, D., Hill, P., & Hanson, G. (1991). Performance of psychomotor skills: A comparison of two teaching strategies. *Journal of Nursing Education, 30*(8), 367-370.

Baldwin, J., & Schaffer, S. (1990). The continuing case study. *Nurse Educator, 15*(5), 6-9.

Bandura, A. (1977). *Social learning theory*. Englewood Cliffs, NJ: Prentice-Hall.
Barker, E. L. (1985). Neuroscience nursing elective for senior nursing students. *Journal of Neurosurgical Nursing, 17*, 321-326.
Battista-Calderone, A. (1989). Designing interactive video instruction. *Nursing & Health Care, 10*(9), 505-510.
Bell, D. F., & Bell, D. L. (1983). Harmonizing self-directed and teacher-directed approaches to learning. *Nurse Educator, VIII*(1), 24-30.
Bizek, K. S., & Oermann, M. H. (1990). Study of educational experiences, support, and job satisfaction among critical care preceptors. *Heart & Lung, 19*, 439-444.
Blainey, C. A. (1991). Using clinical focus guidelines to emphasize processes of learning. *Journal of Nursing Education, 30*(3), 141-142.
Blenner, J. L. (1991). Researcher for a day: A simulation game. *Nurse Educator, 16*(2), 32-35.
Blood money. (1975). New York: Gamed/Simulations.
Brown, P. A. (1991). Computers in nursing practice. In M. H. Oermann, *Professional nursing practice: A conceptual approach*. Philadelphia: J. B. Lippincott.
Chang, B. L. (1986). Computer-aided instruction in nursing education. In H. H. Werley, J. J. Fitzpatrick, & R. L. Taunton (Eds.). *Annual Review of Nursing Research* (pp. 217-233). New York: Springer.
Clayton, G. M., Broome, M. E., & Ellis, L. A. (1989). Relationship between a preceptorship experience and role socialization of graduate nurses. *Journal of Nursing Education, 28*(2), 72-75.
Cooper, S. S. (1981). Methods of teaching—revisited: The incident process. *The Journal of Continuing Education in Nursing, 12*(6), 22-24.
Cooper, S. S. (1982a). Methods of teaching—revisited: The demonstration. *The Journal of Continuing Education in Nursing, 13*(3), 44-45.
Cooper, S. S. (1982b). Methods of teaching—revisited: Nursing rounds and bedside clinics. *The Journal of Continuing Education in Nursing, 13*(5), 19-21.
Cusack, J. M., Joos, L. J., & Simenc, G. L. (1990). Cooperative education. *Dimensions of Critical Care Nursing, 9*(2), 119-125.
de Tornyay, R., & Thompson, M. A. (1987). *Strategies for teaching nursing* (3rd ed.). New York: John Wiley.
Evans, M. L. (1989). Simulations: The selection and use in developing nursing competencies. *Journal of Nursing Staff Development, 5*(2), 65-69.
Fitzgerald, L. T., & McCurren, C. D. (1988). In pursuit of accreditation. *Nursing & Health Care, 9*(3), 143-145.
Hanna, D. R. (1991). Using simulations to teach clinical nursing. *Nurse Educator, 16*(2), 28-31.

Hassett, M. R. (1984). Computers and nursing education in the 1980s. *Nursing Outlook, 32,* 34–36.

Hsieh, N. L., & Knowles, D. W. (1990). Instructor facilitation of the preceptorship relationship in nursing education. *Journal of Nursing Education, 29*(6), 262–268.

Hughes, O., Wade, B., & Peters, M. (1991). The effects of a synthesis of nursing practice course on senior nursing students' self-concept and role perception. *Journal of Nursing Education, 30*(2), 69–72.

Into aging. (1978). Thorofare, NJ: Charles B. Slack (developed by T. L. Hoffman & S. Dempsey).

Jairath, N., Costello, J., Wallace, P., & Rudy, L. (1991). The effect of preceptorship upon diploma program nursing students' transition to the professional nursing role. *Journal of Nursing Education, 30*(6), 251–555.

Kilcullen, P. B. (1985). A learning experience in independent study. *Journal of Nursing Education, 24,* 30–31.

Koehler, C., Broome, M., Clayton, G., & Morse, J. (1988). Rural preceptorship program for baccalaureate students. *Nurse Educator, 13*(2), 5–6.

Lowdermilk, D. L., & Fishel, A. H. (1991). Computer simulations as a measure of nursing students' decision-making skills. *Journal of Nursing Education, 30*(1), 34–39.

Matthews, R., & Viens, S. (1988). Evaluating basic skills through group video testing. *Journal of Nursing Education, 27*(1), 44–46.

Meyers, C. (1986). *Teaching students to think critically.* San Francisco: Jossey-Bass.

Miller, M. A., & Malcolm, N. S. (1990). Critical thinking in the nursing curriculum. *Nursing & Health Care, 11*(2), 67–73.

Miner, D., & Schuelder, H. (1987). Students to perioperative nurses. *AORN Journal, 45,* 993–998.

Myrick, F. (1988). Preceptorship: A viable alternative clinical teaching strategy? *Journal of Advanced Nursing, 13*(5), 588–591.

Oermann, M. H. (1984a). Analyzing and selecting audiovisual materials. *Nurse Educator, 9*(4), 24–27.

Oermann, M. H. (1984b). An instrument for analyzing curriculum materials in nursing. *Journal of Nursing Education, 23,* 404–406.

Oermann, M. H. (1990a). Psychomotor skill development. *Journal of Continuing Education in Nursing, 21*(5), 202–204.

Oermann, M. H. (1990b). Research on teaching methods. In G. M. Clayton & P. A. Baj (Eds.). *Review of research in nursing education* (Vol. III). New York: National League for Nursing.

Oermann, M. H. (1991a). Effectiveness of a critical care nursing course: Preparing students for practice in critical care. *Heart & Lung, 20*(3), 278–283.

Oermann, M. H. (1991b). *Professional nursing practice: A conceptual approach.* Philadelphia: J. B. Lippincott.

Oermann, M. H., & Gignac, D. A. (1991). Knowledge and attitudes about AIDS among Canadian nursing students: Educational implications. *Journal of Nursing Education, 30*(5), 217-221.

Oermann, M. H., Dunn, D., Munro, L., & Monahan, K. (1992). Critical care education at the baccalaureate level. *Nurse Educator* (in press).

Oermann, M. H., & Navin, M. A. (1991). Effect of extern experience on clinical competence of graduate nurses. *Nursing Connections, 4*(4), 2-9.

Oermann, M. H., & Provenzano, L. M. (1992). Students' knowledge and perceptions of critical care nursing. *Critical Care Nurse, 12* (1), 72-77.

Plunkett, E. J., & Oliveri, R. J. (1989). A strategy for introducing diagnostic reasoning: Hypothesis testing using a simulation approach. *Nurse Educator, 14*(6), 27-31.

Reilly, D. E. (1958). *Nursing student responses to the clinical field.* New York: Columbia University, Department of Nursing.

Reilly, D. E., & Oermann, M. H. (1990). *Behavioral objectives: Evaluation in nursing* (3rd ed.). New York: National League for Nursing.

Rizzolo, M. A. (1990). Factors influencing the development and use of interactive video in nursing education. *Computers in Nursing, 8*(4), 151-159.

Roell, S. M. (1981). Nurse-intern programs: How they're working. *Nurse Educator, VI*(6), 29-31.

Rufo, K. L. (1985). Effectiveness of self-instructional packages in staff development activities. *Journal of Continuing Education in Nursing, 16*(3), 80-84.

Rogers, C. R. (1983). *Freedom to learn for the 80's.* Columbus, OH: Chas. E. Merrill.

Schare, B. L., Dunn, S. C., Clark, H. M., Soled, S. W., & Gilman, B. R. (1991). The effects of interactive video on cognitive achievement and attitude toward learning. *Journal of Nursing Education, 30*(3), 109-113.

Scheetz, L. J. (1989). Baccalaureate nursing student preceptorship programs and the development of clinical competence. *Journal of Nursing Education, 28,* 29-35.

Schön, D. A. (1990). *Educating the reflective practitioner.* San Francisco: Jossey-Bass.

Seidenberg, J. M. (1989). Investing in nursing education: Some evidence of immediate private monetary benefits. *Journal of Nursing Education, 28*(5), 210-214.

Spears, M. W. (1986). The benefits of preceptorships. *JONA, 16*(6), 4-5.

Starpower. (1969). Del Mar, CA: Simile II.

Strength, D. E., & Keen-Payne, R. (1991). Computerized patient care documentation. *Computers in Nursing, 9*(1), 22-26.

Swayne, M. (1986). Why we work side by side with student nurses. *RN, 49*(8), 44-45.
Tanner, C. A. (1986). The nursing care plan as a teaching method: Reason or ritual? *Nurse Educator, 11*(4), 8-10.
Turkoski, B. (1987). Reducing stress in nursing students' clinical learning experience. *Journal of Nursing Education, 8,* 335-337.
Van Dover, L., & Boblin, S. (1991). Student nurse computer experience and preference for learning. *Computers in Nursing, 9*(2), 75-79.
Waite, M. E., Duckett, L., Schmitz, K., Crisham, P., & Ryden, M. (1989). Developing case studies for ethics education in nursing. *Journal of Nursing Education, 28*(4), 175-180.
Waters, V., Limon, S., & Spencer, J. B. (1983). *Ohlone transition: Student to staff nurse.* Battle Creek, MI: W. K. Kellogg Foundation.

BIBLIOGRAPHY

Allanich, B. C., & Jennings, B. M. (1990). Evaluating the effects of a nurse preceptorship programme. *Journal of Advanced Nursing, 15*(1), 22-28.
Allen, B. S., Devney, A. M., & Sharper, D. M. (1986). The effect of practice in detecting technical errors on performance of a simple medical procedure. *Computers in Nursing, 4*(1), 11-16.
Ball, M. J., & Hannah, K. J., Jelger, U. G., & Peterson, H. (Eds.). (1988). *Nursing informatics.* New York: Springer-Verlag.
Billings, D. M. (1984). Evaluating computer assisted instruction. *Nursing Outlook, 32,* 50-53.
Billings, D. M. (1991). Assessing learning styles using a computerized learning styles inventory. *Computers in Nursing, 9*(3), 121-215.
Bolwell, C. (1988). Evaluating computer-assisted instruction. *Nursing & Health Care, 9*(9), 511-515.
Brundenell, I., & Carpenter, C. S. (1990). Adult learning styles and attitudes toward computer assisted instruction. *Journal of Nursing Education, 29*(2), 79-83.
Cooper, S. S. (1982). Methods of teaching—revisited: Experiential diaries and learning logs. *The Journal of Continuing Education in Nursing, 13*(6), 32-34.
Dear, M. R., & Bartol, G. (1984). Independent study as a learning experience in baccalaureate nursing programs: Perceptions and practices. *Journal of Nursing Education, 23,* 240-244.
DiRienzo, J. N. (1983). Before client care—An interactive conference. *Journal of Nursing Education, 22,* 84-86.

Eble, K. (1988). *The craft of teaching* (2nd ed.). San Francisco: Jossey-Bass.
Fuszard, B. (1989). *Innovative teaching strategies in nursing*. Rockville, MD: Aspen.
Goldrick, B., Appling-Stevens, S., & Larson, E. (1990). Infection control programmed instruction: An alternative to classroom instruction in baccalaureate nursing education. *Journal of Nursing Education, 29*(1), 20-25.
Goodman, J., Blake, J., & Lott, M. (1990). CAI: A strategy for training minority and academically disadvantaged students. *Nurse Educator, 15*(2), 37-41.
Itano, J. K., Warren, J. J., & Ishida, D. N. (1987). A comparison of role conceptions and role deprivation of baccalaureate students in nursing participating in a preceptorship or a traditional clinical program. *Journal of Nursing Education, 26*(2), 69-73.
Mitchell, C. A., & Krainovich, B. (1982). Conducting pre- and postconferences. *American Journal of Nursing, 82*, 823-825.
Olson, R. K., Gresley, R. S., & Heater, B. S. (1984). The effects of an undergraduate clinical internship on the self-concept and professional role mastery of baccalaureate nursing students. *Journal of Nursing Education, 23*, 105-108.
Parkinson, C. F., & Parkinson, S. B. (1989). A comparative study between interactive television and traditional lecture course offerings for nursing students. *Nursing & Health Care, 10*(9), 499-502.
Peirce, A. G. (1991). Preceptorial students' view of their clinical experience. *Journal of Nursing Education, 30*(6), 244-250.
Pigors, P., & Pigors, F. (1966). The incident process—A method of inquiry. *Nursing Outlook, 14*(10), 48-50.
Plasterer, H. H., & Mills, N. (1983). Teach management theory—Through fun and games. *Journal of Nursing Education, 22*, 80-83.
Sasmor, J. L. (1984). Contracting for clinical. *Journal of Nursing Education, 23*, 171-173.
Sinclair, V. G. (1989). Addressing challenges in nursing informatics instruction. *Journal of Nursing Education, 28*(2), 82-84.
Sleet, D. A., & Hileman, L. (1981). *Guide to health instruction: Simulations, games, and related activities*. Irvine, CA: Human Behavior Research Group.
Stuart-Siddall, S., & Haberlin, J. M. (Eds.). (1983). *Preceptorships in nursing education*. Rockville, MD: Aspen Systems.
Wilson, B. A. (1991). Computer anxiety in nursing students. *Journal of Nursing Education, 30*(2), 52-56.
Zerbe, M. B., Lachat, M. F. (1991). A three-tiered team model for undergraduate preceptor programs. *Nurse Educator, 16*(2), 18-21.
Zimmer, E., & Hawkins, M. E. (1991). Quality videotapes with the help of a computer. *Computers in Nursing, 9*(3), 113-115.

7

Cognitive Learning in the Clinical Setting

Individuals function as total integrated beings in all human experiences. The learning process engages the learner in a holistic way along cognitive, psychomotor, and affective dimensions. In education, there is reference to these three areas, i.e., cognitive, psychomotor, and affective, as domains of learning. Although most learning involves a composite of behaviors from all three domains, teachers have found it helpful to consider the domains separately for instructional purposes. Because of the special characteristics of performance for each domain, this chapter and chapters 8 & 9 address separately the specific theoretical constructs and teaching processes of each area. Although each domain of learning is emphasized as a separate entity, the teacher must constantly bear in mind that the domains are interrelated, and indeed, this interrelationship may be essential for expert performance of any one skill.

Knowledge has always been recognized as essential to nursing, but how has the term knowledge been generally used? Does it mean "know about something?" or does it refer to an inherent action, "knowing how?" Today's nursing practice must encompass both "knowing about" and "knowing how," for nursing is a discipline that practices in concert with other health professionals, all influenced by the impact of exploding knowledge and technology. The expanding boundaries of knowledge create the need for disciplines like nursing to reexamine its roles and responsibilities and the nature of preparation of its practitioners.

Historically, nurses were receivers of information from others. This information then served as a basis for nursing knowledge. The discrepancy between nursing and medical knowledge occurred as a result of medical education moving into the university, where it began to develop its scientific base, while nursing maintained the practice mode of apprenticeship learning. Nursing then "adopted" the physician's knowledge and incorporated it into nursing knowledge. The usual learning experiences entailed lectures by the physician on a given pathologic phenomenon followed by a class on nursing of that phenomenon. Nursing knowledge was predominantly prescriptive for the medical state of the patient. The authoritarian structure of the hospital setting, modeled from the religious and military influences of nursing's beginnings, left little margin for creative thinkers among nurses in terms of designing nursing care or patterns by which the care was delivered.

Indeed, nursing still does borrow theories, but a new direction is underway as nursing research is generating nursing knowledge. In pursuit of this knowledge, "knowing how" has become a significant factor. This "knowing how" entails the cognitive processes of concept learning, problem solving, decision making, critical thinking, and clinical judgment, which address skills in using and validating both nursing and borrowed knowledge. Emphasis is now on cognitive skill development which considers knowledge as a dynamic factor to be developed and constantly tested. Solutions to problems in patient care and the delivery of this care are more complex and require different cognitive skills than in the past. In this chapter, each of these cognitive processes is explored and its relationship to teaching in the cognitive domain in nursing is demonstrated.

CONCEPT LEARNING

Although the acquisition of facts and specific information relevant to nursing practice represents an important outcome of a nursing education program, it certainly is not the primary goal of teaching. The fragile nature of facts in an information society requires that students learn concepts and theories of knowledge domains pertinent to nursing. The use of this knowledge depends upon the development of intellectual skills for analyzing and evaluating situations encountered in the practice field. Concepts provide a means for individuals to group together facts and organize their perceptions and experiences. Through the learning of concepts, students are able to categorize new information. Since theories consist of concepts, concept learning is a prerequisite to the acquisition of theories for use in practice.

There are many concepts to be learned for the practice of nursing. Some concepts relate to the client, such as health, aging, and pain; others pertain to nursing actions, for instance, nursing process and more specifically, positioning and touch. Still others reflect the physical, social, and symbolic environment, such as territory, social support, and power (Kim, 1983).

Learning would be a difficult process if information was acquired through memorization alone. Students, especially in the health fields, are continually faced with a mass of details to be learned, and the management of this can only be accomplished through the learning of concepts. Concept learning refers to the placing of events or objects into a group or category (Child, 1986, p. 135). The process of conceptualization, placing events or objects into categories, serves to reduce the complexity of the environment, enables learners to identify different events, and gives direction as to actions to be taken (Bruner, Goodnow, & Austin, 1956). For example, once students have learned the concept of pain, they do not have to relearn this concept with each client and instead only need to assess whether or not the essential defining properties are present. If the patient exhibits these defining properties, then "it" is pain. To know that the patient is in pain also provides direction as to appropriate nursing actions to be taken. Concepts enable learners to relate different classes of events and objects to one another to form systems. Bruner and colleagues (1956) write:

> For we operate . . . with category systems—*classes of events that are related to each other in various kinds of superordinate systems. We map and give meaning to our world by relating classes of events rather than by relating individual events.* (p. 13)

Concepts refer to a general *idea* reflecting a group of events or objects that share common characteristics. These characteristics, sometimes referred to as attributes, are the identifying features of a concept. The concept of patient refers to someone receiving health care. Whether or not such a person is male or female or is young or old is irrelevant to the concept of patient. In learning a concept, one identifies the relevant characteristics and learns to ignore irrelevant ones.

Exemplars are positive instances or examples of the concept, while nonexemplars are negative instances. Exemplars carry important information to assist the learner in identifying what the concept is. Research indicates that individuals learn more efficiently from positive instances of the concept than from negative ones (Glaser, 1969). Learning the concept of empathy proceeds more efficiently if examples of empathy are given emphasis rather than instances of a lack of empathy.

Some concepts are more difficult to learn than others. For instance, the concept of nursing team is relatively easy to learn. Essential characteristics of this concept are that it consists of a group of persons who represent nursing personnel. In contrast, the concept of pain is difficult to learn because instances of pain vary and sometimes there is not a clear distinction between pain and a lack of it.

Concept Attainment

Concept attainment involves learning what characteristics are relevant for grouping events or objects into categories. It is the search for defining characteristics to identify a particular concept. Concept attainment, then, is the process of learning a concept invented by someone else. In contrast, concept formation occurs when learners develop concepts of their own.

Nursing diagnosis is an example of a concept attainment task in that the nurse groups characteristics or cues into a diagnostic category. Characteristics such as inability to move, limited range of motion, decreased muscle strength, and impaired coordination may be grouped together and identified as the nursing diagnosis impaired physical mobility. Nursing diagnoses are complex concepts because of the number of cues that need to be interpreted and then grouped together, their variability, and their probabilistic nature. Identification of one nursing diagnosis does not necessarily exclude others.

In teaching students about concepts relevant to nursing practice, case studies, simulations, CAI, and other related teaching strategies may be developed around the concept to be learned. Goosen (1989) describes use of a model case which represents the concept as presented by the teacher. The model case provides enough information about the concept "to simulate a mental image of the concept" (p. 35). In addition to cases which provide an example of the concept, other types of cases may be developed to demonstrate characteristics and clinical situations not representative of the concept. In this way learners begin to differentiate examples of the concept from nonexemplars. Goosen (1989) describes the use of contrary cases, not representative of the concept, for this purpose.

Heims and Boyd (1990) describe a clinical teaching strategy, Concept-Based Learning Activity (CBLA), for assisting students in learning about concepts in the clinical setting. In the CBLA clinical objectives are written specific to the concept, and learning activities are proposed to assist in transfer of learning and facilitate inquiry regarding the concept (p. 251). The clinical experiences are designed around the concept to be learned. This is important in facilitating learning about the concept since it provides experience with real clinical problems in which the student needs to identify characteristics and decide whether or not they represent a particular concept.

Concepts assist learners in categorizing events and objects they deal with in the practice setting. They enable learners to give meaning to what they perceive. There are many concepts to be learned for effective practice in nursing.

PROBLEM SOLVING

In the clinical setting, students are continually confronted with problems, either client- or setting-oriented, demanding resolution. Some of these are relatively easy to solve, but most tend to represent difficult tasks for the learner because of the complexity and uniqueness of the problem, lack of clear solutions, or the learner's unfamiliarity with them. The development of problem-solving ability is an important outcome of a nursing education program.

Problem-Solving Process

Problem solving has been viewed as a process commencing with definition of the problem and proceeding through the gathering of data relative to the problem, formulation of solutions, and testing and evaluation of the solutions chosen. It involves developing and then testing hypotheses that represent possible solutions to the problem. Once the hypotheses have been formulated, the learner deduces the logical implications of each. The hypotheses are then tested until the problem is solved:

Parnes (1984) writes that in problem solving:

The problem-solver goes from an examination of "what is" to an explanation of "what might be" to a judgment of "what should be" to an assessment of "what can be" to a decision of "what will be" to action that becomes a new "what is." (p. 30)

"What is" refers to an understanding of the data relative to the problem; "what might be" implies the development of solutions; "what should be" involves decisions as to the solutions; "what can be" refers to adaptations of approaches into usable solutions; and "what will be" indicates the best plans for solving the problem (Parnes, 1984).

Problem solving is influenced by the learner's knowledge of concepts and theories and past experiences with similar problems. Knowledge is essential for both understanding the problem and arriving at solutions. Familiarity with the subject matter influences the learner's ability to identify the problems and make decisions about possible solutions. Kintgen-Andrews (1991), in a review of the literature on critical thinking, reports that an understanding of the content is a significant factor in problem solving (p. 155). Past experience with a clinical situation influences a practitioner's perception of the situation and predisposition to act in a certain way. Expert nurses and beginners differ in their problem solving in that the expert perceives the clinical situation as a whole, in comparison with the beginner who tends to focus on pieces of information, and uses past concrete situations as paradigm cases for approaching the present one (Benner, 1984). Individuals facing a problem new to them do not have past situations to refer to and use as a guide for action. They approach problems primarily from a theoretical perspective which does not take into account the context and variables associated with the specific case, thus limiting their understanding of the situation and ability to identify possible responses. Through experience the learner comes to know what to expect typically in regard to a particular problem and what actions are appropriately taken.

Problem solving is also influenced by the learner's stage of cognitive development, the ability to think and reason. Theories of cognitive development propose that problem-solving abilities and thinking differ according to the stage the learner is at. With advanced stages of development, individuals are able to solve more complex problems (Stonewater & Stonewater, 1984) because they have a greater repertoire of knowledge and ability to manipulate it and have a different perspective about the nature of knowledge and truth.

In professional practice, not all problems lend themselves to resolution through application of theory and a technical approach. Some problems faced by the practitioner defy technical rationality. They may be difficult to identify, presenting themselves as unique cases, and may have no clearly defined solutions. Schön (1990) refers to these problems as ones in a swampy lowland, not lending themselves to resolution through a technical rationality approach. In comparison, on the high ground, practice problems are able to be solved with solutions based on theory and research, a technical rationality (Schön, 1990).

In nursing practice, many problems faced by students and practitioners do not present themselves as well defined problems to which previously learned rules may be applied. Neither problems nor solutions are clearly defined. There is not an obvious fit between theories and the clinical situation. Instead, the problems require new strategies for analysis, new methods of reasoning, and new kinds of action. For these clinical situations, the learner devises new approaches for dealing with them.

Schön (1990) differentiates professional knowledge in terms of facts, rules and procedures which may be applied nonproblematically to problems with professional knowledge which reflects thinking like a professional. The former represents a technical training. When learning to think like a professional, students develop new ways of reasoning and problem solving. With experience and knowledge, students will develop the expertise that leads to a knowing-in-action skill in problem solving.

Students in nursing are faced with the need to solve different kinds of problems, some for which a technical rationality approach will lead to problem resolution and others which require new ways of thinking. In clinical practice students develop an awareness that existing knowledge does not fit every clinical situation and every client problem does not have one right answer. Many problems faced by the student in the clinical setting are uncertain and unique; for these problems students construct and test "new categories of understanding, strategies of action, and ways of framing problems" (Schön, 1990, p. 39).

Intuition

Not all problem solving involves use of a conscious and logical sequence of steps to identify the problem and arrive at a solution. Problems are also solved through intuition, an understanding in which the individual is unaware of how it occurred. Bruner (1963) views intuition as "the intellectual technique of arriving at plausible but tentative formulations without going through the analytic steps by which such formulations would be found to be valid or invalid conclusions" (p. 13). Intuition refers to an immediate awareness of "events without the conscious use of linear reasoning" (Miller & Rew, 1989, p. 85). It is a sense of knowing without a preceding rational analysis. Intuitive thinking does not follow a careful sequence of steps toward problem solution but instead reflects the process by which an individual arrives at an answer without awareness of how that answer was reached. Bruner emphasizes the importance of intuitive thinking. "Through intuitive thinking the individual may often arrive at solutions to problems which he would not achieve at all, or at best more slowly, through analytic thinking" (p. 58). Miller and Rew (1989) emphasize that nursing requires both analytical and intuitive thinking processes. Problems and solutions arrived at through intuition can often be confirmed later through an analytic approach.

Benner (1984) acknowledges the role of intuition in solving clinical problems and making nursing judgments. Often the nurse begins with vague hunches, not arrived at through a conscious and rational thought process, which then direct the practitioner in obtaining evidence to confirm them. A hunch is not sufficient but leads to confirming data. Benner writes, "Experts dare not stop with vague hunches, but neither do they care to ignore those hunches that could lead to early identification of problems and the search for confirming evidence" (p. xix).

Miller and Rew (1989) call upon nurse educators to encourage students to use intuitive processes as well as analytical ways of thinking. They propose greater emphasis on the processes of learning, more awareness of the unique qualities women bring to the learning situation, and use of experiential forms of learning "with emphasis on the problem and process rather than on the solution" (p. 86). Group discussions which are open and encourage reflective thinking and use of teacher behaviors which reinforce the thinking process rather than seeking the one right answer encourage students to develop their intuition.

DECISION MAKING

Decisions are made throughout the problem-solving process—decisions as to the nature of the problem, whether or not a solution is necessary, types of data to be collected, potential solutions, and the best one for that particular problem. The very nature of nursing practice requires that nurses make decisions relative to clients, staff, and activities in the clinical setting which are not based on problems but indicate a course of action. For these reasons, decision making represents another essential cognitive skill to be developed in a nursing education program.

Decision making involves a series of steps in which information is gathered, "integrated, weighed and valued" to arrive at a decision on a course of action from a number of alternatives (Prescott, Dennis, & Jacox, 1987, p. 58). Decision making requires choosing among alternatives. This notion of choice is the important element in the process, for in decision making the individual chooses a course of action following consideration of alternatives. Making a choice involves examining different alternatives and the consequences of each and weighing them against criteria to arrive at a judgment as to the best one.

Although there are different theoretical perspectives to decision-making, the process, in general, addresses the following phases:

1. Collection of information about the situation in which a decision is required and analysis of the situation to identify the problem.
2. Generation of alternatives and consideration of the possible consequences of each if selected.
3. Selection of one of the alternatives for implementation.

Selection of the best alternative, in terms of its benefits, represents a rational decision. In a rational decision, the individual analyzes the situation, alternatives, and their consequences and then judges which alternative is preferable. Yet, there are limits to rationality in decision making since rarely does one make a decision based on knowledge of all possible alternatives and consequences.

Decisions are affected by one's values and biases and by cultural norms. These influence the individual's perception and analysis of the situation, alternatives considered, and ultimate choice. What seems rational to one individual may not be so to someone from a different cultural group. Decisions are made *with* clients and/or staff, not *for* them. Participatory decision making is important so the decision is congruent with the values, beliefs, and culture of the recipient of the decision and has a greater likelihood of acceptance.

Decisions may be categorized according to the degree of risk faced in making the choice which is dependent on the extent of objective knowledge about the possible consequences for a given alternative action. There is less risk in making a decision when the person has sufficient knowledge about the actions and consequences. Few decisions as to nursing problems or actions to be taken are made with complete certainty. More commonly, decisions in the clinical setting are made under conditions of uncertainty.

In decision making, as with problem solving, the learner's knowledge base is important, for learners must be able to analyze the situation in which a decision is required and know which alternatives to consider and the possible consequences of each. This knowledge refers

CRITICAL THINKING

Thinking may be creative or critical (Yinger, 1980). Creative thinking results in the development of new ideas and products, whereas critical thinking involves the evaluation of ideas. Critical thinking is rational thinking. It includes ability to (1) evaluate a statement and (2) identify reasons, for instance, evidence on which to base that evaluation. "A critical thinker is one who recognizes the importance, and convicting forces, of reasons. When assessing claims, evaluating procedures, or making judgments, the critical thinker seeks reasons on which to base his or her assessment, evaluation, or judgment" (Siegel, 1980, p. 8). Siegel suggests that critical thinking is also principled thinking which entails making judgments that are nonarbitrary, impartial, and objective. Halpern (1984) views critical thinking as purposeful and directed toward goals, compared to thinking associated with one's everyday routine.

Learners who engage in critical thinking do not accept statements outright but instead seek reasons for supporting them. Through evaluation they decide for themselves which ideas to accept and which to reject, and they can provide reasons underlying their decisions. Kitchener (1983) proposes that students at the college level "need more help in actively applying the tools of evaluation and the rules of inquiry to the critical examination of . . . [different perspectives]" (p. 92).

Meyers (1986) suggests that critical thinking is discipline-specific, therefore, varying across disciplines. Nurses, for instance, may engage in critical thinking differently than philosophers and historians. Critical thinking differs across fields of study because the core ingredient of critical thinking is the foundational knowledge of the discipline (Meyers, 1986). One cannot think critically about nursing without a basic knowledge of its concepts, theories, and content. The teacher presents a framework for critical thinking within nursing and encourages development of an attitude of inquiry (Reilly & Oermann, 1990).

Critical thinking represents the thought process that underlies problem solving and decision making; both intellectual processes require rational thinking. According to Yinger (1980), problem solving and decision making serve as tasks to be accomplished through critical thinking.

The ability to think critically is essential to the practice of nursing and functioning effectively within the health care system. Nurses need to think critically to be "safe, competent, and skillful practitioners" (Miller & Malcolm, 1990, p. 67). Development of critical thinking skills has always been important but is particularly acute today considering the types of decisions required for practice, complexity of client needs, and amount of information the nurse is faced with in practice. Meyers (1986) suggests that critical thinking is more important now than in the past because the amount of information exceeds ability to think critically about it (p. xi).

Skill in assessing claims and making judgments on the basis of reasons is not sufficient, for critical thinking also requires a certain set of attitudes. A critical thinker is one who is inclined to search for reasons, exhibits a questioning attitude, and avoids judgments that are arbitrary, partial, and subjective. "It is not enough for a student to be able to evaluate claims on the basis of evidence . . . to be a critical thinker, a student must be *disposed* to do so" (Siegel, 1980, p. 9). Miller and Malcolm (1990) believe that "attitudes set the tone for inquiry" (p. 69). Both the teacher's and student's attitudes are important in the process. The student explores ideas, considers different perspectives, struggles with issues, and examines problems and solutions in a new way; and the teacher promotes and supports such thinking.

The teacher presents a framework for critical thinking and assists students in developing an attitude for engaging in such thought (Meyers, 1986). The teacher is crucial in promoting this type of thinking in clinical practice. Students must be encouraged and supported in expressing ideas and questioning long-standing approaches to problems (Reilly & Oermann, 1990, p. 64). Encouraging learners to ask questions, examine problems, consider different perspectives, and pursue alternate lines of thinking about their clients becomes an important role for the teacher in the clinical setting.

Development of critical thinking ability is vital to effective nursing practice, particularly considering the influence of expanding knowledge and technology on health care and political, economic, social, and ethical decisions affecting care delivery. The complexity of nursing practice demands competent and independent judgments. Competent judgments are made on the basis of reasons; such reasoning represents critical thinking.

Cognitive Development

Ability to think and reason develops over time through a series of stages. The developmental stage the student is at in thinking influences the ability to solve clinical problems, make independent decisions and judgments, and deal with ambiguity, as well as the willingness to accept diverse points of view and commitment in personal and professional life. Perry (1970) has developed a theory of cognitive development which postulates how students evolve in their thinking about the nature of knowledge, truth, and values and meaning of commitment.

According to Perry, students move from thinking that is simplistic and categorical to where they recognize and can accept diverse perspectives. Development is represented along a continuum of nine positions, which may be grouped into four categories:

1. Dualism (Positions 1 and 2): At this level students view knowledge and values in terms of absolute and concrete categories. They are unable to deal with multiple points of view. In dualism, the right answer is determined by the teacher and other authorities. In the clinical setting, the student seeks the one "correct" problem and approach and accepts that those suggested by the teacher and others are the only appropriate ones.
2. Multiplicity (Positions 3 and 4): In this stage of development, learners acknowledge different perspectives to a given problem or situation although they are unable to evaluate them. There exists an acceptance of uncertainty and, therefore, diversity of opinion.
3. Relativism (Positions 5 and 6): Whereas multiplistic thinkers only acknowledge that different perspectives and solutions to problems exist, relativistic thinkers, in contrast, have acquired the ability to evaluate these perspectives and solutions. In relativism, learners are able to analyze situations with which they are faced and evaluate their own ideas and judgments and

those of others (King, 1978). Decision making often becomes difficult at this point in cognitive development because of the learner's improved understanding of the alternatives and possible outcomes of each if chosen.

4. Commitment in Relativism (Positions 7 to 9): The most advanced stage of cognitive development, representing commitment in personal and professional life, reflects the willingness of learners to act according to their values and beliefs. At this point, learners have established their own identities. Commitment in relativism "entails a readiness to tolerate paradox, take risks, embrace irony, and identify oneself with chosen notions, even when perfectly plausible alternatives exist and are acknowledged" (Hursh, Haas, & Moore, 1983, p. 46).

Learners do not necessarily progress through these nine positions. Some temporize or remain at a particular position, explicitly hesitating to move on; others escape and stay in relativism to avoid commitment; and still others retreat to dualism and absolute thinking.

The Positions of deflection (Temporizing, Escape, and Retreat) offer alternatives at critical points in the development. A person may have recourse to them whenever he feels unprepared, resentful, alienated or overwhelmed to the degree in which his urge to conserve is dominant over his urge to progress. (pp. 57–58)

Perry's theory has applicability to nursing education since the learner's stage of development influences the cognitive processes used in practice. It also provides a theoretical framework for interpreting student behavior in response to situations arising in the clinical setting. Dualistic thinkers view knowledge in terms of absolute categories, unable to recognize differing perspectives and solutions to problems. Because of their authoritarian thinking, students at this level depend on the teacher or someone else in authority to tell them the right answer or procedure to follow and make decisions and judgments for them. Complexity in thought and problem solving, acceptance of diverse perspectives, ability to deal with ambiguity, willingness to take risks, independence in practice, and commitment to be responsible, all important in nursing practice, develop at advanced cognitive levels. Valiga (1983) reports, from a study of 123 baccalaureate nursing students, that while students generally increase in cognitive development through their program, they still remain in the category of dualism at graduation. Her research suggests that the learning experiences in which students engage and faculty with whom they work may be ineffective in assisting them to move forward in their cognitive development.

Frisch (1987) evaluated the level of cognitive development of junior-level baccalaureate students using Perry's theory. Students were evaluated at the beginning and end of an academic semester in which they completed specific learning activities geared to improving cognitive development. In one group, students were also taught specific strategies to enhance their cognitive reasoning skills. Findings indicated that the majority of students were operating at Perry's position 3; only one of the 42 subjects who participated in the study attained Perry's position 4 (p. 27). Frisch suggests that nursing students do not graduate at a level of professional commitment, and cognitive development takes time.

The teacher in the clinical setting plays an important role in the cognitive development of the student. Do faculty encourage divergent thinking or do they instead look for one right answer? Are students asked to examine multiple solutions to clinical problems and solve those problems independently? Are they encouraged to take calculated risks and experiment with care? Dualistic thinking is incompatible with professional nursing practice. "Professional nursing in any setting requires individuals to consider events from multiple points of view and to make independent judgments" (Frisch, 1987, p. 27). Nurse educators are challenged to listen to what students say in response to clinical situations and assist them in moving toward a level of cognitive development more compatible with the complexity of nursing practice.

CLINICAL JUDGMENT

In the setting, practitioners continually make decisions as to nursing diagnoses and courses of action for these diagnostic problems. Through the process of clinical judgment, the nurse decides on data to be collected about the client, makes an interpretation of the data (an inference) to arrive at the diagnosis, and identifies appropriate nursing actions. Judgment, which emphasizes the evaluation of phenomena, is used throughout the process as are problem-solving, decision-making and critical thinking skills. del Bueno (1990) proposes that clinical judgment, a complex skill involving several cognitive and integrative activities, is an important, if not the most important, dimension of nursing practice (p. 290).

Clinical judgment has been viewed according to three theoretical perspectives: (1) information processing theory, (2) decision theory, and (3) phenomenology.

Information Processing Theory

Information processing theory as applied to clinical judgment describes the process by which the practitioner addresses client-oriented problems. The process is similar across health care disciplines although the types of judgments made differ. Problem solving, within an information processing framework, represents an interaction between the nurse, as the information processing system, and task environment. Initially, the nurse attends to cues, i.e., sensory input, in the clinical situation. Cues include signs, symptoms, and other data about the client and environment (Oermann, 1991, p. 159). The nurse then associates an appropriate diagnostic label with these cues. Students are not as attentive to cues as are expert practitioners because of their lack of knowledge and experience. Tentative hypotheses as to the diagnosis (problem presenting in the clinical situation) are then generated from these cues. Between four and seven hypotheses are considered at any one time (Elstein et al., 1972).

Studies in clinical judgment have indicated that these tentative hypotheses are generated early in the interaction with the client (Elstein et al., 1972; Elstein, Shulman, & Sprafka, 1978; Itano, 1989; Putzier, Padrick, Westfall, & Tanner, 1985; Tanner, 1987). The hypotheses define the problem space of possible diagnoses. Arriving at early hypotheses, it is postulated, limits the size of the space that must be searched. Data can then be gathered in relation to these specific hypotheses which provides a means of managing the data. Elstein and colleagues (1978) comment that without such a strategy, a diagnostic work-up could never be completed within a reasonable time. This strategy is believed to represent one that all health care practitioners use as a way of coping with the limitations in the amount of information they can process relative to the client.

The finding as to early hypothesis generation in clinical judgment is important since frequently students are taught in the clinical setting not to decide on the diagnosis until all data are collected. Research suggests, however, that practitioners develop hypotheses early in their interaction with the client and then use them to guide further data gathering. It is also important that learners as well as practitioners consider multiple hypotheses to avoid disregarding a diagnosis.

Hypotheses that are related to each other aid retention in short-term memory (Carnevali, 1984). Arranging them in a hierarchy, from general to specific, allows for better storage of cues (Elstein et al., 1978; Tanner, 1984b). It also directs data collection toward the most general hypotheses, enabling the practitioner to avoid focusing data gathering on specific ones which then may not be accepted. Another way of retaining hypotheses and data in short-term memory relates to the development of competing hypotheses (Carnevali, 1984). Recording data also serves as a way of retaining information in short-term memory.

Generation of hypotheses depends on the possession of an adequate knowledge base stored in long-term memory. With this knowledge, the learner and practitioner alike identify a diagnosis to reflect the cues. The difference between a learner's and an expert's knowledge base is apparent, making it easier for experts to select appropriate diagnoses from long-term memory.

Once early hypotheses are formed, subsequent data gathering focuses on these tentative hypotheses until a diagnosis is made (Elstein et al., 1978; Gordon, 1980; Itano, 1989; Kassirer & Gorry, 1978; Putzier et al., 1985). The nurse collects information to evaluate each hypothesis in order to decide which ones to maintain or modify and which to reject. Evaluation involves comparing the new data collected against each hypothesis in terms of its probability of occurrence given these data. Because of their knowledge and experience, expert nurses are more efficient in collecting specific data to accept or reject a hypothesis than are students, who are often nonselective in the data gathered and tend to collect more information before deciding on a hypothesis (Tanner, 1984a). After arriving at the diagnosis, the nurse then decides on an appropriate course of action.

While clinical judgment is conceptualized as following a logical sequence from data collection through identification of the diagnosis, practitioners, particularly those with expertise in nursing practice, may decide on a client problem without awareness of how they arrived at that problem. Intuition, therefore, enters into the process of clinical judgment.

Decision Theory

Another approach to understanding clinical judgment involves the use of mathematical models for arriving at the diagnosis and course of action. These models attempt to reflect the probabilistic nature of clinical decision making.

Bayesian Model. The Bayesian model is a mathematical formula for determining the probability of a diagnosis following the introduction of new information. In this view of clinical judgment, the decision as to the diagnosis is based on the probability of occurrence of the diagnosis with the addition of a new cue. Often with the Bayesian model, a decision tree or flow chart is used which includes possible diagnostic hypotheses and their probabilities. The nurse moves through the tree to decide if the cues present are associated with a particular diagnosis. Aspinall (1979) examined the effectiveness of a decision tree in improving the accuracy of nurses in making a diagnosis. With a decision tree, accuracy in diagnosis did improve for many of the nurses, although some did not benefit from its use. Jones (1988) believes that decision analysis aids the nurse in identifying the sequences of decisions needed for a client and consequences of each possible decision (p. 190).

Lens Model. The lens model uses correlations to express the relationship between cues and diagnosis. As indicated in Figure 7-1, cues are viewed as the center of the lens. On the left-hand side is the criterion state, or state of the patient, unknown to the practitioner; and on the right is the judgment or inference made about this state from the cues. The patient state and cues represent the task system or environment. Cues and the inference form the cognitive system. Each cue is individually correlated with the patient state and inference (Elstein et al., 1978). Inferences are made from the cues considering their probabilistic

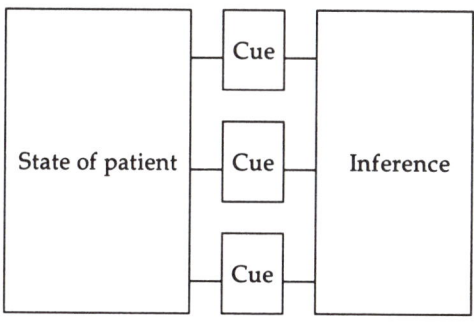

Figure 7-1
Lens Model

relationships to the patient state. The lens model has been applied to inferential judgment in nursing through studies by Hammond and associates (Hammond, Kelly, Castellan, Schneider, & Vancini, 1966; Hammond, Kelly, Schneider, & Vancini, 1966a, 1966b).

Studies conducted using decision theory as a framework for clinical judgment have indicated that often practitioners do not make the same decisions as prescribed by a mathematical formula (Tanner, 1983). Human error and biases not accounted for in a mathematical model enter into clinical judgment.

Phenomenologic Approach

The phenomenologic approach to clinical judgment views decision making in context. Such an approach emphasizes how judgments are made in real practice and how they are influenced by the clinical situation. Benner (1984) describes five levels of competency in clinical nursing practice, following the Dreyfus model of skill acquisition and development, and characteristics of performance at each level.

Stage 1: Novice—Beginners, i.e., nursing students or practitioners entering a new clinical area, function as novices using context-free rules learned in the classroom to guide their actions. Because of their lack of practical knowledge and experience, learners at this level have only these principles on which to base their actions which do not reflect the particular clinical situation encountered. Beginners focus on individual pieces of information and lack a unified framework for approaching the situation.

Stage 2: Advanced Beginner—Advanced beginners have had enough clinical experience to identify meaningful characteristics, referred to as aspects, of the clinical situation. Identifying these aspects requires previous experience with related situations.

Stage 3: Competent—The competent level of performance indicates ability to plan in a conscious way considering a projected future situation. Such a plan reflects long-term goals and "is based on considerable conscious, abstract, analytic contemplation of the problem" (Benner, 1984, p. 26). To become competent, the nurse needs at least two years of experience in practice with similar clinical situations.

Stage 4: Proficient—Proficiency represents the ability to view the clinical situation in terms of the gestalt rather than specific aspects within it. At this level, the nurse, because of prior experience with similar situations, has learned what to expect typically in a particular clinical situation. Benner proposes that this ability to view the clinical situation as a whole promotes clinical judgment because the nurse can more clearly identify which aspects in the present clinical situation are most significant.

Stage 5: Expert—The expert practitioner, because of extensive experience in the clinical field, "has an intuitive grasp of each situation and zeroes in on the accurate region of the problem without wasteful consideration of a large range of unfruitful, alternative diagnoses and solutions" (Benner, 1984, p. 32). Expert nurses have an indepth understanding of the meaning of a clinical situation and actions to be taken. Judgments by proficient and expert nurses are based on a perception of the clinical situation as a whole and the use of past concrete situations as paradigm cases for approaching the present one.

Three major theories represent different perspectives of the process of clinical judgment. In information processing theory, emphasis is placed on how the nurse adapts to limits in the amount of information able to be processed. Clinical judgment within this perspective begins with an identification of cues from which tentative diagnostic hypotheses, generated early in the process, are derived. Data are then collected to evaluate each hypothesis and decide on the diagnosis. Decision theory describes through mathematical formulas how the practitioner arrives at a diagnosis or action. In a phenomenologic approach, clinical judgment is viewed as it is actually used in clinical practice. Regardless of the theoretical approach, clinical judgment is recognized as a complex process by which nurses arrive at diagnoses from cues and decide on appropriate courses of action. Itano (1989) suggests that although making judgments about clients seems "quite obvious, the complexity of the act may be hidden in its familiarity" (p. 120).

TEACHING

The framework for teaching in the cognitive domain is derived from theory and research on how individuals learn concepts, problem solve, make decisions, and arrive at sound clinical judgments as well as the influence of critical thinking and the learner's stage of cognitive development on these processes. An understanding of these cognitive skills provides a basis for teaching them in the clinical field.

Concepts

What is known about concept learning may be used as a framework for teaching concepts in the clinical setting. Principles for teaching are organized in five areas:

1. Definition of Concept—Teaching concepts begins with a definition of the concept or category to be learned. This definition specifies the characteristics of an object or event relevant for grouping it into the category. An understanding of these characteristics is critical in learning the concept, for it provides the basis for distinguishing examples from nonexamples of that concept in clinical practice. This knowledge is therefore essential for students to begin to conceptualize in the practice setting.
2. Emphasis on Relevant Characteristics—For instructional purposes, the relevant characteristics of the concept should be emphasized, particularly as they compare with irrelevant ones. A major task of the teacher is to highlight (verbally or through student experience) relevant features of the concept.

Asking learners to describe these characteristics in their own words not only promotes learning them but also decreases the chance of memorizing the definition without comprehending the concept.

3. Use of Examples—A concept has been learned when the student can differentiate examples from nonexamples of that concept. In teaching concepts, emphasis should be given to examples of the concept, since individuals learn more efficiently from positive instances than from negative ones, although nonexamples should also be presented for comparison of the two. In teaching the concept of narcotics, for instance, examples of different types of narcotics serve to illustrate relevant characteristics of medications for placing them in this category. Comparing examples of narcotics with ones of nonnarcotic substances assists students in focusing on the relevant characteristics. Differences between examples and nonexamples should be made explicit for learners. In addition, learners should be asked to cite new examples of a concept which aids in refining their understanding of it and promotes retention.

In addition to these teaching strategies, cases may be developed, in print form, CAI, simulations, or discussions with students, around the concept particularly as represented in clinical practice. Through the case, examples of the concept and its defining characteristics may be emphasized, and illustrations can be provided of related concepts and differentiating features.

4. Variety of Examples—A variety of examples of the concept should be presented, particularly in terms of different clients and varying clinical situations.

5. Experience with Concept—Concept learning is enhanced with experiences that enable the learner to become actively involved with an example of that concept. Clinical practice provides these experiences with concepts. For example, students can learn about immobilization through experiences with clients in the immediate postoperative period, in a comatose state, following cerebral vascular accident, or who have a fracture or other problems resulting in immobilization.

Problem Solving

Development of skill in problem solving requires experience in using it with real practice problems. The teacher should be alert to problems, client- or setting-oriented, that relate to the objectives of the experience and are within the level of knowledge and skill of the learner. Principles for teaching problem solving in the clinical setting are organized in seven areas:

1. Compatibility with Level of Learner—Solving problems requires ability to use concepts and theories in practice, so the nature of the problems selected for student involvement needs to be at an appropriate level in terms of the learner's knowledge base.

2. Identification of Problems—Learners, because of their limited practical knowledge and experience in clinical practice, need assistance in identifying and delimiting problems. The teacher should make explicit for learners aspects of the clinical situation significant in identifying the problem, whether client- or setting-oriented. Students may be asked to describe the problem, reflecting their levels of understanding, and provide supporting data for its identification. Assisting learners to develop new strategies for analysis of the clinical situation and new methods of reasoning is an important aspect of teaching problem solving in the practice setting.

3. Identification of Multiple Solutions—It is vital in teaching problem solving that learners be assisted in identifying multiple solutions for problems and developing new strategies for action. This is important in terms of their cognitive development and promoting divergent thinking. Explanations, verbal or written, by learners as to the solutions considered and a rationale for the decision made provide a means of assessing the thought process used by students and assisting them in identifying other possibilities. Discussions such as this encourage learners to examine own biases and values that may influence problem solving.

Sometimes the solution proposed may not be part of the accepted practice in the clinical setting, and the teacher may need to assume an advocacy role for the learner so the approach may be implemented. This support on the part of teacher and staff is necessary to provide for experimentation with care and opportunity for calculated risk taking, within the realm of safe practice, in the clinical field.

4. ==Integrity of Process==—Although in reality the problem-solving process does not always follow a linear sequence of steps from definition of the problem through evaluation of solutions, in developing skill in problem solving, it is important for learners to proceed through these steps so the integrity of the process is maintained.

5. ==Focus on Process==—The emphasis in teaching problem solving is on the *process* by which problems are identified and solutions are proposed and tested, rather than on the outcomes.

6. ==Use of Intuitive Thinking==—Learners are also taught the importance of ==recognizing hunches and searching for evidence to confirm them==. Group discussions which are open and support reflective thinking are important in encouraging students to express their intuition.

7. ==Acceptance of Individual Differences Among Learners==—The teacher needs to be supportive of differences among learners in their approaches to problem solving. A fundamental difference between field-independent and field-dependent learners, for instance, relates to their analytic ability which influences problem solving in the setting. Field-dependent learners, because they do not readily use a hypothesis testing approach to problem solving, may require additional guidance from the teacher in analyzing clinical situations, identifying problems, and proposing and testing solutions for them.

Decision Making

Similar to problem solving, decisions relative to practice require an adequate knowledge base for analyzing the situation in which a decision is required, generating possible alternatives, determining consequences of each, and making a judgment as to which alternative to select. The decisions students are involved in making need to reflect their levels of understanding.

Consideration of different alternatives and consequences of each is vital to rational decision making in clinical practice. Learners, because of their limited knowledge and experience in the specific area of practice, often need assistance in exploring these alternatives.

Discussion of decisions with others provides a means of assessing the thought process used to arrive at the decisions and improving understanding of alternatives that might have been considered. Encouraging learners to examine their own beliefs and values that may influence their decision making and those of the recipient of the decision is also important.

Critical Thinking

Critical thinking cannot be developed in one course or through one clinical assignment. Development of this skill requires sustained learning activities over a period of time and teachers who in their interactions with learners encourage and support the critical thinking of students. Students are challenged to think critically in all of their clinical experiences.

In conferences with students about their patients and other clinical experiences, the teacher encourages open discussion of client problems and solutions. Different perspectives to care are examined and evaluated. The teacher seeks through questioning of students the underlying thought processes used to arrive at decisions. The process of thinking becomes of greater importance than the outcomes at this developmental stage. Student participation in discussions and meaningful dialogue is essential in this process. Encouraging students to think aloud as they progress through the critical thinking process may be helpful (Kintgen-Andrews, 1991).

Meyers (1986) suggests beginning a discussion with questions which have no simple answers. These questions give the learner a chance to offer own hypotheses before the teacher presents his or her view. Discussions of different opinions regarding some aspect of clinical practice are important in promoting critical thinking. Students need to struggle with issues and dilemmas about client care. In these discussions, students search for alternate meanings and explanations. Students cannot learn to think critically until they can "set aside their own visions of the truth and reflect on alternatives" (Meyers, 1986, p. 27).

In teaching critical thinking, it is important to assist students to distinguish relevant from irrelevant data, draw clinical inferences from the data, recognize unstated assumptions, weigh findings, and examine the basis of generalizations (Miller & Malcolm, 1990, p. 72). In clinical practice students need opportunity to try out different approaches to care with support from the teacher. For some faculty changes may be needed in own way of thinking and interacting with students. In many areas of nursing practice, there is no "right" way; students are encouraged to examine alternate modes of care and develop their own approaches. Faculty, in turn, avoid their biases of looking for the one correct answer or approach, for the nature of nursing practice demands varied approaches in solving problems.

Strategies for teaching critical thinking in nursing require an attitude of inquiry on the part of both student and teacher. There is a spirit of critical thinking which the teacher is instrumental in developing within the practice setting.

Clinical Judgment

Development of skill in clinical judgment requires: (1) relevant knowledge for application to the clinical situation, (2) skill in data collection, and (3) knowledge of strategies for effective problem solving with clients. Judgment is influenced by the learner's stage of cognitive development and critical thinking ability. These elements provide direction for faculty as to teaching clinical judgment in the field.

Knowledge Base of Learner. Effective clinical judgment requires an adequate knowledge base for analyzing the clinical situation, gathering and interpreting data, generating tentative hypotheses, considering alternative actions and consequences of each, and deciding on actions to be taken. Clinical judgment cannot proceed without this store of knowledge for retrieval from long-term memory. For this reason, experiences in practice in which the learner is called upon to make a clinical judgment need to reflect the learner's level of knowledge and skill.

Skill in Data Collection. Clinical judgment depends on comprehensive data gathering, for it is from these data that diagnostic hypotheses are generated and then tested and decisions relative to the client and others are made. Teaching for clinical judgment involves assisting students to develop their skill in various means of data collection.

Strategies for Problem Solving. Teaching is directed toward assisting students to understand the process of clinical judgment and strategies for effective clinical problem solving. Four strategies and related teaching implications are presented:

1. Early Hypothesis Generation—Research has indicated that practitioners generate hypotheses early in their interaction with clients and proceed to gather data to test each hypothesis. Traditional instruction in nursing, however, often teaches students to complete all of data collection and then analyze the data to determine nursing diagnoses. Instead, students should identify tentative diagnostic hypotheses early in assessment of the client and then focus subsequent data collection on these hypotheses.
2. Multiple Competing Hypotheses—Learners may need assistance in generating multiple competing hypotheses that might be possible given the data instead of accepting the first diagnosis that comes to mind which may prove to be incorrect. Generating several possible diagnostic hypotheses improves the chance of identifying the correct one.
3. Hypothesis Testing—Teaching includes helping students to search for and evaluate data that assist in eliminating tentative hypotheses as well as that which facilitates confirmation. Skill in directing data collection toward specific hypotheses needs to be developed.
4. Relevant and Irrelevant Data—Learners need assistance in distinguishing relevant from irrelevant data, identifying cues in the data, and clustering them.

Cognitive Taxonomy

Important in teaching the cognitive processes inherent in practice is assisting learners in the progressive development of these skills. The taxonomy of the cognitive domain views intellectual abilities within a development perspective and, therefore, is valuable for this teaching.

The taxonomy represents a system for ordering cognitive behaviors from simple recall to the complex processes of analysis, synthesis, and evaluation. The taxonomy is thus organized according to the principle of increasing complexity. Reilly and Oermann (1990) describe the use of the cognitive taxonomy by Bloom (1956) for the progressive development of intellectual skills in nursing education.

There are six levels in the cognitive taxonomy, each with specific sublevels except for one of the categories, application. The levels in the taxonomy are presented in Table 7-1.

Use of Taxonomy. The cognitive taxonomy provides a framework for selecting the appropriate level of learning behavior and for writing objectives. The decision as to the level of learning desired is based on the faculty's professional judgment considering the level of the learner, complexity of the phenomenon, and experiences available for achieving the objectives. In using the taxonomy, the teacher first decides on the desired level in the taxonomy, then develops objectives to reflect learning at that level.

Cognitive skill development at the lower levels of the taxonomy, knowledge and comprehension, is oriented toward an understanding of concepts, principles, and theories but not to an ability to use them in practice. Objectives written at the lower levels reflect the student's acquisition of the knowledge base needed for problem solving and decision making in the practice setting. These behaviors are important for development of cognitive skill. Problem solving begins at the comprehension level in which students learn to interpret data and extrapolate meaning.

Objectives written at the application level reflect ability of the learner to problem solve using knowledge that relates to prescriptive solutions. At the analysis level, the learner is able to problem solve and make decisions in a clinical situation through the analytical process. Learning at this level addresses both known and unknown solutions. It reflects ability to analyze data, compare different alternatives and their consequences, search for evidence to support claims and conclusions, and determine how ideas relate to one another. Problem solving and decision making at this level are needed for professional nursing practice. Learning at the synthesis level is important in developing new and creative products. At the evaluation level, the learner makes judgments about value based on criteria and standards.

Once faculty determines the cognitive level desired as the outcome of the nursing program and writes objectives to reflect this learning, the outcome objectives for each level in the program are designated to

Table 7-1
Taxonomy of Cognitive Domain

C1.00 **Knowledge**
Knowledge involves the recall of specific facts and information. Learning at this level represents the process of remembering information, not ability to understand its meaning.

1.10 Knowledge of Specifics	Recall of specific pieces of information
1.11 Knowledge of Terminology	Recall of terms
1.12 Knowledge of Specific Facts	Knowledge of dates, events, persons, and other facts
1.20 Knowledge of Ways and Means of Dealing with Specifics	Recall of ways of organizing, judging, and criticizing ideas
1.21 Knowledge of Conventions	Knowledge of ways of presenting ideas
1.22 Knowledge of Trends and Sequences	Knowledge of processes and directions in relation to time
1.23 Knowledge of Classifications and Categories	Recall of classes and divisions considered to be fundamental for a specific discipline, argument, or problem
1.24 Knowledge of Criteria	Recall of specific criteria
1.25 Knowledge of Methodology	Recall of methods of inquiry and techniques employed in a discipline
1.30 Knowledge of the Universals and Abstractions in a Field	Knowledge of major ideas and patterns by which ideas are organized, such as theories
1.31 Knowledge of Principles and Generalizations	Recall of abstractions that summarize observations of phenomena
1.32 Knowledge of Theories and Structures	Recall of a body of principles and generalizations and their interrelationships

C2.00 **Comprehension**
Comprehension indicates understanding, an ability to translate or interpret information and extrapolate beyond that given. At this level, the learner grasps the meaning sufficiently well to relate it to other material or to use it in solving a problem without recognizing its fullest implication. Bloom (1956) considers this category as the first level of intellectual skills.

2.10 Translation	Expression of communication in other terms, another language, or another form of commumication
2.20 Interpretation	Explanation of a communication reflecting a new perspective of the material
2.30 Extrapolation	Extension of trends beyond given data

Table 7-1 *(Continued)*

C3.00 Application
Application, the only category in the cognitive taxonomy without sublevels, refers to *use* of concepts, theories, and other abstractions in concrete situations. Ability to apply requires comprehension of that which is applied.

C4.00 Analysis
The fourth level, analysis, pertains to learning that involves a breakdown of material into its constituent parts and determination of the relationships among them.

4.10 Analysis of Elements	Identification of elements of a communication
4.20 Analysis of Relationships	Identification of relationships among elements and parts of a communication
4.30 Analysis of Oganizational Principles	Identification of the organization, systematic arrangement, and structure holding a communication together

C5.00 Synthesis
Synthesis means the development of a new product through a combination of specific elements and parts. Of the categories in the cognitive taxonomy, this one most clearly provides for creative learning.

5.10 Production of a Unique Communication	Development of a communication reflecting the learner's perspective about some idea
5.20 Production of a Plan or Proposed Set of Operations	Development of a plan of work
5.30 Derivation of a Set of Abstract Relations	Development of a scheme for classifying or explaining certain data or phenomena

C6.00 Evaluation
Evaluation, representing the most complex learning behaviors, reflects the ability to make judgments about value in terms of internal and external criteria.

6.10 Judgments in Terms of Internal Evidence	Evaluation of a communication based on its logical accuracy, consistency, and other internal criteria
6.20 Judgments in Terms of External Criteria	Evaluation of a communication with reference to selected criteria, such as comparing a work against known standards in its field (pp. 48–53)

(Modified from Reilly, D. E. & Oermann, M. H. (1990). Behavioral objectives: Evaluation in nursing (3rd ed.). New York: National League for Nursing.

indicate progressive development. There are two ways to level objectives. The cognitive behavior itself may be changed to a higher taxonomic level, thereby representing greater complexity. Ability to *analyze* an interaction is more complex than ability to *use* principles in interacting with clients and others in the clinical field. This leveling may be illustrated as follows:

Level 1
C3.00 *Uses* principles in interacting with clients and others in the clinical field.
C4.10 *Analyzes* interactions with clients and others in the clinical field.

A second way of leveling involves keeping the cognitive behavior at the same level and making the variables with which the behavior is carried out more complex. Ability to analyze interactions within a *group* is more complex than skill in analyzing interactions with an *individual client*. An example of this leveling is:

Level 1
C4.10 Analyzes interactions with *clients*.

Level 2
C4.10 Analyzes interactions with *groups of clients*.

In some instances, both the behavior and variables may be changed.

The taxonomy provides a system for ordering cognitive behaviors to be acquired along a continuum of simple to complex. It enables faculty concerned with teaching cognitive skills to plan and sequence instruction to allow for their progressive development.

TEACHING METHODS

There are a variety of clinical teaching methods appropriate for teaching in the cognitive domain. Problem-solving strategies, such as written problem-solving and decision-making situations or ones combined with media, assist learners in applying concepts and theories to a clinical situation; identifying, from their assessment of the situation, problems to be solved or decisions to be made; and examining alternate courses of action and their consequences. They provide for practice in solving simulated problems and improving skill in problem solving, decision making, and clinical judgment.

Conference represents another teaching method particularly appropriate for cognitive skill development. In relation to concept learning, students can discuss examples of a concept and its relevant characteristics. They can share clinical problems and decisions made, discuss issues and problems affecting nursing practice, and receive immediate feedback on their approaches and underlying rationale.

Conference provides a means for learners to examine data collected, inferences made, and the course of action chosen which assists in the development of clinical judgment skill. It is important that students have an opportunity to discuss the process used in arriving at nursing diagnoses and deciding on actions. A written care plan or other type of written assignment students might complete does not reflect the underlying thought process used by them. Through interaction with others the learner can discuss the diagnostic hypotheses considered, supporting data, and why an inference was made, and can describe the alternate actions considered and consequences of each. These discussions also provide a means for learners to examine problems which are ambiguous and have no defined solutions. This outcome is important in assisting students to realize that professional knowledge is evolving and uncertain.

Conferences also provide opportunity for learners to reflect on their decisions and evaluate those of others, important in critical thinking. Group discussion promotes cognitive development in that learners are exposed to multiple perspectives relative to care and diverse points of view. A multidisciplinary conference could also be used to compare approaches of different disciplines to problem solving.

A debate about a clinical topic or issue is another strategy for promoting critical thinking skills. To argue or debate requires inquiry and development of reasoned arguments for or against an issue (White, Beardslee, Peters, & Supples, 1990, p. 17).

Clinical assignment is particularly valuable in promoting cognitive skill development. Through clinical practice, students experience examples of concepts, important in their attainment of them. They develop skill in problem solving and decision making, learn to accept multiple perspectives, and have an opportunity to experiment with care, make independent judgments, and develop commitment to be responsible in professional practice.

A written assignment, such as nursing care plan, assists learners in deciding on nursing actions and examining alternate approaches. Short papers addressing clinical problems also may be used for this purpose. With these papers, students can be directed to describe a clinical problem, possible nursing diagnoses and supporting data, and alternate nursing actions and consequences of each. For the purpose of promoting critical thinking, Meyers (1986) recommends short papers which deal with real problems and issues completed over a period of time rather than one long paper.

Case studies, which provide a holistic view of a client's problem, promote problem-solving learning. Simulations, games, and simulation games enable students to practice problem solving and decision making in a safe environment representing a real-life encounter in the field. They provide a vehicle for development of critical thinking skills through the questions asked of learners and related discussion. Role play assists learners in recognizing the value of participatory involvement in problem solving and decision making.

With media, faculty can present client situations similar to ones found in clinical practice for students to identify possible problems and propose different solutions for them. Plunkett and Olivieri (1989) describe use of videotaping and simulation designed to assist students in developing skill in clinical judgment. In this strategy students are asked to generate possible diagnostic hypotheses with supporting data from the simulated case. Each hypothesis is explored instead of arriving at one correct hypothesis or stating a specific nursing diagnosis.

Similar to media, computer-assisted instruction and particularly computer simulations and interactive video provide a means of presenting a case situation for students to analyze, identify problems or decisions to be made, select approaches, and evaluate outcomes. With these strategies, students can be led through the diagnostic reasoning process. They can be asked to identify cues in the assessment data and cluster them, generate tentative hypotheses, evaluate each hypothesis, and decide upon nursing diagnoses. Most importantly, the student and teacher can discuss the underlying thinking process used to arrive at these decisions. The process of thinking can be emphasized rather than a specific diagnosis or course of action.

There is a wide range of teaching methods appropriate for cognitive skill development. Through real or simulated clinical situations, learners are able to attain concepts and develop skill in solving problems and making decisions relative to practice. Critical thinking may also be promoted through use of these teaching strategies if geared to this outcome by the faculty. The key is how the teacher uses the methods and the standards set relative to the thinking process so the responses of learners represent depth of understanding, inquiry, and willingness to search for more effective answers to clinical problems.

SUMMARY

Cognitive skill development is a significant goal of clinical practice and must be of major concern to the teacher in the clinical setting. It is separate from but interrelated to the affective and psychomotor domains of learning. Cognitive skills essential for nursing practice encompass concept learning, problem solving, decision making, critical thinking, and clinical judgment.

Concepts provide a means of categorizing information which reduces the complexity of the environment, enables individuals to identify different events and objects in it, and reduces the need for constant learning. Concept learning involves understanding the characteristics of events or objects relevant for grouping them into categories. A concept has been learned when the student can differentiate examples from nonexamples of that concept.

Students also need to develop skill in problem solving, decision making, and clinical judgment. Problem solving is viewed as a process beginning with identification of the problem and proceeding through gathering data in relation to the problem, generating solutions, and evaluating the solutions chosen.

The very nature of nursing practice requires that nurses make decisions relative to clients, staff, and activities within the clinical setting. Decision making involves choosing among alternatives after considering the possible consequences of each if selected and choosing the best one in terms of achieving the goal.

The decisions and judgments made in clinical practice are influenced by the learner's stage of cognitive development. Complexity of thought and problem solving, acceptance of diverse perspectives, ability to deal with ambiguity, independence in practice, and willingness to assume responsibility, all important in nursing practice, develop at advanced stages of cognitive development. It is important in nursing education that students are moved toward higher levels of cognitive development.

Teaching cognitive skills inherent in practice involves a number of principles. Important in this teaching is providing for the progressive development of skills. The taxonomy of the cognitive domain views intellectual skills within a developmental perspective and, therefore, is valuable as a guide for determining the level of skill development at any particular point in the nursing program.

Methods for promoting cognitive learning in the clinical field include problem-solving strategies, conferences, debates, clinical assignments, written assignments, simulations, games, simulation games, role play, media, and computer-assisted instruction. These strategies provide for student involvement in clinical situations which requires learners to engage in the cognitive processes leading to decisions and clinical judgment.

Faculty has the responsibility not only to assist learners in using concepts and theories relevant to practice and in developing skill in clinical judgment, but also to encourage them to accept diverse points of view, challenge and question, and develop commitment as responsible and self-directed learners and professional practitioners. Teachers need to demonstrate these same behaviors themselves—acceptance of diverse points of view among learners and with their own perspective, support for challenging and questioning by learners, and recognition of the self as learner.

REFERENCES

Aspinall, M. J. (1979). Use of a decision tree to improve accuracy of diagnosis. Nursing Research, 28, 182–85.

Benner, P. (1984). *From novice to expert: Excellence and power in clinical nursing practice*. Menlo Park, CA: Addison-Wesley.

Bloom, B. S. (Ed.). (1956). *Taxonomy of educational objectives: Handbook I: Cognitive domain*. New York: David McKay.

Bruner, J. S. (1963). *The process of education*. New York: Vintage Books.

Bruner, J. S., Goodnow, J. J., & Austin, G. A. (1956). *A study of thinking*. New York: Wiley.

Carnevali, D. L. (1984). The diagnostic reasoning process. In D. L. Carnevali, P. H. Mitchell, N. F. Woods, & C. A. Tanner (Eds.), *Diagnostic reasoning in nursing*. Philadelphia: Lippincott.

Child, D. (1986). *Psychology and the teacher* (4th ed.). New York: Holt, Rinehart & Winston.

del Bueno, D. J. (1990). Experience, education, and nurses' ability to make clinical judgments. *Nursing & Health Care, 11*(6), 290-294.

Elstein, A. S., Kagan, N., Shulman, L. S., Jason, H., & Loupe, M. J. (1972). Methods and theory in the study of medical inquiry. *Journal of Medical Education, 47*, 85-92.

Elstein, A. S., Shulman, L. S., & Sprafka, S. A. (1978). *Medical problem-solving*. Cambridge, MA: Harvard University Press.

Frisch, N. A. (1987). Cognitive maturity of nursing students. *Image: Journal of Nursing Scholarship, 19*(1), 25-27.

Glaser, R. (1969). Learning. In *Encyclopedia of educational research* (4th ed.). New York: Macmillan.

Goosen, G. M. (1989). Concept analysis: An approach to teaching physiologic variables. *Journal of Professional Nursing, 5*(1), 31-38.

Gordon, M. (1980). Predictive strategies in diagnostic tasks. *Nursing Research, 29*, 39-45.

Halpern, D. (1984). *Thought and knowledge*. Hillsdale, NJ: Lawrence Erlbaum Associates.

Hammond, K. R., Kelly, K. J., Castellan, N. J., Jr., Schneider, R. J., & Vancini, M. (1966). Clinical inference in nursing: Use of information-seeking strategies by nurses. *Nursing Research, 15*, 330-336.

Hammond, K. R., Kelly, K. J., Schneider, R. J., & Vancini, M. (1966a). Clinical inference in nursing: Analyzing cognitive tasks representative of nursing problems. *Nursing Research, 15*, 134-138.

Hammond, K. R., Kelly, K. J., Schneider, R. J., & Vancini, M. (1966b). Clinical inference in nursing: Information units used. *Nursing Research, 15*, 236-43.

Heims, M. L., & Boyd, S. T. (1990). Concept-based learning activities in clinical nursing education. *Journal of Nursing Education, 29*(6), 249-254.

Hursh, B., Haas, P., & Moore, M. (1983). An interdisciplinary model to implement general education. *Journal of Higher Education, 54,* 42–59.

Itano, J. K. (1989). A comparison of the clinical judgment process in experienced registered nurses and student nurses. *Journal of Nursing Education, 28*(3), 120–126.

Jones, J. A. (1988). Clinical reasoning in nursing. *Journal of Advanced Nursing, 13,* 185–192.

Kassirer, J. P., & Gorry, C. A. (1978). Clinical problem-solving: A behavioral analysis. *Annals of Internal Medicine, 89,* 245–55.

Kim, H. S. (1983). *The nature of theoretical thinking in nursing.* Norwalk, CT: Appleton-Century-Crofts.

King, P. M. (1978). William Perry's theory of intellectual and ethical development. *New Directions for Student Services, 4,* 35–51.

Kintgen-Andrews, J. (1991). Critical thinking and nursing education: Perplexities and insights. *Journal of Nursing Education, 30*(4), 152–157.

Kitchener, K. S. (1983). Educational goals and reflective thinking. *Educational Forum, XLVII*(1), 75–95.

Meyers, C. (1986). *Teaching students to think critically.* San Francisco: Jossey-Bass.

Miller, M. A., & Malcolm, N. S. (1990). Critical thinking in the nursing curriculum. *Nursing & Health Care, 11*(2), 67–73.

Miller, V. G., & Rew, L. (1989). Analysis and intuition: The need for both in nursing education. *Journal of Nursing Education, 28*(2), 84–86.

Oermann, M. H. (1991). *Professional nursing practice: A conceptual approach.* Philadelphia: J. B. Lippincott.

Parnes, S. J. (1984). Learning creative behavior: Making the future happen. *The Futurist, 18*(4), 30–32.

Perry, W. G., Jr. (1970). *Forms of intellectual and ethical development in the college years.* New York: Holt, Rinehart & Winston.

Plunkett, E. J., & Olivieri, R. J. (1989). A strategy for introducing diagnostic reasoning: Hypothesis testing using a simulation approach. *Nurse Educator, 14*(6), 27–31.

Prescott, P. A., Dennis, K. E., & Jacox, A. K. (1987). Clinical decision making of staff nurses. *Image: Journal of Nursing Scholarship, 19*(2), 56–62.

Putzier, D. J., Padrick, K., Westfall, U. E., & Tanner, C. A. (1985). Diagnostic reasoning in critical care. *Heart & Lung, 14*(5), 430–437.

Reilly, D. E., & Oermann, M. H. (1990). *Behavioral objectives: Evaluation in nursing* (3rd ed.). New York: National League for Nursing.

Schön, D. A. (1990). *Educating the reflective practitioner.* San Francisco, CA: Jossey-Bass.

Siegel, H. (1980). Critical thinking as an educational ideal. *Educational Forum*, *XLV*(1), 7-23.

Stonewater, J. K., & Stonewater, B. B. (1984). Teaching problem-solving: Implications from cognitive development research. *American Association of Higher Education Bulletin*, *36*(6), 7-10.

Tanner, C. A. (1983). Research on clinical judgment. In W. L. Holzemer (Ed.), *Review of research in nursing education*. Thorofare, NJ: Slack.

Tanner, C. A. (1984a). Diagnostic problem-solving strategies. In D. L. Carnevali, P. H. Mitchell, N. F. Woods, & C. A. Tanner (Eds.), *Diagnostic reasoning in nursing*. Philadelphia: Lippincott.

Tanner, C. A. (1984b). Factors influencing the diagnostic process. In D. L. Carnevali, P. H. Mitchell, N. F. Woods, & C. A. Tanner (Eds.), *Diagnostic reasoning in nursing*. Philadelphia: Lippincott.

Tanner, C. A. (1987). Theoretical perspectives for research on clinical judgment. In K. J. Hannah, M. Reimer, W. C. Mills, & S. Letourneau (Eds.), *Clinical judgment and decision making: The future with nursing diagnosis* (pp. 21-28). New York: John Wiley & Sons.

Valiga, T. M. (1983). Cognitive development: A critical component of baccalaureate nursing education. *Image*, *XV*, 115-19.

White, N. E., Beardslee, N. Q., Peters, D., & Supples, J. M. (1990). Promoting critical thinking skills. *Nurse Educator*, *15*(5), 16-19.

Yinger, R. J. (1980). Can we really teach them to think? In R. E. Young (Ed.), *Fostering critical thinking*. San Francisco: Jossey-Bass.

BIBLIOGRAPHY

Agan, R. D. (1987). Intuitive knowing as a dimension of nursing. *Advances in Nursing Science*, *10*(1), 63-70.

Bauwens, E. E., & Gerhard, G. G. (1987). The use of the Watson-Glaser Critical Thinking Appraisal to predict success in a baccalaureate nursing program. *Journal of Nursing Education*, *26*, 278-281.

Benner, P. (1982). From novice to expert. *American Journal of Nursing*, *82*, 402-7.

Benner, P., & Tanner, C. A. (1987). Clinical judgment: How expert nurses use intuition. *American Journal of Nursing*, *87*(1), 23-31.

Brooks, K. L., & Shepherd, J. M. (1990). The relationship between clinical decision-making skills in nursing and general critical thinking abilities of senior nursing students in four types of nursing programs. *Journal of Nursing Education*, *29*(9), 391-399.

Chickering, A. W. (1976). Developmental change as a major outcome. In M. T. Keeton & Associates (Eds.), *Experiential learning*. San Francisco: Jossey-Bass.

Corcoran, S. (1986). Planning by expert and novice nurses in cases of varying complexity. *Research in Nursing and Health, 9*(2), 155-162.

DeBack, V. (1982). The relationship between senior nursing students' ability to formulate nursing diagnoses and the curriculum model. In B. J. Brown & P. L. Chinn (Eds.), *Nursing education: Practical methods and models*. Rockville, MD: Aspen Systems.

Dreyfus, H. L. (1979). *What computers can't do: The limits of artificial intelligence*. New York: Harper & Row.

Ennis, R. H. (1962). A concept of critical thinking. *The Harvard Educational Review, 32*, 81-111.

Gilligan, C. (1982). *In a different voice: Psychological theory and women's development*. Cambridge, MA: Harvard University Press.

Glaser, R. (1968). Concept learning and concept teaching. In R. M. Gagne & W. J. Gephart (Eds.), *Learning research and school subjects*. Itasca, IL: F. E. Peacock.

Gross, Y. T., Takazawa, E. S., & Rose, C. L. (1987). Critical thinking and nursing education. *Journal of Nursing Education, 26*, 317-323.

Holbert, C. M., & Abraham, C. (1988). Reflections on generic thinking and problem solving. *Nurse Education, 13*, 23-27.

Jacobs-Kraemer, M. K., & Huether, S. E. (1988). Curricular considerations for teaching nursing theory. *Journal of Professional Nursing, 4*(5), 373-380.

Kissinger, J. F., & Munjas, B. A. (1981). Nursing process, student attributes, and teaching methodologies. *Nursing Research, 30*, 242-46.

Kitchener, K. S., & King, P. M. (1981). Reflective judgment: Concepts of justification and their relationship to age and education. *Journal of Applied Developmental Psychology, 2*, 89-116.

Klassens, E. L. (1988). Exploring use of computer simulation to teach critical decision-making skills to pediatric nursing students. *Journal of Pediatric Nursing, 3*, 202-205.

Laschinger, H. K., & Boss, M. K. (1989). Learning styles of baccalaureate nursing students and attitudes toward theory-based nursing. *Journal of Professional Nursing, 5*(4), 215-223.

Lowdermilk, D. L., & Fishel, A. H. (1991). Computer simulations as a measure of nursing students' decision-making skills. *Journal of Nursing Education, 30*(1), 34-39.

Matthews, C. A., & Gaul, A. L. (1979). Nursing diagnosis from the perspective of concept attainment and critical thinking. *Advances in Nursing Science, 2*(1), 17-26.

Norris, S. P. (1985). Synthesis of research on critical thinking. *Educational Leadership, 42*(8), 40-45.

Nuernberger, P. (1984). Mastering the creative process. *The Futurist, 18*(4), 33-36.

Pardue, S. F. (1987). Decision-making skills and critical thinking ability among associate degree, diploma, baccalaureate, and master's prepared nurses. *Journal of Nursing Education, 26,* 354-361.

Perry, W. G., Jr. (1981). Cognitive and ethical growth: The making of meaning. In A. Chickering (Ed.), *The modern American college.* San Francisco: Jossey-Bass.

Rew, L., & Barrow, E. M. (1987). Intuition: A neglected hallmark of nursing knowledge. *Advances in Nursing Science, 10*(1), 49-62.

Tanner, C. A. (1987). Teaching clinical judgment. *Annual Review of Nursing Research, 5,* 153-173.

Tversky, A., & Kahneman, D. (1981). The framing of decisions and the psychology of choice. *Science, 211,* 453-58.

Widick, C. A. (1977). The Perry scheme: A foundation for developmental practice. *The Counseling Psychologist, 6,* 35-58.

Williams, R. A. (1988). The relationship of cognitive styles and stress in nursing students. *Western Journal of Nursing Research, 10*(4), 449-462.

Young, R. E. (Ed.). (1980). *Fostering critical thinking.* San Francisco: Jossey-Bass.

8

Psychomotor Learning in the Clinical Setting

Psychomotor skills are an integral part of nursing practice in most settings where nurses participate in the delivery of care. They are found in both the assessment and implementation steps of the nursing process. They constitute a significant portion of nursing interventions. Lack of competency in these skills on the part of new graduates is the subject of much criticism of nursing education, which often is of such vehemence that it takes on a pervasive quality as an indictment of all nursing education.

The teacher of psychomotor skills raises such questions as: How should they be taught? What processes are involved in the learning? What criteria are used in judging the efficiency of a student's performance? A search of current nursing literature provides little assistance in answering these questions. Nursing research in this area, scarce as it is, addresses primarily the comparison of teaching strategies or the scientific rationale underlying the execution of some techniques. A perusal of the indexes of nursing textbooks concerned with teaching or curriculum evidences, in most instances no heading *psychomotor*.

What factors account for this dearth of material in nursing literature on the teaching of psychomotor skills? At an earlier stage in nursing history, excellence in performing psychomotor skills was *nursing*, and the teaching of these skills monopolized much of the curriculum. Other dimensions of care were discussed in classes, but one's expertise in carrying out procedural skills in nursing was the critical evaluative criterion. In one school, students were told by the director of the school, "If your patients tell you that you are a good nurse, don't necessarily believe the praise, for the patient does not know how perfectly you carried out your nursing techniques."

Much has happened since that era as nursing began to redefine its scope of practice and incorporate bodies of knowledge derived from other disciplines' research into its practice. Even more significant changes are underway because nursing is now evolving into a science. For example, remarkable advances in the field of psychiatry during World War II resulted in new directions in the health field where therapeutic use of the self through communication, interpersonal relationships, and other human interactions skills became paramount. Nurses returning to universities through the G.I. Bill developed the knowledge and skills inherent in the behavioral fields and incorporated them in nursing practice. The nurturing role of the nurse moved in new directions and caring took on different meaning with a broader concept of "doing."

The emphasis on the teaching of these new knowledges and skills in nursing programs relegated psychomotor skill teaching to the background. Little concern has been expressed about the teaching processes entailed, in spite of the shift in learning theories from the conditioning and trial-and-error concepts of Thorndyke to the concepts in field theory that emphasize principles and the relationship among phenomena. Today, with emphasis on cognitive skills as inherent in decision making, clinical judgment, and diagnosing, the concern in nursing education relates to the learning and teaching of these skills. Once again, psychomotor skill development is in the background.

CONCEPTS RELEVANT TO PSYCHOMOTOR SKILL DEVELOPMENT

Psychomotor skills in nursing are those dimensions of nursing practice that entail the ability to behave efficiently in an action situation that requires neuromuscular coordination. Singer (1975) states, "Activities that are primarily movement oriented and that emphasize overt physical response bear the label psychomotor" (p. 23). A wide variety of skills is inherent in nursing practice; it is the focus on body or muscular movement patterns which designate psychomotor skills.

Psychomotor skills in nursing are purposeful, complex actions based on principles; they entail cognitive skills in decision making and judgment relative to their use and desired effect. Yet, psychomotor skills are not cognitive skills. They are "doing" skills which result in a performance of a specific act. The teaching of psychomotor skills recognizes skill in practice as an integrated phenomenon comprising cognitive, psychomotor, and affective learning. In teaching, however, emphasis is placed on the performance skill that requires particular teaching, learning, and evaluation strategies. Although the movement component is the focus of the teaching, other cognitive, perceptual, and affective processes interact so that the total act is integrated, meaningful, and successful.

This chapter addresses the teaching of the movement component. It is assumed that relevant cognitive and affective knowledges and skills are being developed concurrently through other strategies. Their synthesis with psychomotor skills will be demonstrated later in the chapter.

Several concepts are essential to understanding the approach to teaching psychomotor skills. Performance and learning are not the same processes. *Performance* is an action, transitory in occurrence, in response to specific cues in the situation. Learning, however, is of more permanent nature resulting from practice or past experience, which is stored in the memory of a learner and subject to retrieval on cue. In motor skill learning, the amount of learning is inferred from the performance of the learner, and the process of learning is inferred from the change in learner behavior that is observed as the task is carried out. Kerr (1982) refers to performance as the end product or behavior that we see; learning is represented by an internalized model that allows us to repeat the performance of the skill.

Ability and skill, likewise, are not the same phenomenon. Skill relates to a specific task and refers to the ability to execute that task efficiently. *Ability* suggests the notion of a generality of a trait the learner possesses and is influenced by heredity and learning.

Skill is an important concept in this discussion and refers to the ability to carry out efficiently and effectively, in terms of speed and accuracy, muscular or body movements required for the act. Skill is relative; its definition for a specific task is determined by the nature of the task and the circumstances in the situation in which it occurs. Three classifications of skills are noted in the literature:

1. Fine motor skills: muscular coordination involves precision-oriented tasks. Nursing skills include: injections, arterial line manipulation, surgical dressings requiring instrumentation.
2. Manual skills: manipulative tasks that are fairly repetitive and usually involve eye-arm action. Nursing skills include: physical assessment, body hygiene, suctioning, chest drainage, touch.
3. Gross motor skills: involve large muscles and movement of the body. Nursing skills include: cardiopulmonary resuscitation (C.P.R.), ambulation, range of motion, patient positioning.

Singer (1975) proposes the following characteristics of the skilled person:

1. Performance is fairly consistent regardless of factors present that might cause the "average person's" performance to fluctuate.
2. Performance coincides with high degree of spatial precision and timing.
3. Responses to stimuli are set in appropriate sequential order.
4. Performances are executed within certain time limitations.
5. Ability to anticipate quickly is present and there is more time to react.
6. Performance has less variability since there is no need to respond to every potential cue in the environment.
7. Ability to receive maximum information from minimum number of identifiable cues is developed. (p. 29)

Johnson (1961) adds two other behavior characteristics:

1. Form of the activity represents economy of effort.
2. Is adaptable, i.e., performs proficiently under varying and even unpredictable conditions. (p. 163)

The goal of psychomotor skills development is more than the ability to perform; it is the ability to perform in a consistent manner within an appropriate time and spatial context irrespective of environmental variations. In education, it is not only the performance of the skill that is the goal, it is the learning of the skill as reflected in the consistent quality of the skill performance.

One other concept essential to understanding this approach to teaching psychomotor skills is the notion of the word *cognitive*. The word has several different meanings in psychomotor skill learning. Cognitive may refer to the *content* of the skill, i.e., its purpose, principles, and consequences. Cognitive also refers to the *intellectual processes* that the individual goes through between receiving the stimulus from the environment and the response. It is the latter notion of cognitive that is particularly relevant in the learning process entailed in psychomotor skill attainment.

LEARNING PROCESS FRAMEWORK FOR PSYCHOMOTOR SKILL DEVELOPMENT

How does psychomotor skill learning occur? What processes are involved? Until the sixties, this skill learning was primarily perceived within the conditioned or behavioristic paradigm: stimulus-response (S-R) or response-stimulus (R-S), and teaching was directed to this modality. As fields of cybernetic and information processing theory evolved with the advent of computers, many educators, who had been disenchanted with the simplistic mechanistic concept of psychomotor learning, sought answers in these new fields of knowledge. This pursuit has been undertaken by engineers, psychologists, and physical educators and since the 1970s much research has been generated and reported in the literature. Inquiry thus addressed was not limited to the outcome of learning but included the means by which muscles are coordinated and controlled so that accurate and efficient motor behavior results. Questions for educators now address process as well as outcome; the notion of motor-skilled performance as a conditioned reflex is no longer acceptable to many researchers and teachers. As Kerr (1982) states, "the current definition of psychomotor learning says we control with the head, not the muscles" (p. 18).

Theoretical Models

A comprehensive presentation of current research into psychomotor learning process is beyond the purview of this chapter. Selected findings perceived to be particularly relevant to this domain in nursing education are presented. The reader is encouraged to explore the literature in the field of motor learning in greater depth.

Theory development of motor learning is evolving primarily from the perspective of three major models: behavioral cybernetics, information processing, and adaptation.

Behavioral Cybernetic Model. This model is a systems approach to psychomotor behavior that defines a new level of experiential study of body motion and psychologic functions in terms of their variable feedback characteristics and determinants (Smith, 1972). Motor skills are perceived as a closed loop system relying on feedback to make the essential adjustments for efficient motor skill. Sensory input from the motor performance, whose origins may be from proprioceptors, stimuli arising within the organism or sense organs or both, provide feedback to the system controlling the output. In turn, the system makes the modifications in the output as indicated. The feedback system is in essence a detection mechanism which provides for a means of correcting motor performance.

The sensory input signifies the individual's ability to "know about" the status of the performance and thus, through one's own internal mechanism can control errors or make the necessary adaptations to variations in the requirements for motor action in the situation. Singer (1975) notes that all body movements are space structured and that learning is a process of establishing new spatial relationships in patterns of motion. Smith (1972), a researcher in behavioral cybernetics, reminds us that "learning is not determined directly by environmental stimuli, but by self-governed selection and control of all levels of environmental stimuli and psychophysiologic function in energy production and response" (p. 345). Researchers who have pursued the cybernetic model as a basis for understanding motor skill learning include Adams (1968), Keele (1968), Bernstein (1967), and Smith (1967).

Information Processing Model. This model represents a descriptive communication theory which addresses the mental processes of attention, perception, memory, and decision making involved in the motor act response to environmental stimuli. This model is not unlike the cybernetic one but is concerned additionally with the processes involved in the transmission of information received by cues in the situation and their resultant response. Of particular concern in this model is the ability of the individual to discriminate among critically relevant and irrelevant cues, select the pertinent and meaningful information, transmit it at a rapid rate, and retrieve desired information from the long-term memory. Each individual has a channel capacity for handling information and any information above that capacity cannot be transmitted. An overloading of the channel capacity results in motor skill decrement with an increasing number of errors.

Singer (1975) identifies three major mechanisms in the information processing model:

1. Perceptual mechanism—receives and identifies information sent from a sense organ.
2. Translation mechanism—decides choice of action.
3. Effector mechanism—coordinates and phases the action. (p. 3)

It is feedback from the latter mechanism that controls information in the perceptual-transmission process.

Stelmach (1982, pp. 66-67) sees three processing stages that occur from the stimulus to response and notes that each stage is sequential and operates only on the basis of information transmitted to it. He diagrams the process in Figure 8-1.

In this paradigm, he identifies two time periods.

1. *Reaction time:* the period between stimulus presentation and the beginning of the response. Keele (1982) found that reaction time is influenced by the number of possible situations that

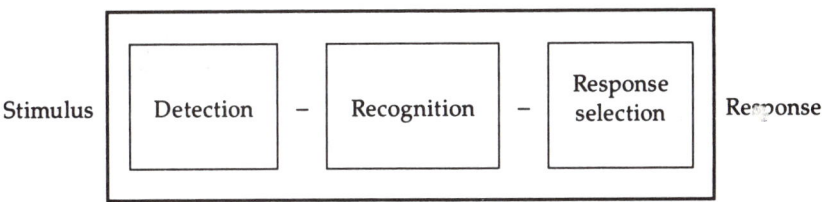

Figure 8-1

can arise and the number of possible responses that could be made in the situation. The greater the uncertainty, the longer the reaction time to decide upon the response.

2. *Movement time*: refers to psychomotor response, and its efficiency is a function of the speed and precision of the movement. (pp. 70-71)

Schmidt (1976) diagnosed two sources of error in the response process: (1) Error of response selection which could result from misperceptions of the environment, so that selection of the wrong response occurs, or the perception and selection seem acceptable. A fluctuation in the environment after the response had been selected, however, could result in an incorrect response; and (2) Error of response execution in which the chosen pattern was not followed, possibly due to unexpected environmental fluctuation, fatigue, or "neural noise."

Welford (1968) theorizes that movement is determined more by central processes controlling movement than by factors of muscular effort involved. Researchers involved in pursuing the information processing model in understanding motor skill learning include: Fitts (1964), Stelmach (1969), Schmidt (1976), Keele (1968), and Poulton (1972).

Adaptation Model. This model views motor skill development from a hierarchical perspective with higher and lower operational processes. It is based on the notion that complex motor skills are composites of subskills which must be mastered before the performance goal can be achieved.

In describing this model, Singer (1975) likens it to a computer plan in which man functions with higher order (executive) programs or routines and subroutines or subprograms. Subroutines, which often function in sequential patterns, are perceived as the "foundational building blocks" for the executive routine, and the mastery of each is essential for efficient and effective performance. Singer describes the essence of the model as follows: "The executive program can be thought of as the plan, idea or goal in a situation. The subroutines are the processes, e.g., movements that enable the plan to be executed" (p. 85). The plan in the organism is the basis of human activity.

Psychomotor skill learning is perceived from the perspective of a hierarchical plan of skill development by which goal attainment is achieved through mastery of subacts, each in sequence with increasing complexity as the act gets nearer the ultimate goal. It is the relationship of each of these subacts to each other that is the focus of study in this area. Theorists addressing this model and its saliency to motor learning are Paillard (1960) and Miller, Galantin, and Pribran (1960).

There are areas of similarity in all of these three models, and newer models are evolving from these three classifications. Model development with the intent of psychomotor learning theory development is progressing, as emphasis is placed on the physiologic, psychologic, and cognitive processes that occur within the organism as it responds to cues from the environment with a coordinated and effective performance. To the teacher of psychomotor skills, these movements are of significance, for such learning can no longer be viewed as a mechanistic process in response to environmental stimuli.

PRACTICE

Motor skill learning requires practice, i.e., the opportunity to "try out" and eventually refine all processes essential for a smooth coordinated performance. The nature of practice and its subsequent results are functions of the goal to be achieved, the degree of complexity of the skill to be mastered, the individual characteristics of the learner, and situational variables which have impact on the learning process. Research into the role of practice in motor skill learning has pursued numerous directions and is reported extensively in the literature. Findings of significance to the teaching of psychomotor skills in nursing are presented.

Variations in Individual Response

As with any learning, there is considerable variation in individual response to a practice learning situation and in the ultimate results of such experiences. Singer (1975) suggests that "variations in performance levels between students throughout practice may be due to the relative ease of gaining insight into the problem; the transferability of related learning skills to the task at hand, which might be of special advantage in the early stages of practice; and various psychological, physiological, intellectual, and emotional adjustments" (p. 373).

The readiness factor is an important one as the learner enters into the practice session for new motor skill development. Readiness relates to motivation to learn, the mind set toward the experience, meaningfulness of the new learning to one's own goals, acknowledgment of need for perseverance in pursuit of mastery learning, and a grasp of the goal to be achieved and the processes entailed in achievement. Motivation, although a recognized positive force in responding to demands of new learning of new motor skills, can also be a discordant force if too intense. Research suggests that an excessively intense level of motivation may impede progress in complex skill attainment. The finding that a moderate degree of motivation results in the greatest success suggests that there may be an optimum level of motivation for each skill.

Readiness to achieve mastery in psychomotor skill learning is also a function of the development of integrated neuromuscular and cognitive processes which must result in coordinated movement. Research by Marteniuk (1969) and Henry (1958) indicates that there is no such element as a generalized motor ability, but rather, that motor learning ability is task-specific and dependent upon such factors as innate ability, previous learning, motivation, and other variables. Henry (1958) states, ". . . it is no longer possible to justify the concept of unitary abilities such as coordination and agility, since the evidence shows that these abilities are specific to the test or activity" (p. 126).

Perceptual Variation and Patterns of Practice

A variation in individual response to learning which was previously discussed is the cognitive style of an individual, field-independent or field-dependent. This characteristic is directly related to the perceptual component of motor skill learning as reflected in the current cybernetic and information processing theories which are identified with such learning. The ability to respond to stimuli and select relevant cues from external and internal environments is perceived to be a function of the individual's perceptual style, for sensory input is essential in controlling and regulating motor activity (Fleishman, 1972; Kelso, 1982; Singer, 1975).

Bruton (1976) explored the influence of the perceptual style of learners in using three patterns of practice when learning the fine complex skill of subcutaneous injection. Three patterns of practice were identified: mental (visualizing the task), physical, and a combination of mental and physical. Students were assigned randomly to each of the three groups and then the cognitive style of each student was identified through the Rod and Frame Tests.

Results indicate that field-independent students learn the task, regardless of the pattern used, more readily than do field-dependent students. This is especially true of the physical-mental pattern where it was noted that performance of the field-dependent students deteriorated. Bruton (1976) explains the success of the field-independent student with this pattern. "In learning skills, perceptual awareness of bodily kinesthetic cues and appropriate response to these contributes to mastery of skill regardless of type of practice used" (p. 73). The intelligence variable of the different cognitive styles and its relationship to learning of perceptual motor skills has not been explored sufficiently, but questions are raised to the possible greater intellectual capacity of field-independent persons who are adept at cue selection and hypothesizing problems and solutions. Data from all groups, regardless of cognitive style, suggest that the most effective practice modality is physical practice followed by mental practice.

Length and Frequency of Practice Periods

Lawther (1977) identifies six factors that need to be considered in answering questions as to the length of the practice session and the spacing of rest intervals.

1. Age of learner
2. Complexity and strenuousness of the skill
3. Specific purpose of the particular practice
4. Level of learning already attained
5. Experiential background of the learner

6. Total environmental conditions including other demands and distractions, activity between practices, and other factors. (p. 139)

Distribution of Practice Sessions. Two general classifications of practice sessions are (1) massed and (2) distributed. Massed practice refers to a pattern in which the rest interval is less than the trial length. Distributed practice refers to a pattern in which the rest interval is equal to or greater than the trial length. Practice occurs over a longer period of time, which may include no practice days. The actual practice time may be the same for both patterns; it is the distribution of time that differs. Research studies by Whitley (1970) and Stelmach (1969) noted no difference in the amount of learning between distributed and massed practice, and Stelmach concluded that learning a motor task is a function of the number of trials and is independent of conditions of practice distribution.

Length of Practice Session. Lawther (1977) summarizes the available evidence on the length of practice sessions:

1. In early stages of gross motor skill learning, relatively short practice sessions are more profitable in terms of minutes of practice. Practices can be too long or too short and only experience with the skill and the learner will indicate the most profitable length.
2. Constant lengths of practice sessions have been reported to produce more learning than regular increases and decreases in length in succeeding sessions.
3. Short, interspersed rest periods within the practice session seem to increase the amount of learning.
4. Adults who are in need of acquiring a skill in a short time can practice profitably many hours per day if it is not an activity that demands great physical effort and entails much fatigue. (pp. 141–42)

The short length of time for beginning learners may be based on their shorter attention span, which increases as practice progresses. Keele (1982) notes that "as practice proceeds, not only is decision time less, but some decisions drop out all together as they become redundant when a pattern of movement can be made" (p. 161). The attention of the learner is freed to address more global decisions relative to the task.

Research suggests that gross skills are learned more efficiently and rapidly with more numerous practice periods spaced over a period of time. It is generally acknowledged that a reasonable degree of achievement in most motor skill learning is accomplished with relatively few practice periods.

Overlearning/Repetition

Overlearning refers to any practice, often referred to as drill, which follows one perfect trial, a generally accepted criterion of success. In psychomotor skill learning, overlearning usually results in greater retention. However, there is a point at which overlearning loses its benefit and actually results in performance decrement. Singer (1975) notes that research indicates a 50 percent overlearning is advantageous. While 100 percent overlearning may produce better performance, the gain is not sufficient to warrant the costs involved in extending practice.

Lawther (1977) sees two significant purposes to be achieved by overlearning: (1) to ensure greater retention over longer periods of time and (2) to generalize the skill so that its adaptability to innumerable changes in the environment is increased, i.e., automatic response to environmental cues.

The decisions regarding the degree of repetition or drill are dependent upon the purposes to be served by acquiring the psychomotor skill. Too much drill results in no increment in skill performance, possibly due to the onset of fatigue, boredom, or frustration when time might be perceived to be better used in other learning.

Retention and Reminiscence

Retention refers to the persistence of learning over a period of time devoid of overt practice periods. Reminiscence refers to significant improvement in performance after periods of considerable lapse of time in which no practice occurred. The latter may be a function of a low level of learning in the initial period as a result of fatigue, boredom, pressure, or other similar factors; or it may mean that the individual has been mentally practicing the skill even though no overt action was evident.

Retention is closely related to the previously discussed matter of overlearning. Fleishman (1972) reports on a study he conducted which indicated that the most powerful variable operating in a study of retention of a perceptual-motor skill was individual differences in the level of the original learning. Rather than retention being a function of pretask abilities, it is a function of specific habits acquired in the original practice of the task. Singer (1975) postulates that retention of motor skills can be achieved with less practice than verbal skills because of the unique nature of each skill. Its uniqueness means that there are not many other learned skills that can interfere with the originally learned skill.

Transfer of Learning

Closely related to the retention variable is the matter of transfer of one psychomotor skill learning to the new task to be accomplished. The closer the new task or its component parts are perceived by the learner to resemble previous learnings, the more quickly and more efficiently it will be learned. The transfer activity, however, may be primarily evident in the early stages of the motor skill learning. As the skill reaches the complex level, task specificity becomes the focus of the learner, and there is less potential for task similarity.

Singer (1975) suggests four factors which may influence the transfer process:

1. Amount of practice of prior skill
2. Motivation to transfer skill
3. Method of training
4. Intent of transfer (p. 47).

Practice is a process during which the learner has the opportunity to master psychomotor skill learning. In addition to multiple variables, which account for the individuality of each learner response, task specificity is a significant factor in motor skill learning and thus influences the patterning of practice sessions, amount needed, retention for long-term use, and potential for transferability.

TEACHING

The theoretical basis for teaching psychomotor skills finds its roots in theories of learning acknowledged as fundamental to psychomotor skill learning. A teaching model based on the S-R or R-S paradigm differs significantly from one that represents the process as well as the outcome, S-O-R, where "O" signifies processes within the organism that influence response. In the latter model, the teacher becomes more cognizant of what is occurring in the learner during the learning process as well as how the learner is performing and thus is able to assess and direct more effectively the learner's progress during skill development.

The directions that theory development in psychomotor learning are taking have significant implications for nursing education. Periodically, questions are raised about the relevancy of psychomotor learning to professional nursing practice. Nursing involves "hands on" activities whose skills are essential in assuring quality care. The present emphasis on physical assessment skills, touch, and nursing management in a highly technical health care setting suggests that psychomotor skills will continue to be an essential part of the assessment and implementation stages of the nursing process.

The teaching of psychomotor skills is a significant component of the education of nurses. Tisdale (1984), a 1983 baccalaureate graduate nurse, affirms this position when she comments on state board examinations and her beliefs about what the new graduate should know. She states:

I have been working since graduation, long enough to see some of the virtues and defects of my education; what I am glad I learned, what I wish I had been offered or listened to more carefully. I'm sorry now that I let my anxiety about more sophisticated topics and my teachers' nonchalance about practical abilities get in the way of perfecting basic skills. My communication skills are put to use every day, and every situation is unique, but it was skills like I.V. calculations and bladder irrigations that threw me as a new graduate. (p. 166)

Can a nonchalant posture of a faculty member be acceptable in teaching any domain of learning that is pertinent to the practice?

Setting

Differences exist between the two practice sites which greatly influence the objectives and teaching strategies used. The learning laboratory is a predictable, unipurpose environment where learning experiences can be controlled and the learner's energy can be focused on the learning task within a designated time frame. Learning activities include the use of resource material, i.e., videotapes, references, and the manipulation of objects. The clinical setting, however, is a nonpredictable multipurpose environment where learning experiences are selected from a large reservoir of options. The continuing distractions inherent in a busy patient care environment place added stress on the learners as they practice their designated tasks. Learning experiences entail direct involvement in the care of clients, which adds a reality dimension for the student. Time allocated to a learning task in this environment cannot be assured because of pressure of other variables in the area which may impinge on the student's ability to focus directly on the learning task to be accomplished.

Gomez and Gomez (1987) report on their study of teaching the blood pressure skill in either the learning laboratory or the practice setting. Students, whose experience was in the clinical area scored higher on the accuracy and confidence index and there were no differences between the groups on the index of discernment. The skill studied was a straightforward one which could be taught in the practice site under reality circumstances. A more complex skill would require use of both settings for practice.

Learning Resources Laboratory. The laboratory with appropriate equipment provides a setting where the learner can learn to manipulate equipment with a sense of its process and intended outcome. The environment provides the necessary situational cues and enables the student to respond to the cues in a nonthreatening milieu. This environment contains the necessary multimedia, including both hard- and software, for use in explaining the process and critical elements of the skill and the models essential for practice.

Psychomotor skill learning is an egocentric process. The learner's sense of self as a coordinated being with control over the skill process is essential before one uses the skill in a more public setting. The time necessary to spend in the laboratory is specific to the task and the individual learner. Since no set time can be designated for a particular skill practice, a learning laboratory needs to be available and accessible to learners on their own terms. Such a laboratory might be perceived for psychomotor learning as the library is perceived for cognitive learning an open environment where the learners practice skills according to their own needs to the point of an agreed upon level of achievement. The laboratory, under the direction of a preceptor skilled in the psychomotor domain, provides a milieu where learners can receive formative evaluation as they progress through the practice experience.

Baldwin et al. (1991) report on their study to determine if the mediated instruction provided in the laboratory, reference books, videos, etc. was sufficient for students to practice and feel confident in their ability to perform the designated skill. One group of students, who was provided with faculty assistance as well as the mediated instruction within the laboratory, demonstrated significantly more confidence in their ability than those who had no faculty contact while learning in the laboratory.

Such a laboratory also serves an important testing function, which will be presented in more detail later in this chapter relative to the use of a taxonomy. The use of the laboratory for practice and for monitoring the performance as the learning process proceeds is to facilitate retention, since retention is a function of the effectiveness of the initial learning.

Clinical Area. This setting places the individual in the world where nurses practice, including the hospital, community, nursing home, and client's home. The nature of the milieu has a bearing on skill performance. The concern here is how that milieu is used in teaching psychomotor skills.

The clinical setting for practice needs assessment in relation to the goal of the practice. Whereas earlier periods of nursing education emphasized psychomotor skill development and used the clinical area for such practice, today the clinical field is established on the basis of care of the patient. Psychomotor skill development should occur without the learner being concerned about the other care activities germaine to the environment. Thus, it is not the setting that determines what the learner will experience, but rather, the needed experience will determine the practice setting.

Teachers will be challenged to reexamine the notion that the learner needs to "know the patient" before performing a psychomotor skill on the patient. Knowledge of the patient is a function of the faculty. It means that faculty, who are in a setting where there is ample opportunity for practice with a particular skill, may invite their colleagues to send their students to the setting for practice. It also means that when learners reach the predetermined level of skill attainment in the laboratory, they will proceed to the clinical field for immediate practice; for learning of a skill is more meaningful and economical when it is linked to application.

Whole versus Part Approach to Teaching Psychomotor Skills

The decision to teach the skill as a whole or to teach it in terms of its parts is often a reflection of the teacher's belief about how psychomotor skills are learned. For clarification, it is important to define the terms whole and part. Gates and colleagues (1953) offer the following definitions:

Whole: a definitely segregated, independent pattern which possesses unity, coherence and meaning in itself above that implied by its parts.

Part: an element in a total situation which is essential to the meaning as a whole, but which loses its peculiar meaning when isolated from the whole. (pp. 371–372)

Part teaching is based on a behavioristic mode which considers learning to be additive; i.e., as each part is learned, a new one is introduced and added to the previously learned one once it is mastered. Whole learning is compatible with gestalt or field theory, which views the whole as greater than the sum of its parts and the parts related to each other and to the whole. Learning is integrative.

Naylor and Briggs (1961) identify two aspects of a psychomotor skill that need to be considered in making the decision as to teaching the skill holistically or partially:

Task Complexity: refers to demands made on a person's memory and is a function of information processing.

Task Organization: indicates the nature of interrelationships of several task dimensions or organization.

Their studies and those of others suggest that part practice is more effective in skills that are highly complex and have low organization (few independent components in the task). Whole practice is more effective with high organization where there is an increase in component interaction. Generalization from this notion is still tentative, and analysis of the task to be learned continues to be an essential action.

Singer (1975) poses questions to be asked in relation to the complexity criterion of a skill:

1. How difficult does the learner perceive the task to be?
2. How many things does the learner have to think about; remember from previous related experiences?
3. To what extent is it possible to forget the task over time and therefore pose a challenge for the learner to remember it? (p. 383)

If part teaching is to be used, the units must be large enough to represent a total phenomenon in themselves. Too small a unit fosters boredom and lack of challenge; too large a unit leads to frustration when repeated practice does not produce success and withdrawal results from loss of interest.

In general, the whole approach to learning is more effective because it does enable the learner to see the goal, that is, what the outcome looks like; gain insight into the total process; and see the relationship of the parts to each other and to the goal. It is more economical because the learner can identify those parts that need more practice for an efficient performance of the total and can emphasize their refinement in relation to the whole. Practice is specific to the learner.

In additive learning, each step is developed in terms of the selected criteria, but at the conclusion the learner still needs time to learn how the parts are related in order to produce an efficient performance. McGuigan and MacCaslin (1955) add another dimension to the issue of whole versus part teaching when they report their study which indicated that the more intelligent subjects responded more favorably to whole learning. This finding may be a function of their cognitive ability in information processing or their ability to learn more and thus have a greater repertoire of experience to draw upon.

Knowledge of Results

Knowledge of results as the learner progresses through the psychomotor practice is essential if skill development is to occur. Bilodeau and Bilodeau (1961) summarized studies as to the role of knowledge of results in skill development and state: "Studies of feedback or knowledge of results show it to be the strongest, most important variable controlling performance and learning" (p. 250). Singer (1975) refers to the two general types of feedback:

Intrinsic: proprioceptive activity and tactile sense inform learner as to "feel" of the response while visual feedback provides data on accuracy of response.

Augmented: the special cues added to the learning situation
(artificial) such as verbal cues, supplementary or artificial visual or kinesthetic cues. (p. 47)

Verbal cues are significant factors in adding to skill performance increment, but the learner's reliance on these cues must be avoided, for performance in skill learning is dependent upon the learner's ability to judge his or her own performance. Feedback only on outcome may influence the performance but not facilitate the process of learning. Lawther (1977) notes that "the feedback should be visual and perhaps quantitatively precise in verbal description" (p. 137). In reference to augmented feedback he suggests that it should be as closely adapted to individual learner needs as possible.

Some skill learning can occur without augmented feedback as learners draw upon their own repertoire of knowledge and rely upon intrinsic feedback. Augmented feedback does facilitate the learning process when there is continuity, yet selectivity in terms of the learner's particular needs. When neither intrinsic nor augmented feedback occurs or is discontinued during the learning process, there is a decrement in psychomotor skill performance and learning.

Occurrence of Two Different Learnings Simultaneously

As was noted earlier, psychomotor skill learning is concerned with the three domains of learning: cognitive, affective, and psychomotor. It was suggested that the cognitive element needs to be viewed from two perspectives: the theory and principles underlying the purpose, process, and outcome of the skill, and the information processes that occur within the individual from the stimulus to the actual performance. The discussion of the research and concepts pertaining to psychomotor learning indicates that the advancement process from novice to expert requires the coordination of all cognitive processes relative to cue selection, interpretation, and the appropriate response in an efficient manner. The theoretical bases underlying the skill are most important but need to be addressed outside the actual performance so that the learner can focus on the coordination processes essential for a coordinated response.

In nursing education there is a tendency to interject the theoretical component of psychomotor skill learning while the process of cognitive information processing is being developed. For example, as the nursing student is going through the process of learning to administer a drug by injection, the teacher says, "What are the actions of that drug you are going to administer?" The student's psychomotor learning is interfered with because of the need to respond to a "knowledge" question. When learning to drive an automobile, what would be the response of the novice if the instructor interrupted the concentration on the driving activity with the following type of question, "What is the purpose of the sparkplugs in the engine?"

Brown, Tickner and Simmonds (1969) examined this dual activity phenomenon in a study of the interference between concurrent tasks of driving a car through a designated gap and making a telephone call, where the effects of divided attention on judgments of clearance, control skills, and checking auditory messages were explored. Results of this study demonstrated that the driver made reliably more wrong decisions while driving and answering questions than while driving in a controlled condition without questions. Questions were also answered reliably less correctly and took longer for response than in the control situation where questions were asked during the time when the car was not in motion. Poulton (1972) concurs that it is possible to carry out two tasks simultaneously, but in order for a person to accomplish this feat one task must have been practiced sufficiently to the point of being automatic.

In a field study, Cairy (1981) examined the effect of cognitive teaching during nursing students' learning of two skills: intramuscular injection and intravenous insertion. The experimental group received its teaching of the cognitive component of the skill prior to the performance while the control group received its teaching of the cognitive component concurrent with the skill performance. The finding supported the hypothesis that those students who experienced teaching of the cognitive prior to performing the skill carried out the skill with a significantly higher degree of precision. Although the limited sample precludes making generalizations, the findings are in accord with those of Brown and colleagues (1969).

Psychomotor skill learning is a complex activity that requires knowledge of purpose, principles, and anticipated outcome in relation to both the cognitive and affective domains. The knowledge component is discussed in conferences either prior to the actual skill performance or following the performance, where the latter is analyzed and evaluated. It is during the actual performance that the learner needs to be free to follow the sequential pattern of the task without interruption, except in instances where safety is at stake.

TAXONOMY OF PSYCHOMOTOR SKILL PERFORMANCE

During practice of a psychomotor skill, changes occur in the learner's performance that signal movement from novice toward expert practitioner. Fleishman (1972) summarizes results of studies that deal with practice tasks:

1. As practice continues, changes occur in the particular combinations of the abilities contributing to performance.
2. These changes are progressive, systematic and eventually become stabilized.
3. The contribution of "non motor" abilities (e.g., verbal, spatial) which may play a role in learning decreases systematically with practice relative to "motor abilities."
4. There is an increase in a factor specific in the task itself. (p. 98)

The developments occurring in the process are directed toward a systematic, sequential order of activities accomplished with spatial and temporal reality and reflective of a consistent response pattern. The learner develops selective attention to cues, is able to select relevant information while disregarding other data (thus greatly decreasing decision time between stimulus and response), and is able quickly to anticipate variables entailed in the total performance. An expert performer develops skills that are almost automatic as a result of increased speed, accuracy, and coordination. Schneider and Fish (1982) state that "practice leads to apparently resource-free automatic productions for consistent processing, but does not reduce resources needed for varied processing tasks" (p. 11).

Psychomotor Taxonomy

Several taxonomies, i.e., hierarchies of behavior, have been developed to identify the growth process from novice to expert by practitioners such as Simpson (1966), Harrow (1972), Kibler, Barker, and Miles (1970), and Cratty (1967). Dave (1970) has proposed a taxonomy for psychomotor skill performance with an integrating concept of neuromuscular coordination. Reilly and Oermann (1990) demonstrated the use of this taxonomy in nursing which delineates the skill development to the level of professional competence.

Taxonomy includes five levels of performance but does not identify discrete components of each level. The levels are:

P 1.0 Imitation
Skills are learned in the beginning after they have been demonstrated, whether directly by the teacher or by observation of the process on a film, videotape, or slide tape sequence. The performance lacks neuromuscular coordination or control and, hence, is generally in a crude and imperfect form (i.e., impulse, overt repetition).

P 2.0 Manipulation
In this level, the learner follows a prescription as outlined on a procedure sheet, learning to follow instructions, performing selected actions and fixing performance through necessary practice.

P 3.0 Precision
Performance has reached a level of refinement and can be carried out without a set of directions or a model, and performance is characterized by accuracy, i.e., exactness with reduction in errors.

P 4.0 Articulation
Performance is coordinated in a logical sequence of activities that reflects harmony and consistency among the activities. The time dimension is added here, for speed and time must be within a realistic expectation.

P 5.0 Naturalization
Skill represents a high degree of proficiency, which has become an automatic response to appropriate situational cues. Performance is efficient and meets criteria for professional competence.

Performance Criteria for Each Level of Psychomotor Skill

Specific expected behaviors for each level of the taxonomy can be determined from research findings and theoretical perspectives about learning psychomotor skills. The behaviors can be used as criteria in determining the expected level of performance.

P 1.0 Imitation
Observed actions are followed
Movements are gross

Coordination lacks smoothness
Errors are present
Time and speed are based on learner need

P 2.0 Manipulation
Written instructions are followed
Coordination of movements is variable
Accuracy is in terms of the written prescription
Time and speed are variable

P 3.0 Precision
(3.1 or 3.2)
A logical sequence of actions is carried out
Coordination is at a high level
Errors are minimal and do not involve critical actions
Time and speed are variable

P 4.0 Articulation
A logical sequence of actions is carried out
Coordination is at a high level
Errors are generally limited
Time and speed are within reasonable expectations

P 5.0 Naturalization
Sequence of actions is automatic
Coordination is consistently at a high level
Time and speed are within reality
Performance reflects professional competence

The changes in behavior indicated in this taxonomy reflect the evolution of skilled performance. In the first two levels, behavior is generally gross with the accuracy dimension entering the schema in the second level in terms of following a prescribed format. These two levels may be achieved in a learning laboratory.

Level 3 is divided according to setting: P 3.1 is the learning laboratory and P 3.2 is in the clinical field. In both, the performance behavior is the same. The difference refers to performance in a controlled setting in contrast to performance in an uncontrolled setting with real clients. The attainment of a P 3.1 level in the laboratory does not necessarily indicate that the same behaviors will be exhibited in the clinical field where the skill is performed with less control of environmental cues.

Level 3 also makes a statement relative to the nature of the errors that might occur. Every skill has certain activities that are essential for maintaining its integrity, while other actions can be altered without influencing the general effect of the skill. It is essential that the critical elements of the skill be identified and considered to be nonnegotiable; i.e., they must be error free at this level.

It is noted that a logical sequence of actions as specified in a procedure is not a criterion for skill attainment. The sequence of actions may not necessarily be the same as specified on the procedure sheet, but as long as the learner can rationally support the decisions involved in the sequencing the criterion is met. Too often the actions described in the procedure are so detailed that the critical judgment of the learner is denied and the procedure becomes a sequence of unchallenged actions.

Level 4 adds a significant dimension, the matter of speed and timing in the performance of a skill. One is not skillful if the act is not performed within a reasonable time period. One may be most accurate and skillful in obtaining a blood pressure reading, but if an hour is required for the act one cannot be considered to be skilled.

Questions are often raised as to whether speed or accuracy should be emphasized in psychomotor skill development. The taxonomy described in this chapter suggests that accuracy precedes speed. The nature of the skill to be taught, the speed requirement for its execution, and the particular abilities of the learner determine the response to that question. Early emphasis on speed is appropriate in psychomotor skills momentum, but since that is not a characteristic of many psychomotor skills in nursing, early emphasis on accuracy is preferred. Accuracy is specific to speed in practice.

The speed dimension as it relates to skilled performance is best evaluated in the setting where the actual activity will occur in practice. It is there that the adaptability of the skill is demonstrated and the learner's use of decision time is expedited through selective attention to cues in the situation. Although time can be a factor in skill performance in the laboratory, its significance in relation to skilled behavior is best demonstrated in the practice setting.

Level 5 is the point where the skill most reflects automatic behavior. The learner is no longer concerned about the "how to do" of the skill. It is now an integral part of nursing practice and can be retrieved upon appropriate situational cues. The synthesis of cognitive, affective, and psychomotor domains has occurred and the performance reflects the criterion of professional competence.

USE OF A PERFORMANCE TAXONOMY

Nursing faculty must come to the decision that not all psychomotor skills applicable to nursing practice should be developed to the level of naturalization of professional competency. The quantity of skills is too large and the frequency of use is so variable that faculty need to be more discriminating as to the level at which each psychomotor skill should be performed. Decisions are based upon need, frequency of skill in usual practice in the local geographical region, and the availability of experience for practice.

Essential Decisions

Mastery/Competency. Before identifying the appropriate level, faculty need to clarify the concepts of mastery and competency and decide how the terms will be used.

Morgan and Irby (1978) define competency as the knowledge and skills necessary for adequate performance in a profession. This definition is more compatible with level P 5.0 being identified as the level of performance competency. Mastery also has a different meaning. In the mastery of learning concept, mastery is defined in terms of objectives to be attained. In this context, mastery relates to the mastery of the learning implied by the designated level to be achieved, not to the ultimate level possible. Because of different meanings attached to these terms, it is important to include the faculty's definition with documents related to psychomotor teaching. In the proposed taxonomy, the ultimate level is considered professional competency with mastery referring to the designated level of achievement.

Skills to Be Included. Decisions as to what skills are to be included are in accord with the overall curriculum plan as it reflects the demands of generic or specialized nursing practice. The decision is best made in joint discussions with faculty and nursing service administrators who employ the graduates. Sweeney and colleagues (1980) report on a study that identified essential skills of baccalaureate graduates from the perspective of education and service.

The influx of technology into the health care delivery system for both diagnosing and intervening in the course of disease and illness have markedly increased the quantity and sophistication of psychomotor skills in nursing practice. Decisions as to what psychomotor skills need to be included in the curriculum and the level of competency that can be realistically obtained challenge nursing faculty, since curricula must also accommodate the developing knowledge related to the other dimensions of nursing practice.

Several changes in the delivery of health care in our society have forced faculty to reexamine their assumptions about the place of psychomotor teaching in the curriculum. During the recent past, the teaching of hi-tech skills was primarily relegated to experiences in the intensive care units, thus only those students who had practice experience in those settings were able to learn these skills. However, with the advent of a budget-driven policy of health care delivery represented by the DRG (diagnostic-related-groups) payment system, the use of many technical skills formerly the province of in-hospital care, is now found in other patient care settings such as, ambulatory care centers, especially where surgery is performed, long term care facilities, and even in patients' homes. In the latter situation, nurses now need to teach families how to use these hi-tech skills and to monitor the results. With these skills now pervasive throughout the health care system, consideration must be given as to the place for their teaching in the total program. This matter is addressed by Neighbors et al. (1991) in their study which demonstrates inadequate teaching in associate degree nursing programs of these skills, which have now in many instances, become the usual rather than the occasional mode of practice. The re-emergence of psychomotor skills must now be accommodated within the broader context of nursing.

Alavi, Hoh, and Reilly (1991) present the experience of a faculty in an Australian school of nursing answering two critical questions; what psychomotor skills should be included in the curriculum and to what degree of competence should each skill be achieved. Seeking a logical framework for examining these questions, the faculty utilized the list of skills from Reilly and Oermann (1985), which also appears in this edition. Faculty sought input from nursing representatives of the 57 agencies where students had clinical practice as to the relevance and frequency of use of the listed skills in their agencies. Using the frequency rating of 65 percent for each skill, the faculty developed a list of skills to be taught. In a few instances, faculty judgment included some lower-scoring items, believing their use would become more frequent at a later date. Physical assessment skills were emphasized more by faculty than by agency response. This approach meant that some skills previously thought to be essential for practice were eliminated since they were no longer relevant to practice. The list represented response from 81 percent of the agencies, thus enabling faculty to accept their list as compatible with present day practice.

The answer to the second question regarding level of competency was derived through the use of the psychomotor taxonomy previously described in this chapter. The two major criteria for determining level were:

1. The acceptance of the psychomotor skill within the broader scope of nursing practice.
2. Opportunities the student would have to practice the skill in the clinical setting. (Alavi et al., 1991, p. 961)

The decision regarding the level to be attained for each skill was determined relative to what could reasonably be expected of all students, with the recognition that some students could attain higher competency on some skills if the experience was available in the practice area. The process of using the data enabled the faculty to develop a psychomotor grid for the total program modeled after the one presented in this book.

The selection of skills must reflect the criterion of motor behavior performance, not cognitive behavior. Recording, although involving some motor action, is in essence a cognitive skill, for the evaluation is based on the substance of the recording, not the actual process of writing. Interviewing is also a cognitive skill although it does involve some muscular activity.

Location of Practice. Another decision affecting the planning for teaching psychomotor skills is the location of the practice; i.e., learning resource laboratory or the clinical field. Preliminary practice in the laboratory for at least the first two levels is generally facilitative, for it affords the student the opportunity to gain a sense of self and the ability to manipulate equipment and coordinate activities in a relatively risk-free environment that does not put patients or others at risk. The student learning a new skill, regardless of the setting, may feel at risk.

When the student enters the clinical setting for a first-time performance of a skill in that setting, faculty must recognize the egocentric nature of psychomotor learning. Until the learner feels comfortable and secure in the knowledge that body movements are coordinated in working with equipment and the client, the learner will not be able to focus on other events that occur within the context of the procedure. It is unrealistic to expect the learner performing a skill for the first time in the setting to be able to greet the patient, explain the procedure, and respond to other demands in the situation. At this stage in the learning, the teacher's role is to manage all the other aspects that relate to patient care so that the learner can focus on the performance.

Once the learner is asked to perform a skill in the clinical environment, regardless of the level of skill development, teachers must be cognizant of the impact of the situational variables and needs of the learners on the outcome of the performance. Cleland (1965) studied the impact of stress in a clinical setting on the performance of graduate nurses. Although the study addressed cognitive testing, similar results can be anticipated in psychomotor testing. Increased situational stress interfered negatively with cue utilization. An additional variable reflective of the social nature of the clinical field was studied; the relationship of the need for social approval to performance. A high need for social approval requires a low stress situation; increase in stress brings a performer to a maximum level of motivation quickly and then performance deteriorates. Low level of need for social approval requires a moderate level of stress to bring the performer to an optimum motivation level for maximum performance.

The findings of Cleland relative to social approval needs is reflective of the data on field-independent and field-dependent learners. The field-dependent learner has a high need for social acceptance while the field-independent learner relies more on intrinsic acceptance. Both groups approach psychomotor performance in a dynamic environment differently; a fact that must be acknowledged by the instructor in determining the best strategies to use in teaching.

Outcome Level for Each Skill. The outcome level selected for each skill must be realistic in terms of its potential for attainment by all students. This decision is in essence a contract with the learner; the experiences will be provided that enable the learner to reach the designated level and the evaluation will be in accord with the level. It does not guarantee that the learner will reach the specified level, for much learning is still under the control of the learner.

The designation of a level does not preclude students from advancing further if the opportunity permits. Students should be encouraged to advance in those skills not designated at the professional competency level when experience is available. A faculty may feel that a P 3.2 level is most realistic for skill in catheterization, but if the student is in a clinical setting where there is ample opportunity for experience, the student should be encouraged to proceed to the P 5.0 level. The outcome level specified for any course or the total program reflects perceived reality, not the full potential for any one student.

Methods of Testing. Decisions on the testing of the student's performance, particularly from level P 3.0 through P 5.0, must include considerations relative to timing, strategy, and location. Testing in the laboratory generally is a function of limited availability of experience in the clinical setting. If a faculty feels that some level of achievement of some skills is necessary but the clinical setting does not provide sufficient opportunity, simulation testing in the laboratory may occur. Testing is indicated at the P 3.1 level. In the clinical field, testing may involve direct observation or videotape. Regardless of the setting and method, testing time is designated and extraneous variables are controlled as much as possible. Unlike formative evaluation which addresses what is and what can be, the teacher in summative evaluation, which addresses what is, assumes the posture of a tester not a teacher. Intervention is restricted to evidence of clear and present danger. Skill delineation is not a matter of the number of times a skill has been performed, but rather, the ability of the learner to perform in accordance with predetermined criteria.

Psychomotor Performance Grid

A taxonomy provides a framework for decisions about appropriate levels of performance for each skill and for planning for the teaching of the skill in a nursing program. When using the presented taxonomy in concert with the taxonomy of one or both of the other domains, it is essential to recognize that each domain is discrete, thus there may or may not be consistency in the designated levels among the domains. A P 4.0 level on the psychomotor taxonomy does not mean that the other taxonomies will be so designated. The knowledge level of a skill is not necessarily the same as the performance level.

In the development of a grid, i.e., a mapping of the teaching of psychomotor skills, faculty first make decisions relative to the outcome performance level for each skill that is expected at the conclusion of the educational program. The course in which the skill is introduced is noted and the expected level of achievement is designated. Some skills, such as taking an oral temperature, radial pulse, and respirations, may reach P 5.0 within the first course, while other skills may progress over a longer period.

When a designated skill level is reached by the student, he or she will be held accountable for maintenance of that level in all subsequent courses. Faculty in the subsequent courses are responsible for monitoring students' performance on all psychomotor skills relevant to the practice area. This formative evaluation is essential for skill maintenance and addresses the habitual practice of the students within the context of normal activities.

When faculty in subsequent courses note that the student does not perform at the expected level of psychomotor skill, it is appropriate to refer the student to the laboratory for further practice. It is essential that the laboratory recommendation not be perceived as punitive, but rather as an opportunity to review and refine performance. This is another example of viewing the learning resource laboratory from the same perspective for psychomotor learning as the library is viewed for cognitive learning. Cognitive and psychomotor skills must be differentiated during these formative evaluation periods. If the student performs the skill at the appropriate level but is unable to answer questions relative to the theory basis of the skill, the problem is cognitive, not psychomotor, and must be addressed accordingly. A return to the learning resource laboratory would not be an appropriate resolution of the problem.

An example of a grid for teaching psychomotor skills is demonstrated in Table 8-2. The grid represents four terms in which students would be in a clinical field practicing their skills with real clients. The format of the nursing program (Table 8-1) is intended to be general rather than representative of any specific nursing theory so that its

Table 8-1
Nursing Program

	Nursing Care of Clients with Minimal Health Care Needs	Nursing Care of Clients with Moderate Health Care Needs	Nursing Care of Clients with Acute Health Care Needs	Nursing Care of Clients with Long-Term Health Care Needs
Role of Nurse	Supportive Monitoring Maintenance Educative	Supportive Supplementary Educative Palliative	Compensatory Monitoring Protective Consultative Educative	Supplementary Monitoring Educative Protective Consultative
Setting	Ambulatory care setting Convalescent home Nursing home	Hospital Client's home Ambulatory care setting	Hospital Intensive care Acute care Psychiatric hospital	Long-term care facilities Rehabilitation facilities Home for mentally retarded Community agencies Client's home

potential can be demonstrated, regardless of the curriculum framework. In a school setting, faculty would develop its own curriculum and plan the sequence in accord with whatever theoretical framework it chose. The grid would relate to the program sequencing and may well differ from the grid proposed here. The program presented is not necessarily meant to depict a total program. Some programs may include an introductory course in which basic skill development is highlighted. Others may have an additional term that provides for synthesizing practice skills and practice in some of the leadership activities of nursing.

The skills used in the grid are derived primarily from the study of Sweeney and colleagues (1980), which listed the skills upon which there was agreement by faculty and nursing service personnel as expected behaviors of graduates (Table 8-2).

Once faculty have developed a psychomotor grid, there exists a master plan which designates what skills are to be taught, where in the total program they are to be taught, and the desired levels of achievement to

Table 8-2
Psychomotor Grid

Skill	Outcome	Minimal Term I	Moderate Term II	Acute Term III	Long-Term Term IV
Fundamental					
Mobilization	P 5.0	P 3.2	P 5.0		
Range of motion	P 5.0	P 3.2	P 4.0	P 4.0	P 5.0
Bed bath	P 5.0	P 3.1	P 5.0		
Mouth care—general	P 5.0	P 3.1	P 5.0		
special		P 3.2	P 2.0	P 3.1	P 3.2
Hair care	P 5.0	P 3.2	P 5.0		
Back rub	P 5.0	P 3.1	P 5.0		
Positioning	P 5.0	P 3.1	P 5.0		
Feeding a patient	P 5.0	P 2.0	P 3.2	P 5.0	
Occupied bed	P 5.0	P 3.1	P 5.0		
Temperature—oral, rectal	P 5.0	P 5.0			
Pulse—radial	P 5.0	P 5.0			
apical	P 5.0	P 3.1	P 5.0		
carotid	P 5.0	P 5.0			
Blood pressure	P 5.0	P 3.2	P 5.0		
Weight/height	P 5.0	P 5.0			
Assist with bed-pan/ urinal	P 5.0	P 3.1	P 5.0		
Body mechanics	P 5.0	P 3.2	P 5.0		
General Therapeutic and Diagnostic Procedures					
Auscultation					
Heart sounds	P 5.0	P 3.1	P 4.0	P 5.0	
Respiratory sounds	P 5.0	P 3.1	P 4.0	P 5.0	
Neurologic—reflex, etc.	P 3.2	P 3.1		P 3.2	
Ear/nose/throat exam	P 5.0	P 3.1	P 3.2	P 4.0	P 5.0
Specimen collection	P 5.0	P 3.2	P 5.0		
Palpation	P 5.0	P 3.1	P 4.0	P 5.0	
Care of skin—					
Prevention	P 5.0	P 3.2	P 5.0		
Sterile dressings	P 4.0	P 3.2	P 4.0		
Bandage application	P 5.0	P 3.2	P 5.0		
Sterile gloving	P 5.0	P 3.1	P 3.2	P 5.0	
Use of instruments in a sterile field	P 4.0	P 3.1	P 3.2	P 4.0	
Precaution technique (isolation)	P 5.0	P 2.0	P 3.2	P 5.0	

Table 8-2 *(Continued)*

Skill	Outcome	Minimal Term I	Moderate Term II	Acute Term III	Long-Term Term IV
Wound irrigation	P 2.0			P 2.0	
Change IV bottles	P 5.0		P 3.2	P 5.0	
Remove IV needles	P 5.0	P 3.1	P 3.2	P 5.0	
Administration of medications					
Oral	P 5.0	P 3.2	P 5.0		
Topical	P 5.0	P 3.2	P 5.0		
Subcutaneous	P 4.0	P 3.1	P 3.2	P 4.0	
Intramuscular	P 4.0	P 3.1	P 3.2	P 4.0	
Draping a patient	P 5.0	P 3.1	P 5.0		
Cleansing enema	P 5.0	P 3.1	P 5.0		
Assist with coughing/ deep breathing	P 5.0	P 3.1	P 5.0		
Catheterization	P 3.1		P 3.1		
Urine tests	P 5.0	P 5.0			
Specialized Therapeutic and Diagnostic Measures					
Bottle feeding	P 4.0		P 4.0		
Fetal heart reading	P 3.2	P 3.1	P 3.2		
Assist with postural drainage	P 3.1		P 3.1		
Respiratory suction	P 4.0		P 3.1	P 3.2	P 4.0
Tracheostomy suction	P 3.2		P 3.1	P 3.2	
Nasogastric	P 4.0		P 3.1	P 3.2	P 4.0
Ileostomy care	P 3.2		P 3.1		P 3.2
Colostomy care	P 3.2		P 3.1		P 3.2
Traction	P 3.1		P 3.1		
Oxygen therapy	P 3.2		P 3.1	P 3.2	
Maintenance of chest drainage	P 3.2		P 3.1	P 3.2	
Vision testing	P 3.1	P 3.1			
Eye drops	P 3.1	P 3.1			
Measure central venous pressure	P 3.2		P 3.1	P 3.2	
Change total parenteral nutrition lines through volumetric pump	P 3.2		P 3.1	P 3.2	

be reached at any point throughout the curriculum. Such a plan is not static and needs to be subjected to periodic reviews in relation to its relevance to current nursing practices and to the accuracy of faculty judgments in level determination.

Psychomotor Grid and Accountability

The grid has built into it a system for assigning accountability. Faculty in each course are accountable to assure that students are at the designated level of mastery before proceeding to the next course. Although there is provision for the unexpected that interferes with a student's achievement of the goal, subsequent faculty have the right to expect that students have met the expectations so that the new learning demands of the next course can proceed. When changes in practice require alterations in expected accomplishment, this is a matter for faculty deliberation.

Student accountability is also prescribed. If students are given a copy of the grid and informed that the completion of the skills at the designated level is a requirement for the course grade and advancement to the next course, they will need to assume responsibility for obtaining the necessary experience. This demand fosters the development of a self-directed learner and facilitates the establishment of a systematic plan for one's own learning.

Procrastination in scheduling experience obligations may result in student inability to secure faculty assessment time. The lesson is learned. It is not meant to imply that the total responsibility lies with the student; a shared accountability is in order. Periodic formative evaluation conferences with students to determine what performance experiences have been achieved and to propose plans for the remaining skills assist the planning process for both the teacher and learner.

The grid also prescribes accountability for the school when it is used as a communication for future employers of the graduates. Since it identifies the quantity and quality of psychomotor skill attainment at the conclusion of the program, employers have a framework of expectations relative to the new graduate's abilities and future learning needs. Each service area in a health care agency might develop a grid of skills appropriate to nursing care in that area, which would be informative to new employees and provide a basis for monitoring performance of the nursing staff at periodic intervals.

In essence, a psychomotor grid provides a framework for ordering the process of skill development within the context of the total program, for designating persons accountable for the learning attainment, and for assuring the place of psychomotor skill learning in a nursing program.

TEACHING METHODS

Methodology for teaching psychomotor skill from the performance perspective includes demonstration, whether by the presence of the individual in the setting or by single concept films or videotapes. The visual component enables the learner to obtain a general idea of the action pattern and supports the notion of whole learning. Playbacks of videotapes of the learner's performance fosters self-knowledge of the action and facilitates correction of errors or unprofitable actions. The principles for using these methods are described in Chapter 6.

Computer-assisted instruction is being developed in this area of teaching. Combinations of verbal and visual cues enable the learner to participate in the process cognitively. Computer instructions can facilitate the learner's grasp of the theoretical basis of the skill and anticipate its use under varying environmental situations.

Whatever the methods used in the demonstration stage, practice is essential in the development of a coordinated, efficient performance. Cognitive learning, which provides for the knowledge of principles and processes, does not develop the body movements responsive to situational cues.

Some psychomotor skills may be approached from a problem-solving or discovery methodology. However, since many nursing skills have been formalized into a procedure, it is more efficient to use the procedure for initial learning. Because nursing has many psychomotor skills that have been "adopted" from other disciplines, there is a great need for nursing research to establish the validity of present procedures or offer modifications as indicated. Newer developments in nursing and science disciplines might well influence current approaches to some of the skills.

The use of client problem situations in the learning of psychomotor skills is best when the learner has obtained a reasonable degree of self-confidence in skill performance. The student is then in a better position to see the skill within the context of patient care and to hypothesize modifications indicated by specific cues in the patient situation. Once the cognitive information processing has been developed for the skill, the learner is ready to deal with the cognitive processes of judgment, inferential reasoning, and decision making.

SUMMARY

Psychomotor skill learning is a significant domain in nursing, separate from but closely related to the cognitive and affective domain. There is a difference between psychomotor performance, the visible evidence of learning and psychomotor learning, the ability to retrieve the skill upon pertinent situational cues.

Skilled performance is characterized by an efficient coordinated behavior pattern within a realistic time, motion, and speed context which is generally consistent in quality whenever it occurs. Practice enables the individual to develop cognitive informational processes which facilitate the skill through selective attention to cues, thus decreasing decision-making time. Use of practice sessions requires consideration of their frequency, distribution, and length and must address the notions of overlearning, retention, feedback, and transfer of learning.

Psychomotor skills are practiced and learned in two practice settings: the learning resource laboratory and the clinical field, which provide a reality context to the learning. Each setting contributes to the skill development, but it is in the clinical field where the evidence of skill learning, especially in relation to the time dimension, is most persuasive.

Not all psychomotor skills in nursing need to or should be developed to a level of professional competency. A psychomotor taxonomy of performance provides a framework for designating a level of achievement for each skill and for sequencing of psychomotor skill learning in a nursing program. The grid that is developed facilitates accountability by all involved.

Psychomotor learning is an egocentric process and requires that the learner feel comfortable with him- or herself in the performance before the skill can be related on a more sophisticated level to the greater sphere of nursing practice.

REFERENCES

Adams, J. A. (1968). Response feedback and learning. *Psychological Bulletin, 70*, 486–504.

Alavi, C., Hoh, S., & Reilly, D. (1991). Reality basis for teaching psychomotor skills in a tertiary nursing curriculum. *Journal of Advanced Nursing, 16*, 957–965.

Baldwin, D., Hill, P., & Hanson, G. (1991). Performance of psychomotor skills: A comparison of two strategies. *Journal of Nursing Education, 30*(8), 367–370.

Bernstein, N. (1967). *The coordination and regulation of movements.* Elmsford, NJ: Pergamon Press.

Bilodeau, E. A., & Bilodeau, I. (1961). Motor skills learning. *Annual Review of Psychology, 12*, 250.

Brown, I. D., Tickner, H., & Simmonds, D. C. (1969). Interference between concurrent tasks of driving and telephoning. *Journal of Applied Psychology, 55*, 419–424.

Bruton, M. R. (1976). *The influence of perceptual style and various combinations of mental and physical practice in facilitating the learning of a novel, fine, complex perceptual-motor skill.* Unpublished doctoral dissertation, New York University.

Cairy, M. (1981). *The timing of cognitive teaching as it affects the performance of psychomotor skills.* Unpublished field study, Wayne State University, Detroit, MI.

Cleland, V. (1965). The effect of stress on performance. *Nursing Research, 14*, 292–298.

Cratty, B. J. (1967). *Movement behavior and motor learning* (2nd ed.). Philadelphia: Lea & Febiger.

Dave, R. H. (1970). *Psychomotor levels in developing and writing objectives.* Tucson, AZ: Educational Innovators Press.

Fitts, P. M. (1964). Perceptual and motor skill learning. In A. Melton (Ed.), *Categories of human learning.* New York: Academic Press.

Fleishman, E. A. (1972). A structure and measurement of psychomotor abilities. In R. Singer (Ed.), *The psychomotor domain: Movement behavior*. Philadelphia: Lea & Febiger.

Gates, A. I., Jersild, A. T., McConnell, T. R., & Challman, R. C. (1953). *Educational psychology* (2nd ed.). New York: Macmillan.

Gomez, G., & Gomez, E. (1987). Learning of psychomotor skills: Laboratory versus patient care setting. *Journal of Nursing Education, 26*(1), 20-24.

Harrow, A. J. (1972). *A taxonomy of the psychomotor domain: A guide for developing behavioral objectives*. New York: D. McKay.

Henry, F. M. (1958). Specificity vs generality in learning motor skills. *Proceedings of College Physical Education Association, 61*, 126-128.

Johnson, H. W. (1961). Skill = speed × accuracy × form × adaptability. *Perceptual and Motor Skills, 13*, 163-170.

Keele, S. W. (1968). Movement control in skilled motor performance. *Psychological Bulletin, 70*, 387-403.

Keele, S. (1982). Learning and control of coordinated motor patterns: The programming perspective. In J. A. Kelso (Ed.), *Human motor behavior: An introduction*. Hillsdale, NJ: Lawrence Erlbaum Assoc.

Kelso, J. A. (Ed.). (1982). *Human motor behavior: An introduction*. Hillsdale, NJ: Lawrence Erlbaum Assoc.

Kerr, R. (1982). *Psychomotor learning*. Philadelphia: Saunders.

Kibler, R. J., Barker, L. L., & Miles, D. T. (1970). *Behavioral objectives and instruction*. Boston: Allyn & Bacon.

Lawther, J. D. (1977). *The learning and performance of physical skills* (2nd ed.). Englewood Cliffs, NJ: Prentice-Hall.

Marteniuk, R. G. (1969). Generality and specificity of learning and performance of two similar speed tasks. *Research Quarterly, 40*, 552.

McGuigan, F. J., & MacCaslin, E. F. (1955). Whole and part methods in learning a perceptual motor skill. *American Journal of Psychology, 48*, 658-661.

Miller, G., Galantin, E., & Pribran, K. (1960). *Plans and the structure of behavior*. New York: Holt, Rinehart & Winston.

Morgan, M. K., & Irby, D. (1978). *Evaluating clinical competence in the health professions*. St. Louis: C. V. Mosby.

Naylor, J., & Briggs, G. (1961). Long term retention of learned skills: A review of the literature. *Academy of Education Development Technical Report, U.S. Department of Commerce, 61*, 390.

Neighbors, M., Eldred, E., & Sullivan, M. (1991). Nursing skills necessary for competency in a hi-tech health care system. *Nursing & Health Care, 12*(2), 92-97.

Paillard, J. (1960). The patterning of skilled movement. In J. Field (Ed.), *Handbook of psychology: Neurophysiology, 3*. Baltimore: Williams & Wilkins.

Poulton, E. C. (1972). Skilled performance. In R. Singer (Ed.), *The psychomotor domain: Movement behavior*. Philadelphia: Lea & Febiger.

Reilly, D., & Oermann, M. (1985). *The clinical field: Its use in nursing education*. Norwalk, CT: Appleton-Century-Crofts.

Reilly, D., & Oermann, M. (1990). *Behavioral objectives: Evaluation in nursing* (3rd ed.). New York: National League for Nursing.

Schmidt, R. A. (1976). Control processes in motor skills. In J. Koegh & R. S. Hutton (Eds.), *Exercise and Sport Sciences Review*. Santa Barbara, CA: Journal Publishing Affiliates.

Schneider, W., & Fish, A. (1982). Attention theory and mechanisms for skilled performance. *ERIC Reports*, Champaign, IL: Illinois University.

Simpson, E. J. (1966). *The classification of educational objectives: Psychomotor domain*. Urbana, IL: University of Illinois Press.

Singer, R. (Ed.). (1975). *Motor learning and human performance*. New York: Macmillan.

Smith, K. U. (1967). Cybernetic foundations of physical behavioral science. *Quest, 8*, 26–82.

Smith, K. U. (1972). Cybernetic psychology. In R. Singer (Ed.), *The psychomotor domain: Movement behavior*. Philadelphia: Lea & Febiger.

Stelmach, G. E. (1969). Efficiency of motor learning as a function of intertrial rest. *Research Quarterly, 40*, 198–202.

Stelmach, G. E. (1982). Information processing framework for understanding human motor behavior. In J. A. Kelso (Ed.), *Human motor behavior: An introduction*. Hillsdale, NJ: Lawrence Erlbaum Assoc.

Sweeney, M. A., Regan, P., O'Malley, M., & Hedstrom, B. (1980). Essential skills for baccalaureate graduates: Perspectives of education and service. *Journal of Nursing Administration, 10*, 37–44.

Tisdale, S. (1984). Reflections: The nouveau boards. *American Journal of Nursing, 84*, 166.

Welford, A. T. (1968). *Fundamentals of skill*. London: Metheun & Co., Ltd.

Whitley, J. D. (1970). Effects of practice distribution on learning a fine motor task. *Research Quarterly, 40*, 577–582.

BIBLIOGRAPHY

Ackerman, W. (1990). Technology and nursing education: Scenario for 1990. *Journal of Advanced Nursing, 13*, 640–641.

Backman, K. (1990). Using mental imagery to practice specialized psychomotor skills. *Journal of Continuing Education in Nursing, 21*(3), 1252.

Baker, N. C., Cerone, S. B., Gaza, N., & Knapp, T. R. (1984). The effect of type of thermometer and length of time inserted in oral temperature measurement of afebrile subjects. *Nursing Research, 33,* 109-111.

Barsevick, A. M., & Llewellyn, J. L. (1982). A comparison of the anxiety-reducing potential of two techniques of bathing. *Nursing Research, 31,* 22-27.

Bates, B. (1987). *A guide to physical exam* (4th ed.). Philadelphia: Lippincott.

Bauman, K., Cook, J., & Larson, L. (1981). Using technology to humanize instruction: An approach to teaching nursing skills. *Journal of Nursing Education, 20*(3), 27-31.

Bell, M. (1991). Learning a complex nursing skill: Student anxiety and the effect of preclinical skill evaluation. *Journal of Nursing Education, 30*(5), 222-226.

Bount, J. (1985). An exploration of the relationship between nurses' empathy and technology. *Nursing Administration Quarterly, 9*(3), 69-78.

Carnevali, D. L. (1985). Nursing perspectives in health care technology. *Nursing Administration Quarterly, 9*(3), 10-18.

Crow, J. (1980). Using performance testing to determine student achievement and teacher effectiveness in nursing skills lab. In K. Mikan (Ed.), *Learner resource center conference: Proceedings and evaluation* (pp. 78-80). Bethesda, MD: U.S. Department of Human Resources.

Dressler, D. K., Smejkal, C., & Ruffolo, M. L. (1983). A comparison of oral and rectal temperature measurement of patients receiving oxygen by mask. *Nursing Research, 32,* 373-375.

Flynn, K., Norton, L., & Fisher, R. (1987). Enteral tube feeding: Indications, practices, and outcomes. *Image: Journal of Nursing Scholarship, 19*(1), 16-19.

Gilmore, B. (1982). The relationship between fear of failure/anxiety performance trials and errors among associate and baccalaureate degree students while learning a selected perceptual-motor task. *Journal of Nursing Education, 21*(8), 61.

Goldsmith, J. (1984). Effect of learner variables, media attributes, and practice conditions in psychomotor task performance. *Western Journal of Nursing Research, 21*(8), 229-240.

Gomez, G., & Gomez, E. (1984). The teaching of psychomotor skills in nursing. *Nurse Educator, 9*(2), 35-39.

Hawkeness, E., & Halloran, M. (1984). A second look at psychomotor skills. *Nurse Educator, 9*(1), 9-13.

Harris, R. B. (1984). Clean vs sterile tracheostomy care and level of pulmonary infection. *Nursing Research, 33,* 80-91.

Hoding, D. H. (Ed.). (1981). *Human skills.* New York: John Wesley.

Infante, M. (1985). *The clinical laboratory in nursing education* (2nd ed.). New York: Wiley.

Ingham, A. (1989). A review of the literature relating to touch and its use in intensive care. *Intensive Care, 5*(2), 45-51.

Jones, D. A., Lepley, M. F., & Baker, B. A. (1984). *Health assessment across life span.* New York: McGraw-Hill.

Kieffer, J. S. (1984). Selecting technical skills to teach for competency. *Journal of Nursing Education, 23*(5), 198-203.

Larsen, D. (1983). *Computerized nursing skills simulations.* Philadelphia: Lippincott.

Lewis, L. (1984). *Fundamental skills in patient care.* Philadelphia: Lippincott.

Lindberg, J. B., Hunter, M. L., & Kruszewski, A. Z. (1983). *Skills manual for person-centered nursing care.* Philadelphia: Lippincott.

Love, B., McAdams, C., Patton, D. M., Rankin, E. J., & Roberts, J. (1989). Teaching psychomotor skills in nursing: A randomized control trial. *Journal of Advanced Nursing, 14,* 970-975.

Manderino, M. A., Hollerbach, A. D., & Brooks, C. P. (1984). Clinical evaluation of three techniques for administering low dose heparin. *Nursing Research, 33,* 15-19.

McCormick, K. A. (1983). Preparing nurses for the technologic future. *Nursing & Health Care, 5,* 379-382.

McGill, S. L., & Smith, J. R. (1983). *I V therapy.* Bowie, MD: Robert J. Brady.

Mehlman, M., & Younger, S. (1991). *Delivering high technology home care.* New York: Springer.

Nelson, E. J., Morton, E. A., & Hunter, P. M. (1983). *Critical care respiratory therapy: A laboratory and clinical manual.* Boston: Little, Brown.

Newshan, G. (1989). Therapeutic touch for symptom control in persons with AIDS. *Holistic Nursing Practice, 3*(4), 45-51.

Norris, S., Campbell, L., & Brenkert, S. (1982). Nursing procedures and alterations in transcutaneous oxygen tension in premature infants. *Nursing Research, 31,* 330-336.

Oermann, M. (1990). Psychomotor skill development. *Journal of Continuing Education, 21*(5), 202-204.

Oxendine, J. (1984). *Psychology of motor learning* (2nd ed.). Englewood Cliffs, NJ: Prentice-Hall.

Pillar, B., Jacox, A., & Redman, B. (1990). Technology, its assessment, and nursing. *Nursing Outlook, 38*(1), 16-19.

Randolph, G. L. (1984). Therapeutic touch and physical touch: Physiological response to stressful stimuli. *Nursing Research, 33,* 33-36.

Schmidt, R. A. (1982). *Motor control and learning.* Champaign, IL: Herman Kinelus Publ.

Singer, R. (Ed.). (1972). *Psychomotor domain: Movement behavior.* Philadelphia: Lea & Febiger.

Smith, S. F., & Duell, D. (1982). *Nursing skills and evaluation: A nursing process approach.* St. Louis: C. V. Mosby.

Stelmach, G. E. (1978). *Information processing and motor control learning.* New York: Academic Press.

Takacs, K. M., & Valenti, W. M. (1982). Temperature measurement in a clinical setting. *Nursing Research, 31,* 368–370.

Wachtel, P. L. (1972). Field dependence and psychological differentiation. Reexamination. *Perceptual and Motor Skills, 34,* 179–181.

Welford, A. T. (1976). *Skilled performance: Perceptual and motor skills.* Glenview, IL: Scott, Foresman & Co.

Yonkoma, C. A. (1982). Cool and heated aerosol and the measurement of oral temperature. *Nursing Research, 31,* 354–357.

Zielstorff, R. (1987). In high-tech care, the challenge remains: To nurse. *American Nurse, 19*(9), 4, 18.

9

Affective Learning in the Clinical Setting

Affective competencies, including moral reasoning, and value based behavior, are essential elements in skilled nursing practice. They represent those dimensions of nursing that characterize it as a humanistic discipline whose practice is noted for its quality of caring. They transcend all aspects of nursing. Competencies, so critical to a practice discipline, are taught in preparatory programs, and opportunities for their development need to be provided. The development of affective competencies must be subject to the same rigor and pedagogy as are competencies in the other two domains, cognitive and psychomotor.

The notion of teaching the affective domain in a nursing program is surrounded with mythology and confusion, reflective of a lack of understanding of the nature of the affective domain and its relationship to personhood and the profession. Some faculty see the affective domain as primarily concerned with problems of attitude or behavior, especially in relation to students or staff. Others perceive affective behavior to be based on values that are personal and not subject to questioning. Some equate the teaching of values with indoctrination, a practice antithetical to a free society. For many, the idea of teaching values conjures up the image of a teacher "imposing" values on captive students. Interestingly, one never hears fears expressed as to the danger of the teacher imposing cognition or psychomotor skills on the student. No learning can be imposed; it is derived through the student's own experiences. Affective competencies, like the competencies in the other two domains, are developed within the same framework of the teaching-learning process, and the levels of competence are delineated in terms of expected behaviors that are subject to appropriate evaluation processes.

Affective competencies have a more positive connotation than is often associated with them. They relate to the individual's ability to use moral reasoning in decisions for the management of moral and ethical dilemmas and to the development of a value system that guides decisions and activities compatible with the individual's and society's notion of what is good and what is right. Affective competency is more than the affirmation of personal beliefs. It requires cognitive skills of choice and decision making and a pattern of behavior reflective of commitment to the choice made.

The Talmud says:

Let not thy learning
exceed thy deeds
Mere knowledge is not the goal, but action

James Turro (1972) elaborates on this theme:

How laughable
some persons in our midst
make themselves by talking
so glibly of love
and being so obviously
unloving.
Think of
their expressed attitudes
toward established authority
too often
gratuitously hostile.
How incredible

*they make themselves
by their incessant chatter
about community
while being so intolerant
of differing tastes and personality.
We must learn from their failures.
Let it not be said
of us
as, I believe
it can be said
of them
vox, vox, et praeteria nihil
words, words, and nothing else. (p. 63)*

There is no place in nursing for "words, words, and nothing else." It is the fostering of integrity between the nurse's verbal affirmations on positions and beliefs compatible with nursing as a helping profession and the behaviors exhibited in moral and value conflicts that become the charge to teachers of nursing.

The need for affective competencies is particularly evident in contemporary society. The ever-changing technologic world in which nurses practice and live is forcing them to seek those humanistic qualities inherent in their practice which enables them to minister to clients in a manner that is satisfying and fulfilling to the clients and to themselves.

Nursing practice is value laden; indeed it is an ethical enterprise. What do the terms, "value-based practice" and "ethical enterprise" mean to the professional nurse, educators, practitioners, and researchers? The notion that nursing, like other health professions, is scientifically based is acknowledged. What are the implications of stating that they are also value based? Are the two ideas compatible or are they sources of conflict? Can a practice be both scientific and value based?

H. Englehardt (1977) says, "The Holy Grail of modern western thought has been objective truth untouched by uncertainty or value judgment, along with a secular account of values" (p. 1). What has this Holy Grail search meant to educators, practitioners, and researchers in nursing? Does nursing perceive the world of facts as the only world of truth and reality while designating the world of values as primarily one of emotion devoid of truth?

Science implies impersonality and objectivity and is empirical and descriptive. It is perceived to be value free; although this perception is now challenged. But science is not all of health care. Nurses care for and about people. This component of practice is personal and value based. Is it considered to be unscientific? Ayer (1946) supports this position when he says: "In so far as statements of values are significant, they are ordinary scientific statements and in so far as they are not scientific, they are not in the literal sense significant, but are simply expressions of emotions which can be neither true nor false" (pp. 102-103). The fact that the affective domain has not been addressed with the same intensity of teaching as the other domains suggests that Ayer's position may be supported by some nurse educators and practitioners.

Historically in nursing education programs, caring about the patient was stressed as a worthy goal in practice. However, the teaching of this goal was more by fiat and precept. One more or less "caught" the skills pertinent to the *caring about* action of nursing. Professional adjustment was the thrust of the time. Emphasis was on the decorum of the professional nurse in matters of dress, appearance, and actions that reflected the "image of the nurse." Ethical and moral decisions were examined more from a legalistic than an ethical or moral framework.

It is important to recognize that in an earlier period, the necessity for developing other strategies for teaching the affective skills was not present, for a simpler society existed where differences were limited, hidden, or ignored. Many nurses went to school and practiced nursing in their own communities where the same beliefs and value systems were accepted at least tacitly by the majority of the residents of that community. One's patients were of the community and they often attended the same school, church, or community functions as the nurse. These institutions were strong enforcers of community values. Limitation of knowledge presented few challenges to nursing, medicine, and other disciplines. Decisions as to when life began and ended were simplistic and accepted by all; e.g., the failure to obtain an apical pulse was sufficient for the physician to declare a person dead. The advent of mass media and mass travel exposed persons to differing beliefs, values and life styles. The relative homogeneity and absolutism of beliefs and values held by members of a community were displaced and the handling of divergent and contradictory claims became a necessity.

Contemporary world and the portents for the future world indicate an increasingly complex society where moral decisions will be more numerous and intricate and where value conflicts will be more evident. Differences are now more overt, although the institutionalizing of some prejudices (unsubstantiated beliefs) still persists. Knowledge and mechanisms for using that knowledge continue to expand, thus providing society and individuals with extraordinary power to control lives of persons in that society. The very nature of our society and the political processes by which it is governed are regarded with cynicism by many whose trust is shattered by the unethical behavior of leaders they chose to direct the society toward its potential. A democratic society that values individual freedom and rights yet makes decisions more reflective of materialistic values than humanistic ones serves only to confuse its body politic. Dewey (1962), a democratic philosopher, raised the question: "Can a materialistic industrial civilization be converted into a distinctive agency for liberalizing the minds and refining the emotions of all?" (p. 28).

American society is now in the postindustrial era, embarked on an information society overwhelmed by technology. This technology has improved instrumentation, but its use may or may not contribute to the improvement in the quality of life, society, or the care provided by health professionals. Dewey's question becomes even more significant in relation to a materialistic technologic civilization. There are some positive responses to the question as citizens' voices are being heard in the political arena. They are saying "No" to decisions that threaten the quality of the environment, health of a community, or quality of life. The voices of minority groups; i.e., women, elderly, and those of various ethnic persuasions are now raising the issue of justice as decisions not in their interest are being proposed. Political power no longer has a negative value. Justice for the less fortunate, however, is an unstable factor influenced by mood swings of the populace from a humanistic view, which sees these individuals as victims of societal pressures, to a derogatory view, which blames them for their inability to keep pace with society's movements.

Allocation of resources is developing as a major concern of government and citizens with much potential for generating moral and ethical dilemmas. Financial resources are of particular relevance to those in the health field as the realization that there are limits to moneys for health care becomes more apparent. Efforts toward cost-effective health care limit the hospitalization options for individuals receiving Medicare through the use of diagnostic categories as a basis for prospective payment to hospitals. What conflicts will nurses encounter when decisions for early discharge of patients are not congruent with the nurse's judgment? Decisions will need to be made indicating who should receive care, especially the costly diagnostic and treatment modalities. Will some individuals not be eligible because of age, lack of money, or importance to society? Ross (1984) notes that the answer to this question is already in operation with the use of triage in deciding who will be the recipients of the costly medical care. Triage, a decision-making method in times of war is predicated on the notion that human life can be selected for distinction if it lacks quality. The triage used in this situation is referred to as *economic triage,* a decision available to persons with economic resources to avail themselves of the advances in health care. As care becomes more costly and financial resources become more restricted, a period of hard moral choices awaits nurses and other health care providers.

Nurses will be challenged to promote humanistic values and to be ever sensitive to the changes instigated by technology and societal decisions that threaten the rights of the individual. Nurses are already involved with moral conflicts as technology is imposed in the patient care setting. Reilly and Behrens-Hanna (1991) note some of the conflicts encountered by perioperative nurses in their practice such as, surgery performed on individuals that is not perceived to be in accord with the best interest of the client and the process of harvesting organs from brain-dead persons. The advent of computers challenges the notion of the client's right to privacy in a way never anticipated by those who saw gossip, for example in elevators, public transportation, and other similar situations, as the primary means of violating this right. Although the legalistic approach to problems will be ever present, decisions for action must also be on the basis of moral reasoning in terms of the ethical or moral concepts inherent in the dilemma.

The question today is not should the affective competencies of moral reasoning and value development be taught, but rather the question is in terms of how they should be taught. Of particular concern is how one uses the rich resources of the clinical practice field in fostering the development of those affective skills so central to the evolution of the individual from a novice to an expert practitioner.

The Phenomenon of Care in Relation to Nursing

As the 1990s proceed, a significant movement which emphasizes the phenomenon of care as the core of nursing is evident in the literature by nursing scholars, Benner and Wrubel (1989), Leininger (1988a), Stevenson (1990), Gadow (1990), Watson (1985), Noddinger (1984), and Fry (1989). The direction of the dialogue, study and research is toward an analytic examination of the concept of care and its relationship to nursing. Some scholars see care as a basis for a theory of nursing, others see it as a critical element of a theory of nursing ethics. The scholarly efforts are resulting in a theoretical perspective of care within the context of nursing which demands more rigorous study on the part of nursing students and practitioners than has heretofore been acknowledged. Its depth in permeating the very nature of nursing itself and the nurse-patient relationship as evidenced by the analysis thus far, challenges the notion of caring as a natural, expected, emotional response to the nursing of individuals. Caring is a desired transcendental quality of all helping professions; the questions being raised relate to its particular bond to nursing and its substantive nature.

The relationship of care to nursing ethics is of concern to nursing scholars. Watson (1985) believes that "caring is the moral ideal of nursing, whereby the end is protection, enhancement and preservation of human dignity" (p. 29). Fry (1989) challenges the notion that nursing ethics is derived or closely allied to the model of biomedical ethics. She examined three caring models, Noddinger (1984), a model of caring stressing ethics and morality from a feminist perspective; Pellegrino (1988), a moral obligation model of caring; and Frankena (1983) a moral point of view model of caring. She proposes five major recommendations to consider in developing a theory of nursing ethics:

1. Nursing needs a moral view of person rather than a theory of moral action of behavior.
2. The moral point of view focus is directly on the nurse-patient relationship.

3. Value of caring ought to be central to any theory.
4. Morality ought to turn on a philosophical view of caring that posits caring as a foundational rather than a derivative value among persons.
5. A moral, point of view should not be defined by reference to any external system of justification. (pp. 20-21)

The pursuit of the phenomenon of care in nursing whether as a theory of nursing, as the core of nursing ethics or as a critical dimension of practice is affirming that care is not sentimentality, but is a deliberate mode of behavior directed toward the welfare of the client. Norris (1989) sees care as "the fusion of thinking, feeling and acting" (p. 554) and recognizes that in a professional service it "requires a vast amount of knowledge, experience, wisdom and expertise" (p. 550).

Care may be acknowledged by most nurses as an inherent part of their nursing, but in reality, is it more an ideal than a reality? Caring requires commitment; it is contextual, relational, and subjective. Its referent is the nurse's perception of actions, not the action itself nor the client. Caring is different from caring about, for caring implies action whereas caring about may or may not entail action.

Several authors address the notion of caring as an invisible and potentially undervalued dimension of nursing. Benner (1990) sees invisibility as a function of society's ambiguity toward care with preference for technical fix (p. 16). Roberts (1990) relates the invisibility of caring to the very nature of caring; its virtue in protecting human dignity. Caring's identity with feminist behavior may be another reason for its perceived invisibility, thus it lacks the status for study and analysis that accompanies more dramatic medical therapies.

As the analysis of care in nursing progresses, Norris (1989) posits some interesting concerns about its implementation in practice to be pondered. Can care actually be practiced in a hospital environment characterized by short stays and high technology? Can care be conceptualized by those nurses whose preparation emphasizes concrete approaches when care demands a holistic, abstract as well as a concrete perspective. Care demands of nursing a value system which views the client subjectively with sensitivity to needs and personal dignity, yet the values of the society from which the nurse comes is pleasure driven, money-minded and fast-paced, avoiding dealing with many of life's problems. Can nurses practice against the value mainstream of society? A further question raised is in reference to the marketability of care, i.e., are people willing to pay for care? (Norris, p. 548). These questions are relevant to the discussion of the care phenomenon in nursing and need to be considered. The operationalization of care in general practice of nursing presents a challenge for nurse practitioners, researchers, and educators.

CONCEPTS RELEVANT TO AFFECTIVE SKILL DEVELOPMENT

There are several significant concepts encompassed under the rubric *affective domain*, whose understanding is essential for those teaching in this area.

Beliefs

The terms "beliefs" and "values" are often used interchangeably, but there is a significant difference in their interpretation. Beliefs respond to questions of fact, irrespective of the actual reality of the fact. Beliefs are perceptions of reality that have significant meaning to the individual. Beliefs may be supported by valid and reliable data or they may be unsubstantiated, as occurs in prejudice, which is often a reflection of ignorance due to lack of contact or exposure to the substance of the fact or due to fear of change in behavior necessitated by alterations in belief.

Some individuals maintain beliefs in spite of new information that disputes the claim for the original belief that guided the actions of the individual. Scheibe (1970, p. 91) relates this rigidity of beliefs to the common information tendencies of human beings which act as mechanism of conservation in mind whereby the interpretation of incoming information is in relation to its congruence with the original belief. He cites two ways information is distorted:

> Assimilation—give more support to an entrenched belief than it should

Contrast—deny the relevance of information to the belief if it is sufficiently incompatible with it.

Stated beliefs are not always reliable because of an individual's proclivity for stating one thing while inwardly accepting a very different belief. Statements of belief are particularly vulnerable to social forces operating in a situation at any one particular time. Beliefs, like values, serve as a guiding influence in behavior, but unlike values, the commitment based on rational choice is not apparent. A belief becomes a value when it is rationally examined, freely chosen, and a commitment is made to support the belief in action.

Values

Values are judgments about the worth of an object, person, group, belief, or event. They connote a preference for something, as exhibited in behavior, on a selective basis. Values are viewed contextually within a group or society standard, which may or may not reflect what is good for the total society. Moral values are those that are in accord with ethical and moral standards which refer to the good of the greater society with protection of the individual's rights within that society.

Reilly (1989) conceptualizes a value as an operational belief which an individual accepts as one's own and uses as a basis for behavior. Not only is the value chosen through a deliberative analytic process, it must also be expressed in a relatively consistent manner in the person's behavior. Morrill (1980) defines values as standards and patterns of choice that guide persons and groups toward satisfaction, fulfillment, and meaning. Davis and Aroskar (1983) describe their concept of values thusly: "Values may be considered to be a set of beliefs and attitudes for which logical reasons can be given. Values are significant as they influence perception, guide our actions, and have consequences" (p. 197). Steele and Harmon (1983) perceive a value as an affective disposition toward a person, object, or idea. Values represent a way of life.

Raths and colleagues (1966) define values as those elements that show how a person has decided to use his or her life. They note that values are learned through experience and must meet the criteria of choice, commitment, and action. They introduce the notion of valuing, a process that suggests the action dimension of values and the interrelationship between knowing and doing. The three processes are:

Choosing (1) freely
          (2) from alternatives
          (3) after thoughtful consideration of the consequences of each alternative
Prizing   (4) cherishing, being happy with choice
          (5) willing to affirm the choice publically
Action   (6) doing something with the choice
          (7) repeatedly in some pattern of life. (pp. 28–30)

Raths and colleagues contend that unless these three processes are involved, a value is not present. Interests, aspirations, or attitudes are seen as value indicators. One may affirm an interest or a belief but be unwilling to act in accord with that interest or belief. Likewise, one may act in a pattern reflective of a belief but be unwilling to make the choice that leads to commitment. The general consensus of most authorities is that values are important motivators of actions that are selective and the result of rational choice and commitment.

Attitudes

Attitudes, often confused with values, represent a feeling for or against a person, object, belief, or event. The rationale for the feeling may or may not be understood by the individual, but the responses generated by the feeling greatly influence the individual's ability to maximize the potential from the relationship with the object, person, or event. Positive attitude may be a value indicator and present a signal to the teacher to help the student move through the valuing process toward transforming it into a value. Negative attitudes may be a reflection of ignorance, fear of an unfulfilled need. One must recognize that all behavior is not value based, for needs are powerful forces for action. In general, a need, for example, love, must be fulfilled before one can value love. Reilly (1978) drawing from the work of Raths and colleagues differentiates between the characteristics of value and need.

Needs	Values
1. Start with life	1. Start when child becomes conscious that he is different from what he was
2. Push one into action	2. Pull one toward action
3. Ashamed of	3. Cherish
4. Pervasive	4. Selective
5. Strong visceral component	5. Strong intellectual component
6. Met by others	6. Met by self
7. Deficiency behaviors: aggression, withdrawal, submission, psychosomatic illness symptoms	7. Deficiency behaviors: apathy, flighty, inconsistency, hesitancy, overconforming, overdissenting role playing (p. 38)

Knox (1977) refers to attitudes as the residue of past experiences in the form of inclination or feelings that predispose a person to the choice of activities, companions, and locations. Because attitudes lack the rational choice and commitment, they are vulnerable to external and internal forces in a situation and may shift as the individual interacts with these forces.

Moral Reasoning

Moral reasoning implies the cognitive processes of analysis and interpretation of a moral dilemma as a basis for determining some course of action. Moral reasoning, according to Kohlberg (1981), does not involve knowing or deriving specific ethical rules of conduct; rather, it concerns the structure through which reflection and experience in the moral sphere are first processed and organized. Moral reasoning, dependent upon skills of critical thinking, is called into play when a moral situation is evident for which the usual rules of conduct are not sufficient. Davis and Aroskar (1983) refer to this situation as a dilemma, a difficult situation incapable of satisfactory solution. They further define such a situation as a moral claim conflict when a choice or situation involving choice between equally unsatisfactory alternatives exists. Moral reasoning is a fundamental process in making choices but does not guarantee that moral behavior will result.

Kohlberg (1981) is one of the most noted theorists in the area of cognitive development as it pertains to moral reasoning. He sees justice as the highest moral condition and has developed a cognitive hierarchical schema which moves from the lowest to the highest type of moral reasoning. Basing his work on that of Piaget and Dewey, he identifies three moral levels individuals pass through en route to principled action. Each level encompasses two stages. The literature contains many references to this theory and the characteristics of the stages. A brief summary of the levels is included here.

Preconventional Level. Two stages are included: obedience—punishment orientation and personal interest orientation. Behavior at this level is determined by cultural roles and notions of what is considered good or bad as defined by superior power consequences, punishment, reward, or exchange of favors.

Conventional Level. Two stages are: interpersonal concordance ("Good Boy, Nice Girl") orientation and law and order orientation. Behavior at this level is in terms of maintaining expectations of the individual's family, group, or nation, regardless of immediate or obvious consequences. Attitude is one of loyalty to the prevailing order and conformity to the rules and expectations held by those who are significant.

Postconventional Level. Two stages are: social contract, legalistic orientation and universal, ethical principled orientation. Behavior at this level is internally controlled; the standards conformed to have an internal source and the decision to act is based on an inner process of thought and judgment concerning right and wrong. The universal principles of justice, reciprocity, and equality of human rights and the respect for the dignity of human beings as individuals become the basis for moral decisions.

For purposes of viewing this theory in relation to the development of affective competencies, its assumptions are significant. This theory proposes that there are patterns of moral reasoning behavior associated with each level and that individuals with appropriate stimuli can move to a higher level. The stimulus of moral disequilibrium at the next highest level for the student enables the individual to seek out a more sophisticated level of reasoning. The theory operates on the findings that most people function at one level of moral reasoning most of the time but some regression can occur at intervals. Smith (1978) summarized some of the research in the use of Kohlberg's theory and found general support for it, especially for individuals who complete high school and go on to college.

Holstein (1976) and Gilligan (1982) found evidence of sex bias in the test scoring which favors men. This is a concern since nurses are primarily women. Gilligan's (1982) position that Kohlberg's theory of moral development is deficient where women's moral development is concerned has received the attention of nurse scholars, Cooper (1989), Chally (1990), Cassidy (1991) and Frisch (1987). Kohlberg's theory evolved from study of males using hypothetical situations. The theory is based on the belief that justice is the highest moral value and implies independence of person who relies on universal moral principles in moral decision-making. Gilligan's theory of moral development relates to the connectedness of persons within the context of the care perspective. Cooper (1989) notes that care and justice are not in opposition, but rather they reflect a different organizing principle; justice relates to self and equality, care relates to others, and attachment between them (pp. 11, 13). Chally (1990) sees value in Gilligan's theory based on the moral judgment within the context of care and avoidance of hurt as relevant to nursing and its emphasis on care. It is this moral emphasis that accounts for women's tendency to remain on the third or fourth stage of Kohlberg's moral development taxonomy.

Some questions are raised in relation to the cultural bias of the questions and scoring, although Kohlberg asserts that the theory has no cultural boundaries. Other questions are raised about the emphasis on moral rationality through patterns of thinking to the exclusion of any concern about conduct resulting from these cognitive processes. Morrill (1980) reminds the reader that Kohlberg argues that moral rationality is a precondition for moral action, for one can scarcely choose a good that one does not know.

Perry (1970), another cognitive development theorist, has also developed a hierarchy of stages of ethical development toward the highest level of moral commitment. These stages, previously discussed, are based on the assumption about the way students perceive the nature and characteristics of truth, values, and life goals. The scheme of the stages of development describes the steps by which students move from a simplistic, categorical view of the world to a realization of the contingent nature of knowledge, relative values, and the formation and affirmation of their own commitments.

Ethics

Ethics refers to standards of conduct or "right" behavior based on moral judgment. Churchill (1982) considers ethics as a systematic reflection of moral behavior; morality as the practical activity; ethics as the theoretical and reflective one (p. 305). Stent (1977), in developing his theory of structural ethics, supports Gustafson's notion of ethics "as a human intellectual discipline which develops the principles which account for morality and moral action and the normative principles and values that guide human action" (p. 243). Ketifian (1991) states that ethical theories and principles are concerned with the content of moral choice. These theories are utilitarianism and deontology and the three major principles are autonomy, nonmaleficence and beneficence, and justice (pp. 222–223).

Morrill (1980) differentiates between the traditional study of ethics, *metaethics*, which concerns itself with logical, epistemologic and semantic issues addressed to the question of what *ought* to be done in situations, not the actions themselves, and the current study of ethics, *normative*, which is concerned with classification, analysis, and critique of moral arguments and issues at hand (pp. 44–45). It is normative ethics that relate to the exploration of ethical dilemmas in nursing practice that is the focus in teaching for the development of affective competencies.

Morality

Morality, although concerned with moral judgment and right behavior, is perceived within a social context. It is a system of moral conduct. Societies, whether communities, cultural groups, nations, professions, and even schools of nursing, determine the ethical standards and values to be respected and supported by its membership. Exemplars serve as models of the accepted code of behavior and can be most effective in teaching the behaviors that a group accepts. Sanctions are instituted less by the legal route than by verbal or nonverbal responses of the group members. These sanctions serve to bring the errant or potentially errant individuals into accord with the group's idea of morality. Societies have often attempted to legislate morality, for example, prohibition in the United States in the 1920s, but have generally been less successful than when group pressure is exerted.

Choice

One concept that is fundamental to the other concepts in affective learning and critical in teaching is that of choice. Choice entails making decisions for or about something. In the affective domain, it refers to decisions based on values and moral beliefs. René Dubos (1981) associates choice making with the quality of humanness when he states: "We are human beings, not so much because of our appearance, but because of what we do, the way we do it, and more importantly, because of what we elect to do or not do" (p. 9). He further states: "Intentionality and freedom of choice are at least as important in human life as is biological determination, whether genetic or environmental" (p. 15).

Frankl (1963) attests to the value of choice in maintaining the human quality of persons. He vividly describes his life in a concentration camp where any semblance of value of human life and human dignity was nonexistent and where individuals were robbed of their will and served only as objects to be manipulated by their captors. Frankl raised the question: Does man have no choice of action in the face of such circumstances? He affirms from experience as well as principle that man does have a choice of action. He states: "There is sufficient proof that everything can be taken from a man, but one thing—the last of the human freedoms—to choose one's attitude in any given set of circumstances to choose one's way" (p. 105). Referring to human beings' ability to preserve even a trace of spiritual freedom and independence of mind under such circumstances as he encountered, he concludes that people can decide what will become of them spiritually and mentally and that each individual has the freedom to make a choice between accepting or rejecting an offer.

Both Dubos and Frankl affirm that choice making is essential to the very human nature of the person and is a characteristic of one's freedom. Podeschi (1976) interprets William James' concept of freedom and its meaning in choice making as: "Human freedom does not mean any choice that tempts us, but choices that lead to maturation of our human capacities" (p. 228). He further notes that free choices come in the form of forced options. McBee (1978) refers to self-imposed limitations on freedom of action—a choice among options open to free people. Freedom within this context is not perceived as license where one "does one's own thing." Freedom does not mean freedom from structure, but rather freedom within the structure. It means the individual is free from coercion in making choices.

The making of choices within the concept of the affective domain involves more than expressing a preference, which is often transitory. Competency in choice making is the ability to ponder evidence, examine assumptions, make judgments, and evaluate. When one makes a choice, one takes a position which has been logically and rationally determined. It tells what one will stand up for. Podeschi, drawing upon Wild's (1969) interpretation of James' view of freedom, suggests James' position about the substance of choice making. "The individual who believes that choices really matter will take life seriously. What we freely choose to do makes a difference; real issues are at stake. This means the willingness to live with energy, though energy brings pain" (p. 228). The making of choices can be an uncomfortable experience because it involves dealing with alternatives and then assuming responsibility for the choice made. Dubos (1981) suggests: "The greater freedom of an organism to select where it goes and what it does and how it responds to stimuli, the more complex and creative is the living experience" (p. 31).

Skill in the selection of choices is a critical component in affective learning, but it is only one part of the learning. In teaching, faculty must be concerned not only with the process of choice making, but also with the pattern of behavior that reflects that choice.

AFFECTIVE COMPONENT IN NURSING

The discussion thus far has addressed the processes of affective skill development. What about the content of these competencies? Are there certain values that all nurses must accept as their own? The answer must be in the affirmative if, as stated earlier, the affective domain must be subjected to the same pedagogy as the other domains of learning; i.e., objectives are written, learning experiences provided, and evaluation carried out. This response may be disturbing to those who perceive values only from the personal perspective. The concern of teachers is not the personal values held by students, but rather, those values inherent in the nursing profession. Levine (1977), who sees ethical responsibility in every dimension of nursing practice, notes that the very nature of nursing practice precludes the individual nurse from standing aside from the experience of interacting with human beings (pp. 8-9).

Conflict Sources

Much of the emphasis in the nursing literature that refers to moral, ethical, or value issues relates to those entailed in the interactions of the nurse with the client or with the physician, often reflective of medical ethics. A much broader perspective is needed, for these issues transcend all aspects of nursing practice.

In 1972, the Carnegie Commission on Higher Education published a report on professional education. The challenge to educators addressed their failure to see in this time of rapid social change that new clients and new client systems were evolving that markedly influence the need for greater balance of science and humanism in educational programs. Recognizing that health problems are now too complex for the purview of one health profession, there is a plea for more realistic analysis of health problems and the involvement of multidiscipline approaches.

In the report, Schein (1972) notes that the professional of the future will need to have a different set of skills, a different set of images, and a different set of attitudes from the professional today. According to Schein, six factors of particular significance to nursing are identified as influencing these changes:

1. Change in work setting within which professionals operate
2. Change in fee structure
3. New concept of who is the client
4. Multiple client systems with which professionals must work

5. Availability to client of more basic knowledge and sophisticated technology
6. Change in social values calling for the professional to be an advocate, to improve not just serve society, and to be more an initiator than a responder.

All helping professionals need to think in terms of multiple client systems arising from the increasing bureaucratization of health professionals and thus prepare to work with values and goals of organizations. A concern of this matter was expressed in the Carnegie Report by Schein (1972):

As client systems become more differentiated and as clients become more resourceful and powerful, the professions have a less clear concept of what standards and ethics should govern client relationships and are therefore more vulnerable to a variety of attacks and pressures both from their employers and their intermediate and ultimate clients. (p. 31)

Nagel (1977) identifies five fundamental types of values that give rise to basic conflict, especially in a practice field:

1. Specific obligations to other people or institutions: to patients, one's family, hospital or university at which one works, one's community, or one's country.
2. Constraints on action deriving from general rights that everyone has either to do certain things or not to be treated in certain ways.
3. Utility: the effect of what one does on everyone's welfare and includes all aspects of benefit and harm to all people, not just the recipient.
4. Perfectionist ends or values: the intrinsic value of certain achievements or creations apart from the value to the person.
5. Commitment to one's own projects or undertakings. (pp. 281–283)

The determination of the stance of a profession, such as nursing, must take into account the world in which it practices and the social and political values that motivate the decision makers, especially as they impact on the quality, quantity, and delivery of health care. MacIntyre (1979) sees the overt moral stance of our culture as characterized by a temporary and fragile nature. The indignation expressed over a perceived immoral act is short lived. There is no real endeavor to explore in depth the substance of the indignation as a basis for resolution of the problem.

Currently, conflicts between society and various professional groups are occurring, as flagrant violations of professional behavior threaten the trust accorded by society, and professional groups are challenged to examine the ethical and moral basis of their practice. Reilly and Behrens-Hanna (1991) note that "professional groups, claimants to a highly specialized body of knowledge, are accorded recognition by society and often licensed by society for the services they provide" (p. 11). Schön (1983) refers to the crisis of confidence in professions, "In public outcry, in social criticism, and in the complaints of the professionals, themselves, the long-standing professional claim to monopoly of knowledge and social control is being challenged, first because professionals do not live up to the values and the norms they espouse and second because they are ineffective" (p. 11).

The plurality of citizenry in a society means a plurality of value systems represented in cultural norms, values, and behavior. The loss of significance of the melting pot theory means the acknowledgment of varied culture groups. Since each group has its own value system and seeks to maintain it while bringing it into accord with that of the larger society, nurses are finding that their practice is taking on different meanings. Recognition that concepts of health, illness, and sick role have particular meanings to each group requires that nurses respect these diversities as they provide care. Nursing process, the methodology of practice, facilitates the nurse in providing for these diversities, but the nurse is continually challenged to avoid biases from influencing the assessments or interventions on the basis of the nurse's own value system.

The development of nursing theories of transcultural nursing and care are providing a context within which the varied meanings and practices of different groups can be acknowledged and respected. They can be used to facilitate the progress toward well-being of individuals within these groups rather than create barriers to care when an ethnocentric perspective dominates the nursing care. Leininger's (1988b) theory of cultural care seeks a meaningful relationship of cultural care, beliefs and values, and practice between health care providers and the recipient so as to maintain, protect, or alter the care practices of the client. Marchione and Stearns (1990) identify the significance of ethnic power as a source of power in ethnic families which can be available to the health care provider. This indigenous power has evolved over time and is evident in ways which are symbolic, relational, communicative, and intuitive. Nursing education for the future incorporates knowledge of values, practices, and beliefs of various cultural groups so that nursing care can be recognized as having both cultural and universal dimensions, and care provided is congruent with the life style patterns of the client.

Bonaparte (1979) found in her study of 300 nurses a significant relationship between closemindedness and attitude toward culturally different patients. She depicted the closeminded nurse as unconsciously avoiding culturally different patients with incongruous health-related beliefs and practices that tended to be seen as a conflict with a rational scientific approach and anxiety producing and threatening to the nurse's professional image. Patients received less care. The open minded nurse readily sought out information about culturally different clients relative to their diet, language, inter- and intragroup social patterns, value concepts of health and illness, and other factors helpful in planning care.

As nursing operates within the society where multiple sources of ethical, moral, and value conflicts exist, it must also deal with these conflicts within itself. The pursuit of a value system by which it functions as a discipline and a practice profession is confronted with ambiguity and uncertainty. Gardner (1978) responds to the present decision-making state when he states: "The heart of our problem is not that betrayal of values is more vivid and more acknowledged today. The trouble runs deeper. The disintegration of traditions, customs, and communities has shaken our confidence. Our standards and guiding ideas are in disarray" (p. 23). Nursing has also lost some of its traditions, customs, and sense of community. The charge to nursing educators and practitioners is to clarify the concept of standards and ethics governing nursing practice. A paraphrase of Gardner's statement regarding obligations of society by inserting the word *nursing* for the word *society* would read: The whole structure of values, beliefs, laws, and standards by which *nursing* lives must be continuously restored or they will degenerate. They will survive and flourish only if people continuously renew their values and reinterpret traditions to make them serve contemporary needs.

Gardner calls upon nursing to rebuild. It is not necessary to develop a new set of values. Inherent in nursing are values reflective of the dignity and worth of each human being. The fundamental values have been there, although their interpretation and expression differed in accord with the society's values at any particular time.

Sources of Values

Bill of Rights. What is the source of values that must be accepted by professional nursing? One source would be the Bill of Rights of the Constitution (Figure 9-1) which clearly states those dimensions of an individual's life that must be respected if justice is to prevail. These rights are based on a moralistic premise about the individual in society and reflect the acceptance of the worth and dignity of the individual.

Throughout history, the concept of human rights has been challenged; sometimes resulting in an era of denial, sometimes one of indifference, and sometimes in an era of acknowledgment. Cranston (1983) presents the various historical swings regarding the acceptance of human rights as society policy when he raises the question: Are there any human rights? He defines human rights as ". . . something that everybody has. They are not rights a man acquires by doing certain work, enacting a certain role, or discharging certain duties; they belong to him simply because he is a human being" (p. 11). In response to those who believe that rights are earned, Cranston identifies three tests that confirm the existence of universal rights:

1. It is something that no one, anywhere, may be deprived of without a grave affront to justice.

2. It must be a universal right, one that pertains to every human being as such.

A Bill of Rights

as provided in the Ten Original Amendments to
The Constitution of the United States
in force December 15, 1791

AMENDMENT I
Congress shall make no law respecting an establishment of religion, or prohibiting the free exercise thereof; or abridging the freedom of speech, or of the press; or the right of the people peaceably to assemble, and to petition the Government for a redress of grievances.

AMENDMENT II
A well regulated Militia, being necessary to the security of a free State, the right of the people to keep and bear Arms, shall not be infringed.

AMENDMENT III
No Soldier shall, in time of peace be quartered in any house, without the consent of the Owner, nor in time of war, but in a manner to be prescribed by law.

AMENDMENT IV
The right of the people to be secure in their persons, houses, papers, and effects, against unreasonable searches and seizures, shall not be violated, and no Warrants shall issue, but upon probable cause, supported by Oath or affirmation, and particularly describing the place to be searched, and the persons or things to be seized.

AMENDMENT V
No person shall be held to answer for a capital, or otherwise infamous crime, unless on a presentment or indictment of a Grand Jury, except in cases arising in the land or naval forces, or in the Militia, when in actual service in time of War or public danger; nor shall any person be subject for the same offence to be twice put in jeopardy of life or limb; nor shall be compelled in any criminal case to be a witness against himself, nor be deprived of life, liberty, or property, without due process of law; nor shall private property be taken for public use, without just compensation.

AMENDMENT VI
In all criminal prosecutions, the accused shall enjoy the right to a speedy and public trial, by an impartial jury of the State and district wherein the crime shall have been committed, which district shall have been previously ascertained by law, and to be informed of the nature and cause of the accusation; to be confronted with the witnesses against him; to have compulsory process for obtaining witnesses in his favor, and to have the Assistance of Counsel for his defense.

AMENDMENT VII
In suits at common law, where the value in controversy shall exceed twenty dollars, the right of trial by jury shall be preserved, and no fact tried by a jury, shall be otherwise reexamined in any Court of the United States, than according to the rules of the common law.

AMENDMENT VIII
Excessive bail shall not be required, nor excessive fines imposed, nor cruel and unusual punishments inflicted.

AMENDMENT IX
The enumeration in the Constitution, of certain rights, shall not be construed to deny or disparage others retained by the people.

AMENDMENT X
The powers not delegated to the United States by the Constitution, nor prohibited by it to the States, are reserved to the States respectively, or to the people.

Figure 9-1

3. It must be of paramount importance. It is something that can and from a moral point of view *should* be respected here and now. If it is violated, justice itself is abused.

The significance of these rights within society was recently rediscovered, so that there are now many social movements in society of groups seeking to redress the wrongs caused by violations of these rights. The individual in the health care system is also asserting these rights through active consumer movements. How quickly are these rights taken away from individuals who enter health care agencies? Of particular concern are the rights to know, to participate in decisions about one's own care, and the right to privacy and protection from unwarranted search. The American Hospital Association has published a Bill of Rights for Patients, which is designed to protect the rights of patients while in the hospital. The nurse has a responsibility to see that these rights are implemented in the care setting.

Code for Nursing. The source of values particularly relevant to nursing is the body of professional documents that arise from the professional organization. The Code for Nurses (Table 9-1) is one such document. The first Code for Nurses was endorsed in 1950, and, characteristic of that era, it provided prescriptions for appropriate personal conduct of nurses. As the rebuilding process occurred in revisions of the Code, emphasis moved from the nurse to broader ethical values which are applicable to a variety of situations. The latest revision of the Code, adopted in 1976, provides a guide for the resolution of ethical dilemmas with an underlying theme of moralistic concept of the dignity and worth of each individual. It also addresses issues of accountability of the nurse to the efforts of the profession as it assumes its role in promoting the health and well-being of society.

It is important, however, to recognize the limitations of such a document. Toulmin (1977) recognizes that there is no conflict-free code, for individuals wear many hats and often their obligations are at variance. He says: "Professions organize their procedures and frame their codes of professional responsibility to minimize the risk of recurrent conflicts of obligation" (p. 261). Intraprofessional conflicts are of three types; accountability to group loyalty, accountability for competence, and accountability for respectability. The conflicts nurses face in

Table 9-1
Code for Nurses

1. The nurse provides services with respect for human dignity and the uniqueness of the client unrestricted by consideration of social or economic status, personal attributes, or the nature of health problems.
2. The nurse safeguards the client's right to privacy by judiciously protecting information of a confidential nature.
3. The nurse acts to safeguard the client and the public when health care and safety are affected by the incompetent, unethical, or illegal practice of any person.
4. The nurse assumes responsibility and accountability for individual nursing judgments and actions.
5. The nurse maintains competence in nursing.
6. The nurse exercises informed judgment and uses individual competence and qualifications as criteria in seeking consultation, accepting responsibilities, and delegating nursing activities to others.
7. The nurse participates in activities that contribute to the ongoing development of the profession's body of knowledge.
8. The nurse participates in the profession's efforts to implement and improve standards of nursing.
9. The nurse participates in the profession's efforts to establish and maintain conditions of employment conducive to high-quality nursing care.
10. The nurse participates in the profession's effort to protect the public from misinformation and misrepresentation and to maintain the integrity of nursing.
11. The nurse collaborates with members of the health professions and other citizens in promoting community and national efforts to meet the health needs of the public.

(Reprinted from the American Nurses Association. *Code for Nurses with Interpretive Statements*, Kansas City, MO., 1976, with permission.)

their practice may cause them to choose one of these accountabilities as a priority. The Code for Nurses guides nurses in their decisions, but it does not provide a means of establishing priorities when ethical or value conflicts arise. The nurse must ultimately make the choice for his or her own self.

Standards of Practice. The American Nurses Association has published a set of standards for nursing care in many of the specialty areas of practice as well as general standards which transcend all nursing. These standards, as is true of other documents, reflect the belief in the rights of clients in maintaining their dignity and control in matters affecting them. The meaning and implications of these standards are appropriate subjects for analysis as the learner or practitioner identifies the moral and ethical components of their practice. The reader is referred to these standards for a more detailed presentation.

One standard to be examined refers to rights of patients to appropriate knowledge for making decisions.

> *The client/patient and family are provided with the information needed to make decisions and choices about:*
> *Promoting, maintaining, and restoring health*
> *Seeking and utilizing appropriate health care personnel*
> *Maintaining and using health care resources. (ANA, 1973, p. 5)*

This standard relates to the teaching function of nursing. Consider the dilemma of a nurse whose professional standards require the nurse to teach, yet a physician states that his or her patient is not to be taught by the nurse? If the nurse follows the command of the physician, then teaching is a delegated task, not a professional activity. Of even greater concern is the fact that if the nurse does not teach the client, the nurse is vulnerable both ethically and legally. The issues raised in this dilemma concern the patients' right to know and the nurses' right to tell. This standard, like the others, is a statement of accountability and demands careful analysis.

Social Policy Statement. A significant document was published by the American Nurses Association in 1980. *Nursing, A Social Policy Statement* was prepared by a task force of the Congress of Nursing Practice and addresses three main themes: the social context of nursing, the scope of nursing practice, and the role of specialization in nursing. The document reflects the rebuilding process advocated by Gardner.

The social context statement notes: "Nursing can be said to be *owned* by society in the sense that nursing's professional interest must be perceived as serving the interest of the larger whole of which it is a part" (ANA, 1980, p. 7). The concept of *society ownership* needs to be pondered more fully for it suggests rights that society can proclaim from those it has licensed as practitioners.

The statement of the nature and scope of nursing practice includes the following:

Nurses have the highest regard for self-determination, independence, and choice in decision-making in matters of health. Nurses are committed to respecting human beings because of a profound regard to humanity. Basic commitment is unaltered by social, educational, economic, cultural, racial, religious, or other specific attributes of human beings receiving care, including nature and duration of disease and illness. (ANA, 1980, p. 18)

The significance in present times of this statement regarding the nature and scope of practice is particularly relevant to two evolving classifications of patients, those with AIDS and those in the frailty of aging. Numbers of patients in these two groups are increasing at a remarkable pace and challenge the care competency of nurses. Withdrawal from patient care because of fear of contracting AIDS or limited to addressing only custodial needs of the elderly is not acceptable nursing response. Confidence in one's self as a professional practitioner with requisite knowledge and skills provides the framework by which the scope of nursing practice can meet nursing needs of these and other clients. This document clearly states commitment and responsibilities of nurses to those they serve, individuals, and the larger society. It demands that nurses be open-minded and care about those who place trust in them for quality care.

All three professional documents have a common theme, i.e., a commitment to the dignity and worth of each person and accountability to society for a quality performance. There is a danger that the content of these pronouncements will sound familiar and not receive the careful analysis required. The basic premise is not new; but the interpretation and expression is new within the context of present society. The four documents referred to provide the subject matter of teaching in the affective domain. They provide the subject for objectives to be developed and attained.

APPROACHES TO TEACHING

Two general approaches are entailed in teaching the affective domain. One addresses the valuing process toward the end of developing an integrated value system and the other addresses the skills of moral reasoning when encountering moral or ethical dilemmas.

Values Clarification

Raths and colleagues (1966) and Simon and associates (1972) have developed the values clarification strategy which enables people to identify for themselves the values that guide their own actions. Numerous types of activities, such as games, questionnaires, and role playing, are designed to aid the student through the valuing process. Examples of strategies are found in the previously mentioned two references and those that are relevant to nursing are in Steele and Harmon (1983) and Reilly (1978).

This approach is process oriented and does not concern itself with content, the *what* to value. An unfortunate outcome of the activity is that expressed conscious awareness may be perceived as the goal without any examination of the validity of the expressed belief and the potential consequences. Choices may be superficial and lack the rigorous discipline of intellectual inquiry and commitment. Speaking of the limitations of this approach and its emphasis on personal values, Morrill (1980) states: "The obligatory and normative dimensions of the experience of values are given virtually no direct attention nor does the technique address as ends in themselves the values that inhere in the social and political dimensions of life" (p. 17).

Values Inquiry

This is a process that speaks to some of the weakness in the values clarification method. Its aim is to explore the meanings and possibilities of a human situation by discovering the values that motivate choice and decisions by individuals (Morrill, 1980). Values inquiry is an intellectual activity which is descriptive and seeks to assist the individual in discovering the value and moral connotations in activities or situations encountered.

Although process is an essential component of this method, the content, i.e., values, is also significant. Value choices identified in the inquiry process are examined from a normative perspective in accord with social and moral standards. Morrill (1980) notes two limitations in the value inquiry method when he raises these questions:

> *If one's analysis has depicted a set of competing and conflicting values—as it usually does—is that the final word? To what extent does a full and clear analysis of values affect the development of a student's own values and the exercise of choice? (p. 23)*

In the first question the issue of principles for selecting from competing values is addressed. The second question raises the critical issue of the internalization of the value so that it is an integral part of the student's value system and is exemplified in actions.

Moral Reasoning

The theories of Kohlberg (1972), Perry (1970), Gilligan (1982), and others have been presented as viable approaches to moral development. Kohlberg's work involves moral reasoning relative to hypothetical moral dilemmas. Nursing offers numerous examples of dilemmas drawn directly from real practice situations to which students can relate. Examples may be found in Davis and Aroskar (1983), Steele and Harmon (1983), and Reilly (1978).

The use of this method requires disciplined critical thinking and that inquiry be substantive and methodic. Ketefian (1981) studied 79 practicing nurses relative to their educational preparation, skill in critical thinking, and score on moral reasoning. Higher scores were more evident in nurses with professional preparation in contrast to those with technical preparation. Munhall (1980), using Rest's Defining Issue Test (DIT) based on Kohlberg's theory, found that the average baccalaureate student functioned at the conventional level while faculty were primarily at the principled level. There was no difference according to level of student, but it was noted that students with the higher grade point average scored higher in the levels of moral reasoning. These studies indicate that moral reasoning is a cognitive skill activity dependent upon knowledge and reflective thinking. It is a legitimate concern for faculty teaching the affective domain.

Experience

It must be noted that all of the described methods rely primarily on the cognitive processes of judgment and choice making and do not provide for experiential sequences where the learner develops a pattern of behavior consistent with stated values or moral decisions. The methods can be used appropriately in teaching students providing that the faculty understand the purpose for each and the limitations in terms of outcome.

Provision for experiential learning in addressing ethical, moral and value conflicts is essential if affective skills are to be acquired. However, experiential methods without disciplined cognitive skills are not sufficient. Cross (1975), who sees *reasoning* as the heart of the educational process no less in areas of morality than in other fields of learning, refers to the need of practice when she states: "Just as we do not expect the student in mathematics to become proficient without practice in solving problems; so we should not expect students to develop skills in moral reasoning without practice in thinking about moral dilemmas" (p. 627).

CLINICAL SETTING FOR EXPERIENTIAL AFFECTIVE LEARNING

Much discussion surrounds the teaching of the affective domain in nursing programs. Some proposals include such formal courses as ethics and logic, while other proposals suggest integrating concepts into all nursing courses. Whether or not there is a formal course, provision must be made for the student to work with the issues that are real in practice. Most of that experience is obtained in the clinical field where issues are directly related to nurse-client interactions, nurse–nurse interactions, nurse–other-discipline interactions, or nurse-bureaucratic conflict. Although these conflicts occur within the practice setting, many have much broader implications that incorporate issues of the larger society. Inquiry and analysis need to include all significant dimensions of the issue so that the student's data are qualitatively and quantitatively sufficient for making choices. Once the choice is made, students can experience the choice in action and evaluate the action. Experiences need to be repeated, for consistency in response pattern is the desired goal.

The clinical setting is replete with affective learning experiences. The setting in which students are asked to effect behavior change is a complex one where values and expectations of participants are shared, competitive, or contradictory. The teacher comes to the setting with his or her own perceptions, values, and convictions about the world of nursing, student learning behavior in a practice setting, and how health care "ought" to be delivered in that setting. Likewise, the students bring to the setting their own ideas and values, some of which will be altered in the process of learning. Adult learners in the program bring a reasonably stabilized value system and decision-making process yet may be threatened when alteration is indicated. Regardless of the age of the student and life experiences, there is a need for a supportive, trustworthy, and authentic environment where mistakes or trying out of new selves will occur within a learning rather than a punitive context.

PREPARATION OF OBJECTIVES

As with the other domains, planning for experience is required. Objectives must be prepared, relevant learning experiences and teaching strategies devised, and evaluative methods selected. As with the other domains, affective learning must be a developmental process, proceeding from simple to complex. The student does not enter the practice setting with a *tabulae rasa*; some values inherent in nursing are developed, some are still at the value indicator stage, and some have not been recognized. For those values that have been developed, their expression in nursing may be different from what the students have experienced in their life encounters. This situation is no different from what occurs with the other domains; there are various levels of achievement among students.

Taxonomy

In preparing objectives for the field experience, the level of achievement needs to be identified. Behaviors to be demonstrated in the clinical field must arise out of course objectives. In some instances they may be the same ones, with the cognitive component taught and evaluated in the classroom and the use of the cognitive behavior in a consistent pattern of behavior taught and evaluated in the clinical field.

A taxonomy serves the purpose of identifying the increasingly complex level of value development. Krathwohl and associates (1964) developed a taxonomy of the affective domain which Reilly & Oermann (1990) applied to nursing. The essence of affective learning is internalization, continuity between knowing and doing in a consistent pattern. Internalization is the integrating principle of the taxonomy.

The first two levels relate to the value indicators that Raths and colleagues (1966) mention. It is at the third level where choosing occurs and internalization begins. The levels in the taxonomy are described in Table 9-2.

Use of Taxonomy

Like the other taxonomies, the affective taxonomy provides a framework for selecting the appropriate level of learning behavior and for writing objectives. The desired level is selected in terms of the learner's status in the program, the complexity of the phenomenon, and experiences available for achieving the objective. Preparation of objectives in terms of the taxonomy follows using the nursing standard cited earlier.

> Standard V: Nursing action provides for client/patient participation in health promotion, maintenance, and restoration.
> 2. The client/patient and family are provided with the information needed to make decisions and choices about: promoting, maintaining and restoring health, seeking and utilizing appropriate health care personnel, maintaining and using health care resources. (ANA, 1973, p. 5)

A 1.0 Receiving

1.1 The student acknowledges that nurses provide information for client/family.

1.2 The student listens to client/family express concerns and need for knowledge.

Table 9-2
Taxonomy of Affective Domain

Taxonomy		Behavior
A 1.0	Receiving (attending)	
1.1	Awareness	Knows about, no response offered
1.2	Willingness to receive	Interested in giving attention; may or may not act
1.3	Controlled or selected attention	Differentiates stimuli; selects ones of personal interest
A 2.0	Responding	
2.1	Acquiescence in responding	Responds to authority's command
2.2	Willingness to respond	Voluntary action; likes idea
2.3	Satisfaction in response	Enjoys act; still no commitment
A 3.0	Valuing	
3.1	Acceptance of value	Reasonably certain about belief
3.2	Preference for value	Attaches worth to belief and acts accordingly
3.3	Commitment	High degree of certainty; usually consistent in action
A 4.0	Organization	
4.1	Conceptualization of value	Conceptualization gives value stability; action is consistent
A 5.0	Characterization by a value or value complex	
5.1	Generalized set	Internalization provides means of ordering complex world and acting consistently and effectively
5.2	Characterization	Integration so complete that actions are consistent and compatible

(Adapted from Reilly, D. E., Oermann, M., *Behavioral objectives: Evaluation in nursing* (3rd edition) New York: National League for Nursing 1990, pp. 76–79, with permission.)

1.3 The student listens to comments by client/family which indicate areas where they wish information before making decisions.

A 2.0 Responding

2.1 The student provides information to client/family according to requirements of the care plan.

2.2 The student seeks opportunity to provide client/family with information needed for making decisions.

2.3 The student responds willingly in meeting information needs of client/family.

A 3.0 Valuing

3.1 The student assists client/family in obtaining data relevant to decisions to be made.

3.2 The student supports the right of client/family to be informed about all matters relevant to decisions affecting them.

3.3 The student assumes responsibility for informing client/family on matters pertinent to decisions involving them.

A 4.0 Organization

4.1 The student formulates a position relative to the client/family right to information and the nurse's responsibility to that end.

4.2 The student formulates a plan of action which assures advocacy of client/family rights to be knowledgeable in making decisions irrespective of circumstances.

A 5.0 Characterization

5.1 The student acts consistently both in protecting the information rights of client/family and assuring that they possess sufficient knowledge for making decisions relative to their health needs.

5.2 The student develops a philosophy of life and nursing which manifests itself in practice as a consistent advocacy for the value of client/family knowledge in maintaining control of decisions affecting their lives.

The level of affective competency to be achieved at the end of the program or at any point in the curriculum is a professional judgment decision of the faculty. On any one objective, one must recognize the time it takes to integrate knowing and doing. The higher two levels require considerable commitment and may be beyond the purview of some undergraduate programs. Professional schools may bring the students to the first stage in level four. Graduate programs are directed toward the upper levels for their students.

When the program outcome is determined, the level for each year of the program and courses are designated to show development. As with the other taxonomies, leveling may occur by increasing the taxonomy level, increasing complexity of the variables with which a behavioral level interacts, or by both processes at the same time. An illustration of the use of the taxonomy with the above objectives might appear in a baccalaureate program thusly:

End of program (senior year)	A 4.1
Junior Year	A 3.3
Sophomore Year	A 2.3

A technical program might expect level A 3.3

Reilly (1978) notes that many courses direct evaluation of cognitive learning at the three lower levels (knowledge, comprehension, application) while expectations of affective learning are directed to the complex level of consistency in behavior. She states:

> . . . *for both domains, the lower levels of learning can be evidenced within a reasonable space of time and can be evaluated with rather easily developed appraisal strategies. In both domains, the complex learning behaviors require an extended period of development and require sophisticated appraisal techniques. (pp. 51–52)*

TEACHING STRATEGIES

The principal criterion in selecting teaching strategies in the affective domain is involvement, experiential involvement, cognitive involvement. Hypothetical situations involving ethical, moral, and value conflicts are useful for teaching, but they often lack the reality, i.e., the student can remain outside the conflict. Situations drawn from actual practice enable the student to identify with the individuals dealing with the conflict. Teaching in the clinical field then provides not only the experiential and cognitive learning, but it also adds the reality dimension.

Some strategies are directed at the affective domain specifically; some strategies are an added dimension to other ongoing methods. A teacher attuned to affective teaching keeps an "antenna" focused on all activities in which the student is engaged in the search for affective learning experiences.

Analysis and Confrontation

Decision making is often considered primarily in the cognitive domain, yet almost every decision has an affective component reflective of a belief, value, or moral stance. Examination of the student's decision from a value, ethical, or moral perspective as well as from a cognitive one helps the students to know their own frame of reference. When this analysis of a decision occurs in clinical conferences, then affective questions are explored with input of differing perspectives as viewed by the members of the group. Through divergent thinking, various alternatives are explored and the potential consequence of each is noted. Thompson (1991) recommends the use of ethical case study analysis as a means of assisting students in using various ethical theories and principles in identifying the moral and ethical issues which are included and the types of decisions which were made.

The reliance on cognitive analysis only of students' decisions and actions in the practice setting impedes the development of the students toward an advocacy role in matters of health and welfare for a pluralistic society. The exploration of values, which often means confrontation, can raise consciousness of disharmony and inconsistency of values that are often quiescent. Confrontation is an important strategy for use by the teacher; for with no challenge to one's beliefs no growth will occur. Confrontation can be difficult, even painful for students and teachers. Churchill (1982) sees confrontation as essential and states: "The refusal of a teacher to challenge and even critically evaluate the values of a student, however benevolently motivated, undermines appreciation of the moral life and handicaps the development of students into self-affirming and self-critical moral agents" (p. 302). Shinn (1979) recognizes the disarming effects that may accompany value confrontation as self-images are threatened, but he sees positive results from the experience. "It may also lead a person to confront conflict and to recognize values more coherently. It may be a social and personal healing experience" (p. 30).

Clinical Assignment

In the National Geographic Society's publication *Journey into China,* the following statement occurs: "The Wall (Great) stood for the proposition that unbridgeable cultural differences exist among people, differences so profound that they could be dealt with only by separation" (Smith, 1982, p. 84). Does such a wall exist in nursing practice, whether within a person or within a system? Teaching in the affective domain requires that such a wall be dismantled if it exists, for the respect for the dignity and worth of each person, as stated thematically through all nursing documents, does not mean "persons like me." The ANA Social Policy Statement previously cited declares that nursing's concern is for all individuals, regardless of life style, value system, or appearance.

Confrontation is once again called upon as a method, this time in terms of the clients or situations to which students are assigned. Augmentation of the care component of "different" clients with study of particular mores, values, or behavior patterns of the client's group will help students place the client in the client's own perspective, not in that of the students. Conferences, which are exploratory not only in terms of the client's behavioral responses but also the student's, will foster the student's growth in serving and living in a pluralistic society. Emphasis must be placed on the client's right to his or her own life style and values with the recognition that the acceptance of this right does not mean that the nurse accepts the life style and values for himself or herself.

Teachers' biases in making these assignments require scrutiny so that assignments are compatible with growth needs of students. In urban schools of nursing, faculty are often concerned that suburban students obtain community health nursing experience with city clients in order to broaden their perspective of how nursing care needs are influenced by socioeconomic and cultural factors. However, seldom do they see the need for city students to gain experience with clients in suburban areas on the same premise.

Hands-On Care

Hands-on care is usually taught from the psychomotor perspective with recognition of the student's need to know the underlying principles. The affective domain has much to contribute to expert performance. The domain refers to the nonverbal message the student brings to the client in the process of carrying out a procedure.

Nursing is one of the few professions in which society permits the touching of individuals on any part of their body. How is that touch administered? Literature in nursing is now addressing the therapeutic value of touch. The concern in the affective domain is the way the nurse touches and carries out the procedures so as to connote the message: "I care. I respect your dignity and worth."

Baths can be stimulating and refreshing or they can be uncomfortable and wearisome, resembling more of a dry cleaning. Careless tossing of limbs, ignoring of privacy needs of patients through failure to keep covered those parts of the body not involved in the treatment and/or failure to explain to the client the processes involved in a procedure all reflect a communication that ignores the dignity of the client. Nurses are particularly challenged when caring for clients with body drainage or inability to control bodily functions. At that time, clients already distressed with loss of control and disturbed body image are particularly sensitive to the nurse's response to them and to the nurse's manner in caring for them.

The relationship of touch to the phenomenon of care in nursing has been examined at various levels of study and research. Bottorff (1991) has completed a review of many of these studies, noting several observations in her report. Most research studies have defined touch in relation to physical contact in tactile stimulation whereby it encompasses its communication role. Weiss (1979) identifies five tactile symbols which define qualities of touch as a means of communication—location, pressure, action, duration, and intensity. The review also indicated that most studies on touch were biased toward positive effects (p. 333). Gadow (1990) views touch in a broader perspective. She says, "Among all the forms of human interaction, touch is the reminder that objectivity is not even skin deep; subjectivity exists at the surface of the body" (p. 39). She notes that not all touch is supportive of caring; the instrumental touch as in some surgery where the subjectivity of the person is not engaged, and beneficent touch which is a surrogate for engagement which assumes a basic asymmetry between nurse and patient (p. 29).

Faculty observing students in carrying out psychomotor skills need to note the affective component of the skill. Acceptable performance incorporates not only the quality of the technique and knowledge but also the quality of the touch and caring.

Examination of Verbal Expressions

The human proclivity to use a generalized word to convey a complicated phenomenon is particularly relevant in teaching the affective domain. The word is generally a way of categorizing information and beliefs to simplify the handling of large amounts of data. The teacher in the affective domain listens carefully to the labels the learner uses when referring to clients or others in the practice setting. Such words as uncooperative, culturally deprived, basket case, or lazy may be heard.

Labels do two things. To the one labeled, the label signifies that since what others say is the way it is, there is nothing the person can do about it. To the labeler, the nurse, it means one accepts the fact and need do nothing about it. It is the latter interpretation that is of concern, for there is no attempt on the part of the nurse to seek the cause of the client's behavior and address the cause. One group of students sought data about a group of patients which the nursing staff labeled as uncooperative. Most of these patients were over 50 years of age with a terminal illness and had few visitors. The patients were exhibiting fear of dying alone, but the label accepted by the nursing staff prevented them from recognizing the patients' behavior as need behavior. One might suggest here that teachers need to examine labels they use in referring to students.

In addition to learner use of labels, the teacher needs to note also the way students present their ideas regarding patients in clinical happenings. The frequent or habitual use of global words such as, all, every, or never suggest the student is failing to accept individual difference among people, events, situations, or phenomena. Some students couch their ideas with expressions that take the onus of owner responsibility away from themselves, such as, *"the other nurses say," "the doctor says," "the author says," "the teachers says."* Concern here is that the students do not take a position and accept the inherent responsibility, an essential behavior in the role of advocate.

Other students will not make a statement that reflects a position for or against anything or anyone. If the student is to be able to make decisions in ethical, moral, or value conflicts, the student must be able to clarify his or her own thinking and be prepared to take a stand and accept the consequences. Faculty noting the communication patterns described that reflect avoidance or inadequate inquiry need to confront the students and select experiences in the clinical field that will foster the students' examination of their own behavioral responses and ability to communicate with confidence decisions rationally made.

Model Learning

Modeling, a method of formal learning whereby the learner seeks to imitate a behavioral pattern of another individual who exemplifies an ideal to the student, is often referred to as essential for learning in a practice discipline. It is often noted in reference to affective learning.

Teaching is not value free, regardless of what the teacher thinks or desires. The very approach the teacher uses in teaching within the practice field, selection of learning experiences, interactions with students, interactions with clients and participants in the delivery of care in the setting, and expected performance standards of all students all reflect in some way the moral beliefs and values of the teacher.

What should be the position of a teacher in discussions of moral, value, and ethical issues? Should the teacher remain neutral? Baumgarten (1982) supports a neutral advocacy stance for liberal arts teachers, for he feels that the declaration of a position by a teacher will stifle inquiry by students' unquestioning acceptance of that position and deprive them of creative anguish that comes with thinking through an issue without knowing the ultimate result.

Other authors support the notion that neutrality is not possible and that, indeed, the teacher may in essence only be feigning neutrality

(Casement, 1984; Churchill, 1982; Robertson & Grant, 1982). Even though a verbal statement of a position may not be made, nonverbal messages, e.g., facial and body cues given in directing the discussion, convey the teacher's real beliefs or values. Robertson and Grant (1982) state, "Teachers who are trying to persuade rationally their students should rely on presentation of arguments to accomplish goals rather than on personal charisma in emotional appeals" (p. 349). Shinn (1979) see exhortation as the least effective way of inculcating values. The suggestions of these two authors are particularly relevant to a professional program such as in nursing, where persuasion for accepting a particular set of professional values is in order.

Robertson and Grant (1982) see educational value to the teacher's declaration of a position on an issue when the teacher encourages students to criticize and question the position. When the teacher tells students how that position was originated, what processes the teacher went through in developing the position, what alternatives were considered, and what doubts or questions still persist, the teacher is demonstrating a model of rational and emotional self-searching in preparation for a declared position with which the person can live.

The emphasis in the use of modeling as a teaching strategy entails leading the student through thought and experiences to one's own conclusions. There is danger in the use of models. Adelson (1962) differentiates between the teacher's style and the teacher's skill. He is concerned that the student may imitate the teacher's style, i.e., way of responding to a conflict, rather than the teacher's skill, i.e., process by which the teacher achieved the responses. Imitation may be a form of flattery, but it is dangerous if the student does not examine the teacher's response in relation to its rationale and appropriateness for self. Style follows skill; the imitation of the skill does not mean that the student's style will be the same as the teacher's. Style is personal.

SUMMARY

Since affective learning occurs in the clinical setting it is subject to the same pedagogic demands as the other domains in learning. The goals of affective learning are the development of skill in moral reasoning for managing ethical and moral dilemmas and the development of a value system which incorporates those values espoused by the profession of nursing through its documents, namely the Code of Nursing, Standards of Nursing Practice, and the Social Policy Statement.

Care is the moral core of nursing. It is the human dimension of nursing which serves to preserve the human dignity of each individual. Research in caring within the practice of nursing denotes its contextual and relational nature; i.e., its essence is in the nurse-patient relationship. Research at the present time is directing some nursing scholars toward viewing care as a theory of nursing while others view care as the core of a theory of nursing ethics. Care is the principle concept and action through which the affective domain in nursing is realized.

Affective skills are becoming increasingly essential for practitioners of all disciplines as they are faced with complex decisions where values representing quality of life, justice, and conservation are in conflict with values associated with profit, expediency, and technology. Although professional documents provide guidelines for the responses of practitioners to conflict situations, they do not suggest priorities in competing values nor the means by which values are expressed. It is the individual who ultimately must resolve the question of what response to make in a conflict situation.

Affective learning entails such concepts as: ethics—standards of conduct; morality—systems of moral conduct; belief—individual perceptions of reality; value—judgment of worth arising from choice and demonstrated in action; attitude—feeling for or against; and moral reasoning—cognitive process of analysis and interpretation of moral issues.

Skills in making rational decisions are not sufficient, for affective competency also requires action consistent with stated beliefs or positions. The clinical setting provides an excellent environment, for by its very nature it represents many of the types of conflicts that nurses encounter in practice. The opportunity to experience conflicts, both through cognition and action, enables learners to explore and test out their own choices.

Value clarification, value inquiry, and exercises in moral reasoning where the substance of each is generated by the practice environment are appropriate methods for teaching the affective domain. Clinical conferences or written issue papers are vehicles for addressing the cognitive component implied by these methods. Behaviors of students connoting action of beliefs, values, and moral stances can also be subject to confrontation and examination. Action is evident in the words students use in expressions about people, events, and situations and in the way they carry out their psychomotor skills. The use of clinical conference, selective client or activity assignment, and field placement as well as the use of modeling are appropriate for teaching the affective domain from a clinical perspective.

The ethical and moral values inherent in nursing practice have a significant bearing on the value orientation of nursing and direct the affective behavior of its practitioners as they serve their clients. Donaldson and Crowley (1978) address themselves to the goal of nursing in fostering self-care behavior which leads to individual health and well-being and to nursing's accountability for social needs. "As a result of this value orientation, knowledge of the basis of human choices and of methods for fostering individual independence are sought, rather than knowledge of interventions that control and directly manipulate the person per se into a societally determined state of health" (p. 117). The charge is made to the faculty teaching the affective domain in the clinical field.

REFERENCES

Adelson, J. (1962). The teacher as a model. In N. Sanford (Ed.), *American College*. New York: Wiley.
American Nurses Association. (1973). *Standards: Nursing practice*. Kansas City, MO: American Nurses Association.
American Nurses Association. (1976). *Code for nurses with interpretive statements*. Kansas City, MO: American Nurses Association.
American Nurses Association. (1980). *Nursing: A social policy statement*. Kansas City, MO: American Nurses Association.
Ayer, A. J. (1946). *Language, truth, and logic*. New York: Davis.
Baumgarten, E. (1982). Ethics in the academic profession: A socratic view. *Journal of Higher Education, 53*, 282–295.
Benner, P. (1990). The moral dimensions of caring. In J. Stevenson & T. Tripp-Reimer. (Eds.), *Knowledge about caring: State of the art and future developments* (pp. 5–18). Kansas City, MO: American Academy of Nursing.

Benner, P., & Wrubel, J. (1989). *The primacy of caring: Stress and coping in health and illness*. Menlo Park, CA: Addison-Wesley.

Bonaparte, B. (1979). Ego defensiveness, open-closed mindedness and nurses' attitude toward culturally different patients. *Nursing Research, 28*, 166–171.

Bottorff, J. (1991). A methodologic review and evaluation of research on nurse-patient touch. In P. Chinn (Ed.), *Anthology on caring* (pp. 303–343). New York: National League for Nursing.

Casement, W. (1984). Moral education: Form without content? *Educational Forum, 48*, 177–178.

Cassidy, V. (1991). Ethical responsibilities in nursing: Research findings and issues. *Journal of Professional Nursing, 7*(2), 112–118.

Chally, P. (1990). Theory derivation in moral development. *Nursing & Health Care, 11*(6), 302–307.

Churchill, L. (1982). The teaching of ethics and moral values in teaching: Some contemporary confusions. *Journal of Higher Education, 53*, 296–306.

Cooper, M. (1989). Gilligan's voice: A perspective for nursing. *Journal of Professional Nursing, 5*, 10–16.

Cranston, M. (1983). Are there any human rights? *Daedalus, 112*(4), 1–18.

Cross, K. P. (1975). Learner centered curriculi. In D. Vermilye (Ed.), *Learner centered reform: Current issues in higher education*. San Francisco: Jossey-Bass.

Davis, A. J., & Aroskar, M. A. (1983). *Ethical dilemmas and nursing practice* (2nd ed.). Norwalk, CT: Appleton-Century-Crofts.

Dewey, J. (1962). *Individualism, old and new*. New York: Capricorn Books.

Donaldson, S. K., & Crowley, D. (1978). The discipline of nursing. *Nursing Outlook, 26*, 113–120.

Dubos, R. (1981). *Celebration of life*. New York: McGraw-Hill.

Englehardt, H. T., Jr. (1977). Knowledge, value, and belief. In H. T. Englehardt, & D. Callahan (Eds.), *The foundations of ethics and its relationship to science: Vol. 2. Knowledge, value and belief*. Hastings-on-Hudson, NY: Institute of Society, Ethics, and Life Sciences.

Frankena, W. (1983). Moral-Point-of-View Theories, Bowie, N.E. (Ed.), *Ethical theory in the last quarter of the twentieth century* (pp. 39–79). Indianapolis: Hackett Publishing Co.

Frankl, V. E. (1963). *Man's search for meaning*. New York: Washington Square Press.

Frisch, N. (1987). Value analysis: A method for teaching nursing ethics and promoting moral development of students. *Journal of Nursing Education, 24*, 375–392.

Fry, S. (1989). Toward a theory of nursing ethics. *Advanced Nursing Science, 11*(4), 9–22.

Gadow, S. (1990). The advocacy covenant: Care as clinical subjectivity. In J. Stevenson & T. Tripp-Reimer (Eds.), *The primacy of caring: State of the art and future developments* (pp. 33-40). Kansas City, MO: American Academy of Nursing.

Gardner, J. W. (1978). *Morale.* New York: W. W. Norton & Co., Inc.

Gilligan, C. (1982). *In a different voice.* Cambridge: Harvard University Press.

Holstein, C. B. (1976). Irreversible stepwise sequence in the development of moral judgment: A longitudinal study of males and females. *Child Development, 47,* 51-61.

Ketefian, S. (1981). Critical thinking, educational preparation, and development of moral judgment among selected groups of practicing nurses. *Nursing Research 30,* 98-103.

Ketefian, S. (1991). Moral and ethical dimensions of nursing practice. In M. Oermann, *Professional nursing practice: A conceptual approach* (pp. 217-232). Philadelphia: J. P. Lippincott.

Knox, A. B. (1977). *Adult development in learning.* San Francisco: Jossey-Bass.

Kohlberg, L. (1972). The cognitive-development approach to moral education. *The Humanists, 32,* 12-18.

Kohlberg, L. (1981). *The philosophy of moral development.* New York: Harper & Row.

Krathwohl, D. R., Bloom, B. S., & Masia, B. (1964). *Taxonomy of educational objectives, Handbook 2, Affective domain.* New York: David McKay.

Leininger, M. (1988a). *Care: Discovery and use in clinical and community nursing.* Detroit: Wayne State University Press.

Leininger, M. (1988b). Leininger's theory of nursing, cultural care diversity and universality. *Nursing Science Quarterly, 1*(14), 152-161.

Levine, M. (1977). Nursing ethics and the ethical nurse. *American Journal of Nursing, 77,* 845-847.

MacIntyre, A. (1979). Why is the search for foundations of ethics so frustrating? *Hastings Center Report, 9,* 8-11.

Marchione, J., & Stearns, S. (1990). Ethnic power perspectives for nursing. *Nursing & Health Care, 11*(6), 296-301.

McBee, M. L. (1978). Higher education: Its responsibility for moral development. *Phi Kappa Phi Journal, 58,* 30-33.

Morrill, R. L. (1980). *Teaching values in college.* San Francisco: Jossey-Bass.

Munhall, P. (1980). Moral reasoning of nursing students and faculty in a baccalaureate program. *Image: Journal of Nursing Scholarship, 12*(3), 57-61.

Nagel, T. (1977). The fragmentation of values. In H. T. Englehardt, & D. Callahan (Eds.), *The foundations of ethics and its relationship to science: Vol. 2 Knowledge, value and belief.* Hastings-on-Hudson, NY: Institute of Society, Ethics, and Life Sciences.

Noddinger, N. (1984). *Caring: A feminine approach to ethics and moral education.* Berkeley, CA: University Press.
Norris, C. (1989). To care or not to care. Questions! Questions! *Nursing & Health Care, 10*(10), 545-550.
Pellegrino, E. D., & Thomasma, D. C. (1988). *For the patient's good.* New York: Oxford University Press.
Perry, W. G., Jr. (1970). *Forms of intellectual and ethical development in the college years.* New York: Holt, Rinehart & Winston.
Podeschi, R. L. (1976). William James and education. *The Educational Forum, 40,* 223-229.
Raths, L. E., Harmin, M., & Simon, S. (1966). *Values and teaching.* Columbus, OH: Merrill.
Reilly, D. E. (Ed.). (1978). *Teaching and evaluating the affective domain in nursing programs.* Thorofare, NJ: Charles B. Slack.
Reilly, D. (1989). Ethics and values in nursing: Are we opening Pandora's Box? *Nursing & Health Care, 10*(2), 90-95.
Reilly, D., & Behrens-Hanna, L. (1991). Perioperative nursing: Moral and ethical issues in high-technology practice. *Today's O.R. Nurse, 13*(8), 10-15.
Reilly, D., & Oermann, M. (1990). *Behavioral objectives: Evaluation in nursing* (3rd ed.). New York: National League for Nursing.
Roberts, J. E. (1990). Uncovering hidden caring. *Nursing Outlook, 38*(2), 67-69.
Robertson, E., & Grant, G. (1982). Teaching and ethics: An epilogue. *Journal of Higher Education, 53,* 345-347.
Ross, V. (1984). The right to die debate. *World Press Review, 31*(2), 33-34.
Scheibe, K. E. (1970). *Beliefs and values.* New York: Holt, Rinehart & Winston.
Schein, E. H. (1972). *Professional education: Some new directions.* New York: McGraw-Hill.
Schön, D. (1983). *The reflective practitioner: How professionals think in action.* San Francisco, CA: Jossey-Bass.
Shinn, R. L. (1979). An educational impossibility: The value-free classroom. *Columbia,* 26-30.
Simon, S., Howe, I., & Kirschenbaum, H. (1972). *Values clarification.* New York: Hart.
Smith, A. F. (1978). Lawrence Kohlberg's cognitive stage theory of the development of moral judgment. *New Directions for Student Services, 4,* 53-66.
Smith, G., Jr. (1982). On the trail of the long stone serpent. In *Journey to China.* Washington, DC: National Geographic Society.
Steele, S. M., & Harmon, V. M. (1983). *Values clarification in nursing* (2nd ed.). Norwalk, CT: Appleton-Century-Crofts.
Stent, G. S. (1977). The poverty of scientism and the promise of structuralist ethics. In H. T. Englehardt, & D. Callahan (Eds.), *The foundations of ethics*

and its relationship to science: Vol. 2. Knowledge, value and belief. Hastings-on-Hudson, NY: Institute of Society, Ethics, and Life Sciences.

Stevenson, J. (1990). Quantitative care research: Review of content, process, and product. In J. Stevenson & T. Tripp-Reimer (Eds.), *The primacy of caring: State of the art and future developments* (pp. 97-120). Kansas City, American Academy of Nursing.

Thompson, D., (1991). Ethical case analysis using a hospital bill. *Nurse Educator, 16*(4), 20-23.

Toulmin, S. (1977). The meaning of professionalism: Doctors, ethics and biomedical science. In H. T. Englehardt & D. Callahan (Eds.), *The foundation of ethics and its relationship to science, Vol. 2. Knowledge, value and belief.* Hastings-on-Hudson, NY: Institute of Society, Ethics, and Life Sciences.

Turro, J. (1972). *Reflections.* Paramus, NJ: Paulist Press.

Watson, J. (1985). *Nursing: Human science and human care: A theory of nursing.* Norwalk, CT: Appleton-Century-Crofts.

Weiss, S. (1979). The language of touch. *Nursing Research, 28*(2), 76-80.

Wild, J. (1969). *The radical imperialism of William James.* New York: Doubleday.

BIBLIOGRAPHY

Anderson, S. (1991). Do student preceptorships affect moral reasoning? *Nurse Educator, 16*(1), 14-19.

Aroskar, M. (1987). The interface of ethics and politics in nursing. *Nursing Outlook, 35*(6), 268-273.

Benjamin, A., & Curtis, J. (1986). *Ethics in nursing.* New York, Oxford.

Benoliel, J. (1983). Ethics in nursing practice and education. *Nursing Outlook, 31,* 210-215.

Bevis, E., & Watson, J. (1989). *Toward a caring curriculum: A new pedagogy for nursing.* New York: National League for Nursing.

Bishop, A., & Scudder, J. (1990). *A practical, moral and personal sense of nursing; A phenomenological philosophy of practice.* Albany, NY: State University of New York Press.

Brink, P. (1984). Value orientation as an assessment tool in cultural diversity. *Nursing Research, 33,* 198-203.

Brummer, J. J. (1984). Moralizing and value education. *Educational Forum, 48,* 263-276.

Chinn, P. (Ed.). (1991). *Anthology of caring.* New York: National League for Nursing.

Cunningham, N., & Hutchinson, S. (1990). Myths in health care ethics. *Image: Journal of Nursing Scholarship, 22*(4), 235-238.

Dewey, J. (1975). *Moral principles in education.* Carbondale & Edwardsville, IL: Southern Illinois Press.

Donley, Sr. R. (1991). Spiritual dimensions of health care. *Nursing & Health Care, 12*(4), 178-183.

Dormire, S. (1989). Models for moral response in care of seriously ill children. *Image: Journal of Nursing Scholarship, 21*(2), 101-103.

Felton, G., & Parsons, M. (1987). The impact of nursing education on ethical and moral decision making. *Journal of Nursing Education, 26,* 7-11.

Fenton, M. (1987). Development of the scale of humanistic nursing behaviors. *Nursing Research, 36*(2), 82-87.

Freitas, L. (1990). Historical roots and future perspectives related to nursing ethics. *Journal of Professional Nursing, 6*(4), 197-205.

Fromer, M. (1980). Teaching ethics by case conflicts. *Nursing Outlook, 28,* 604-608.

Garvin, B., & Boyle, K. (1985). Values of entering nursing students: A change over 10 years. *Research in Nursing & Health, 8,* 235-241.

Gortner, S. (1990). Nursing values and science: Toward a science philosophy. *Image: Journal of Nursing Scholarship, 22*(2), 101-105.

Henry, W. (1990). Beyond the melting pot. *Time, 135*(15), 28-31.

Herbert, G. (1988). Moral development and unethical behavior among nursing students. *Journal of Professional Behavior, 4*(3), 163-167.

Human Rights. (1983). *Daedalus, 112*(4).

Hutchinson, C., & Bahr, Sr. R. (1991). Types and meanings of caring behaviors among elderly nursing home residents. *Image: Journal of Nursing Scholarship, 23*(2), 85-88.

Illich, I. (1975). *Medical nemesis.* New York: Pantheon Books.

Johnson, D., & Johnson, R. (1988). Critical thinking through structured controversy. *Educational Leadership, 45,* 51-64.

Kayser-Jones, J., Davis, A., Wiener, C., & Higgins, S. (1989). An ethical analysis of an elder's care. *Nursing Outlook, 37*(6), 267-270.

Keasey, C. B. (1979). Cognitive stages in developmental phases: A critique of Kohlberg's stage—structural theory of moral reasoning. *Journal of Higher Education, 8,* 168-181.

Kelly, L. (1988). The ethics of caring: Has it been discarded? *Nursing Outlook, 36,* 17.

Ketefian, S. (1981). Moral reasoning and moral behavior among selected groups of practicing nurses. *Nursing Research, 30,* 55-58.

Kohlberg, L. (1978). The cognitive-development approach to moral education. In P. Scharf (Ed.), *Readings in moral education.* Minneapolis: Winston Press.

Leininger, M., & Watson, J. (1990). *The caring imperative in education.* New York: National League for Nursing.

Murphy, C., & Hunter, H. (1983). *Ethical problems in nurse-patient relationships.* Boston: Allyn & Bacon.

Nokes, K. (1989). Rethinking moral reasoning. *Image: Journal of Nursing Scholarship, 21*(3), 172-175.

Parker, R. (1990). Measuring nurses' moral judgments. *Image: Journal of Nursing Scholarship, 22*(4), 213-218.

Pereson, C., Duckett, I., & Maruyanna, G. (1990). Using structured controversy to promote ethical decision making. *Journal of Nursing Education, 29,* 150-157.

Piaget, J. (1965). *The moral judgment of the child.* New York: Free Press.

Pence, T., & Cantrall, J. (Eds.). (1990). *Ethics in nursing: Anthology.* New York: National League for Nursing.

Rest, J. (1976). New approaches in assessment of moral judgment. In T. Lickona (Ed.), *Moral development and behavior: Theory, research and social issues.* New York: Holt, Rinehart & Winston.

Reverby, S. (1987). A caring dilemma: Womanhood and nursing in historical perspective. *Nursing Research, 36*(1), 5-11.

Rogers, B. (1989). AIDS and ethics in the workplace. *Nursing Outlook, 37*(6), 254-255.

Stevenson, J., & Tripp-Reimer, T. (Eds.). (1990). *Knowledge about care and caring: State of the art and future developments.* Kansas City, MO: American Academy of Nursing.

Tanner, C. (1990). Caring as a value in nursing education. *Nursing Outlook, 38*(2), 70-72.

Thurston, H., Flood, M., Shupe, S., & Gerald, K. (1989). Values held by nursing faculty and students in a university setting. *Journal of Professional Nursing, 5*(4), 199-207.

Viens, D. (1989). A history of nursing's code of ethics. *Nursing Outlook, 37*(1), 45-49.

Watson, J. (1988). Human caring as a moral context for nursing education. *Nursing & Health Care, 9*(8), 432-435.

Young-Mason, J. (1991). The secret sharer as a guide to compassion. *Nursing Outlook, 39*(2), 62-63.

10

Place of Clinical Practice Within a Nursing Curriculum

Competency in practice develops over a period of time as a result of planned sequential experiences in the clinical setting. In practice professions, experiential learning in selected clinical settings is essential if the requisite skills are to be achieved by the student.

Some practice disciplines view clinical practice as the culminating experience in a program, often designating the last term as a period of concentrated practice. Others view clinical practice as a concurrent experience offered throughout a program which evolves in complexity as the program itself addresses more complex phenomena. Some nursing programs subscribe to the latter, while others modify the latter by requiring a period of concentrated clinical experience to provide the knowledge and skills necessary for practice.

The selection of an educational model that provides a concurrent clinical practice component denotes the belief that the acquisition of knowledge and its use in developing practice competencies requires a carefully thought out plan of instruction which demonstrates the integration of learning experiences in both the classroom and clinical field. This plan of instruction is the curriculum of a school. Its development entails continuous attention not only to requisite classroom learning as specified in the outcomes of the program but also to the practice experiences which enable the student to integrate this learning in the evolution of one's own theory of practice. This synthesis process occurs not only at the program level, but occurs each time a clinical course or unit in that course is planned.

CONCEPT OF CURRICULUM

There are varying conceptions of curriculum. In most instances it refers to some type of educational plan in which learning activities are specified to meet particular goals. The key phrase in this definition is *learning activities or experiences.* Most definitions of curriculum refer to this notion of learning experience, which originated with Dewey's (1944) philosophical concept of experience.

Curriculum development entails the determination of outcomes to be attained by students at the conclusion of the program, selection and organization of learning experiences directed toward achievement of these objectives, and provision for formative and summative evaluation strategies to ascertain their fulfillment. These activities in curriculum development are the responsibility of the faculty, with input from students, administrators, and others involved in the educational process.

COMPONENTS OF THE CURRICULUM

A curriculum in nursing includes a conceptual framework of nursing, a philosophy, a statement of purpose, program and level objectives, and a sequence of courses.

Conceptual Framework of Nursing

The first step in the development of a nursing curriculum is the identification of a conceptual framework of nursing. This action precedes the development of a philosophy of the educational program and its purposes and objectives, for the entire curriculum is influenced by the concept of nursing practice which is its core. Orb and Reilly (1991) indicate that the most critical curriculum decision a faculty makes is selecting the conceptual model of nursing to guide its development. The framework delineates concepts about human beings, environment, health, and nursing and their interrelationships and provides an overall structure for the curriculum. The conceptual framework describes the practice of nursing and serves as the basis for the selection and organization of content to be taught in the curriculum. It is the source of what nursing to teach. The conceptual framework also provides a rationale for the selection of learning experiences and direction for evaluation.

Each framework has a unifying concept, such as adaptation or self care, to which other components are related. The unifying concept, giving direction to the curriculum, is evident in every nursing course with a practice component. If adaptation is the unifying element, then students learn nursing assessment in relation to data gathering about stressors and the nature of the client's adaptation to them. Intervention strategies are directed toward promoting adaptation. The conceptual framework provides a way of viewing nursing practice and the focus of the teaching of that practice to learners.

Philosophy

A nursing school's philosophy represents a statement of beliefs to be honored in the nursing program congruent with those of the parent institution. The philosophy reflects the beliefs of the faculty; as such, it is a crucial step in the development of a nursing curriculum, giving "the curriculum its uniqueness" (Van Ort & Putt, 1985, p. 84). The philosophy usually includes beliefs about the individual, health, society, the concept of nursing, nursing education (including the relationship of academic and professional disciplines), the teaching-learning process, evaluation, and personal and professional development of the learner. The philosophy influences the other curriculum components, and it guides the teacher in planning for and carrying out the educational process. Beliefs about the roles of the teacher in terms of teaching, research, and service (also expressed in this document) are reflective of faculty responsibilities in the educational setting.

Purpose

The purposes of the nursing program are reflected in broad statements of program goals. These goals are usually few in number and include: (1) preparing a practitioner who is able to deliver nursing care to clients in multiple settings, (2) preparing a practitioner who will contribute to society, and (3) providing the basis for further development and continued learning. In advanced nursing programs, other goals pertain to contributing to the body of nursing knowledge and development of nursing theory.

Program Objectives

Program objectives as outcomes of the nursing program are derived from the conceptual framework, philosophy, and purpose and in turn provide the basis for determining objectives at other levels of the curriculum. The program objectives reflect the outcomes of learning at the end of the nursing program. The program objectives represent the senior year objectives since it is assumed that the learner will achieve these at the completion of the program.

Program objectives are broadly stated and encompass behaviors in the cognitive, psychomotor, and affective domains. According to Reilly and Oermann (1990), these objectives generally reflect six areas:

1. Theory framework of the curriculum
2. Nursing's methodology: nursing process
3. Concept of inherent worth and dignity of the individual
4. Interrelationships, including interactions with clients and intra- and interdisciplinary interactions
5. Development of the learner
6. Profession, relating to the responsibility and accountability of the learner to the client, the nursing profession, and society. (p. 107)

Examples of program objectives in each of these areas are presented in Table 10-1. The taxonomic level at which the objectives are written

Table 10-1
Examples of Program Objectives

Theory framework:
The learner relates Orem's self-care model to nursing management of individuals, families, and groups throughout the life cycle and in varying health states.

Nursing process:
The learner uses the nursing process in promoting self-care of individuals, families, and groups.

Inherent worth and dignity of client:
The learner formulates judgments which reflect respect for the inherent worth and dignity of the client.

Interrelationships:
The learner assumes responsibility for developing working relationships with clients, families, colleagues, and members of other health care disciplines.

Development of learner:
The learner assumes responsibility for self-growth and development.

Profession:
The learner identifies the accountability of the nurse and profession in meeting the health care needs of society.

---

is determined by faculty in accordance with the nature of the educational program involved. In a baccalaureate and higher degree nursing program, an additional objective may be included on the competency expected of the learner in terms of research.

Level Objectives

The curriculum provides for progressive development of the learner in terms of knowledge, skills, and values. A level is a point in this developmental process at which certain competencies are to be demonstrated. Level objectives represent the behaviors expected, in relation to each of the program objectives, at a particular point in time in the nursing curriculum. This time dimension is often defined in terms of years in the curriculum but also may reflect the achievement expected upon completion of a group of courses or modules. The level needs to represent an adequate period of time for a learning change to occur.

Leveling of Objectives. As previously described, objectives may be leveled by changing the behavior to a higher taxonomic level, changing the variables with which the behavior is carried out or altering both of these. Leveling begins with determination of the program objectives, reflecting the six areas the objectives address, which indicate the outcomes expected at the end of the curriculum. Based on the number of levels in the curriculum, objectives are written to reflect behaviors to be achieved in relation to these six areas at the completion of each level. Course objectives, more specific than level objectives, represent the outcomes expected at the conclusion of a course. Some courses are divided into units and specify objectives for achievement at the completion of the unit. For nursing faculty who develop lesson plans, objectives, derived from the unit objectives, may be written to indicate the learning outcomes at the end of a particular lesson. Objectives can also be developed for individual learning experiences. The developmental process of deriving objectives for instruction and examples of objectives at each level are illustrated in Figure 10-1. Objectives at any point in the curriculum are leveled according to the process described previously.

Courses

The courses in the nursing curriculum provide the means through which the conceptual framework, philosophy, and objectives become operationalized. Each course contains objectives, content, teaching methods, learning experiences, and an evaluation component.

The content of a course, identified from the objectives, represents the subject matter (cognitive, psychomotor, and affective) to be learned. An objective specifies the *learner, behavior* the learner is to demonstrate to indicate competence and *content* to which the behavior relates. The level of competency is determined by the taxonomic level deemed appropriate by faculty. These three components are identified in the following objective:

The nursing student	describes	the nursing process.
Learner	**Behavior**	**Content**

PROGRAM OBJECTIVES
  Example: Baccalaureate nursing program
  C 4.2   The learner uses the nursing process in promoting self-care
          of individuals, families, and groups

LEVEL OBJECTIVES
  Example: Junior level
  C 3.0   The learner uses the nursing process in promoting self-care
          of individuals throughout the life cycle and in varying
          health states

COURSE OBJECTIVES
  Example: Junior level course:
           Acute health problems: A nursing perspective
  C 3.0   The learner uses the nursing process in promoting self-care
          of individuals with acute health problems

UNIT OBJECTIVES
  Example: Unit in course:
           Self-care of individuals with impaired gas exchange
  C 3.0   The learner uses the nursing process in promoting self-care
          of individuals with impaired gas exchange

LESSON OBJECTIVES
  Example: Lesson in unit
  C 3.0   The learner carries out assessment of the client with
          impaired gas exchange

Figure 10-1
Leveling of Objectives in a
Nursing Curriculum

An analysis of the objectives reveals broad content areas to be included in the course, which are then organized logically. Instruction proceeds according to the way in which the content is sequenced.

Development of a course involves the selection of teaching methods and learning experiences directed toward attainment of the course objectives in the classroom, learning laboratory, and clinical setting. One other component of a course plan is the development of an evaluation protocol for assessing the process and outcomes of the course. Evaluation includes strategies for measuring learning in the classroom, learning laboratory, and clinical setting and addresses the need for both formative and summative evaluation.

PLANNING THE CLINICAL COMPONENT

Clinical practice is an integral part of the total nursing curriculum. Experiences in the clinical setting provide for the development of the learner in terms of the knowledge, skills, and values inherent in the profession's practice. Not all nursing courses in the program require a clinical component, for some contribute experiences in analyzing theoretical knowledge and developing cognitive skills which affect the broader sphere of nursing as a practice discipline.

Clinical Objectives

Each clinical nursing course includes objectives for clinical practice and a systematic plan for learning in the practice setting. Rather than preparing separate objectives on the competencies to be achieved in practice, clinical objectives are those course objectives and behaviors for which clinical practice is required for attainment. An objective represents a composite of behaviors that must be accomplished to demonstrate achievement of the objective. These behaviors often involve two or more domains of learning. To identify the clinical objectives, faculty determine which behaviors are to be accomplished in class, in the clinical setting, or in both class and the clinical setting. Some behaviors may also be identified for attainment in the learning laboratory.

Table 10-2 identifies this process for a unit on chronic pain management. The unit is presented in Tables 10-3A and 10-3B where the objectives and behaviors are coded according to the taxonomies. Table 10-2 demonstrates the process by which these six unit objectives with their specified behaviors are designated according to the locus of activities for attainment. There are 46 behaviors: 7 are allocated only to classroom experience; 33 only to clinical experience; while 6 are attainable in both classroom and clinical settings. The decision as to the designation of behaviors of a course or unit as outcomes of the class or clinical experience represents a professional judgment on the part of faculty. Decisions may be altered at any time when indicated with the consensus of faculty involved.

Table 10-2
Classification of Objectives and Behaviors for a Unit on Chronic Pain Management

Unit Objectives and Behaviors	Class	Clinical
I. Relate Orem's self-care model to nursing management of patients with chronic pain		
A. Analyzes the relationship between theories of pain and Orem's model of self-care	X	
B. Evaluates the biopsychosocial and cultural influences on the individual's ability to manage one's own pain	X	X
C. Identifies criteria for distinguishing use of traditional and nontraditional methods of pain management	X	
D. Analyzes the various nontraditional pain management techniques in terms of the individual's and family's learning needs and self-care potential	X	X
E. Evaluates critically scientific rationale for implementing traditional and nontraditional methods of chronic pain management	X	
II. Use the nursing process in promoting self-care of patients with chronic pain		
Assessment:		
A. Carries out a systematic assessment of patient		X
B. Evaluates impact of chronic pain on patient's life style		X

Table 10-2 *(Continued)*

Unit Objectives and Behaviors	Class	Clinical
C. Identifies patient's strategies for coping with pain		X
D. Appraises the impact of biopsychosocial and cultural factors on the patient's response to pain		X
E. Analyzes the influence of support systems on patient's ability to manage chronic pain	X	X
F. Assumes responsibility for identifying one's own values and biases that may affect the assessment		X
G. Analyzes the learning needs of patient and family in relation to chronic pain management		X
H. Formulates nursing diagnoses based on identified self-care deficits		X

Planning:

I. Develops with patient goals of care congruent with nursing diagnoses		X
J. Plans nursing management related to self-care deficits of patient and family		X
K. Supports the patient in decision making relative to options for pain management		X
L. Selects appropriate traditional and nontraditional methods of pain management		X
M. Provides for use of appropriate resources to assist patient and family		X

Implementation:

N. Implements nursing interventions congruent with a scientific rationale, research, and the mutually established plan of care		X
O. Is competent in the use of traditional pain management techniques		X
P. Demonstrates skill in the use of nontraditional pain management techniques		X
Q. Initiates referrals to health care providers and/or agencies essential in assisting patient to meet optimum self-care agency		X
R. Encourages patient in use of his or her own potential and resources in addressing self-care limitations		X
S. Documents pertinent nursing observations and interventions		X

Table 10-2 *(Continued)*

Unit Objectives and Behaviors	Class	Clinical
Evaluation:		
T. Develops criteria for evaluating the effectiveness of the plan toward a decrease in self-care deficit and increase in self-care agency		X
U. Uses criteria in evaluating patient and family outcomes of care in terms of stated goals		X
V. Uses professional nursing standards as a framework for evaluating the process of the delivery of nursing care		X
W. Modifies plan of care as indicated by the evaluation results		X
III. Formulate judgments which reflect respect for the inherent worth and dignity of the patient with chronic pain		
A. Defends the patient's right to be informed regarding traditional and nontraditional methods of chronic pain management relative to their expected outcomes and inherent risks		X
B. Supports the patient's choice regarding the selection of pain control methods		X
C. Provides care reflective of the patient's own sociocultural preferences, psychologic needs, health beliefs, and perception of degree of self-care deficit		X
D. Protects the patient's rights to privacy and confidentiality		X
E. Acts as advocate for patient and/or family when individuals or situations appear to impede progress toward goal attainment		X
IV. Foster facilitative relationships with patients with chronic pain, families and colleagues		
A. Analyzes own interactive behavior within a therapeutic or collegial relationship	X	X
B. Assumes a liaison role between patient and other persons who have an impact upon the health care of the individual		X
C. Contributes readily to discussions and decisions that have an impact on matters concerning the patient's pain management		X

Table 10-2 (Continued)

Unit Objectives and Behaviors	Class	Clinical
D. Maintains ongoing communication with appropriate health providers regarding the plans, implementation, and evaluation of care		X
V. Assume responsibility for continued development of the knowledge base and competencies essential for promoting self-care agency in the presence of chronic pain		
A. Assumes responsibility for expanding one's own knowledge base regarding care of the patient with chronic pain	X	X
B. Maintains knowledge of current research findings which address the phenomenon of pain and its management	X	X
C. Is accountable for seeking out those learning experiences that enhance the development of competencies		X
D. Analyzes research on chronic pain management	X	
VI. Affirm the accountability of nurses and the nursing profession to contribute to the development of a theory of practice for patients with chronic pain		
A. Takes a position on the responsibility of nurses and nursing to protect the public against quackery and other kinds of deceptive methods purported to alleviate chronic pain		X
B. Analyzes societal, political, economic, legal, and ethical factors affecting management of the patient with chronic pain	X	
C. Takes a position on issues related to care of the patient with chronic pain	X	
D. Evaluates the role of the nurse as a significant health team member in the research and practice domains that address pain management	X	
E. Declares a position on nursing's ethical and moral responsibilities in the various pain management methods used in practice		X

The objectives for clinical practice provide the framework for teaching in the field since they specify the learning outcomes to be achieved and give direction to faculty in the selection of teaching methods and learning experiences. They also serve as the basis for evaluating learning, for evaluation focuses on the learner's progress in meeting and attaining these objectives.

Some of the objectives represent learning outcomes achieved in previous courses but are now being taught within the context of the new course plan. Students are held accountable for competency in using these previously learned skills but may need assistance with their application to a new set of variables in a different clinical context.

Planning for Clinical Practice Experience

Since the objectives for clinical practice are already stated when the course or unit objectives are developed, it can be concluded that planning for the clinical experience should occur concurrently with the classroom experience. Once the content for the course or unit is extrapolated from the objectives and arranged in a logical sequence for presentation, both the class and clinical activities are planned concurrently. Some content will be addressed in the classroom and further developed in the clinical setting. Other content will be the purview of only the class experience or only the clinical experience. The plan, however, should demonstrate the locus and related learning and teaching activities, whatever they may be, in terms of the objectives to be achieved.

The proposal being made here considers the theory and clinical components of a practice course as one holistic phenomenon. It is recognized that some curricula separate these components into two courses which may or may not have the prerequisite of integrated experiences in both settings.

The ideal of maintaining the integrity of the relationship of class and clinical experience may be challenged when the numbers of students and availability of clinical settings preclude all students from receiving experience in the same type of setting at the same time. A conceptually developed curriculum with an emphasis on concepts and theories rather than specific entities, such as diseases, enables faculty to plan more effectively for concurrent theory and clinical experiences under these circumstances. In some courses students may be in a variety of clinical settings; some of the experiences may be with children and others with adults. In situations in which students are in varied clinical placements, all learners may be involved in the same classroom instruction that addresses overall concepts and theories. Specific application of these concepts and theories to the populations in the different clinical settings may be taught separately in these settings and then repeated as new learners enter them. For instance, if three credits of a course are allocated for classroom instruction, two of these credits may involve all students in learning about the concepts and theories. The third credit would be allotted to teaching relevant specifics about the populations with whom the students are currently engaged in practice.

As an illustration, in a course that addresses chronic illness, students at any point in time in the course may be with clients in an outpatient service, acute care facility, or community setting. The concepts of chronic illness from the biopsychosocial, economic, and political perspective constitute the general core of classroom activity. In each setting, these concepts are explored in relation to the specifics as they pertain to the population with whom the students are involved.

Many concepts can be addressed with a wide variety of clients. It is important that when diverse client populations are required, the selection is based on relevancy to the concepts rather than to a geographical setting.

Planning for clinical learning experiences requires consideration of the taxonomic level of the objectives, for the teaching methods and learning activities need to promote learning at the level indicated by the objectives. For example, an objective at the application level requires methods and learning activities that enable the student to use concepts and theories in practice. An experience in which the learner merely describes the meaning of the concept is inappropriate for this taxonomic level in which the experience needs to focus on how the concept may be applied in the clinical situation.

In planning the clinical component, consideration should also be given to the types of clinical settings in which students practice and kinds of activities in which they engage throughout the nursing program. The settings and experiences should reflect the scope of nursing practice within the health care system. Clinical experiences in only an acute care setting are not representative of the health care problems learners will encounter in practice. Without variety in clinical settings and experiences throughout the curriculum, it would be difficult for learners to meet many of the clinical objectives in a nursing program.

MODEL FOR A UNIT OF A CLINICAL COURSE

A design for a unit of a clinical course is proposed in Tables 10-3A and 10-3B to demonstrate the interrelationship of class and clinical practice experiences as they relate to specific objectives. The unit illustrated here is one of five units in a senior level nursing course, in a baccalaureate program, on Chronic Health Problems: A Nursing Perspective. The overview describes the purpose of the course, prerequisites, credit allotment, units in the course, teaching personnel, teaching methods, and evaluation strategies.

Course objectives indicate expected achievement at the completion of the course. Unit objectives and related behaviors represent the learning outcomes at the completion of Unit IV: Chronic Pain Management. The objectives are coded as to taxonomic level.

The components of the model shown in Table 10-3B include:

1. Objectives: This column includes the designated number and letter of the objectives and behaviors to which the content and activities relate. It is recognized that an experience may incorporate one or many behaviors, so the same objective and behavior will often be designated at varied points in the unit plan.
2. Content: Derived from the substance of the objectives, the content is organized in a logical sequence within the time constraints of the unit.
3. Teaching Methods: These columns include the activities used by the teacher in addressing the content. One set of activities takes place in the classroom; the other set of activities in the clinical setting.
4. Learning Activities: The experiences in which the learner is involved are noted in the learning activities columns, one within the classroom and the other within the clinical setting.

A significant factor must be noted in viewing this model. In the classroom setting, the time frame for each class is designated. No time frame is noted for the clinical experiences because of the variability of the clinical environment. The intent is to demonstrate that the clinical experiences as noted will occur within the time allocated to the unit.

SUMMARY

A curriculum in nursing includes a conceptual framework of nursing, a philosophy, a statement of purpose, program and level objectives, and a sequence of courses. Not all courses in the nursing program have a clinical component, although clinical practice is needed for those courses reflecting use of theories in practice. Each clinical nursing course includes objectives for clinical practice and a systematic plan for related learning in the practice setting. Rather than representing separate competencies to be achieved, clinical objectives are those course objectives and behaviors for which clinical practice is associated. Some course objectives and behaviors are accomplished in the classroom setting. Others are achieved in clinical, and still others are identified for attainment in both the class and clinical settings. The objectives for clinical practice provide the framework for teaching in the clinical setting since they specify the learning outcomes to be achieved there and give direction to faculty in choosing teaching methods and learning activities.

Content for a course is extrapolated from the objectives and organized in a logical sequence. Some content is addressed in the classroom and further developed in the clinical setting; other content is taught only in the classroom or in clinical practice.

Development of the plan for learning in the clinical setting involves the selection of teaching methods and learning activities to promote attainment of the clinical objectives and meet individual learner needs. Planning for the practice experience occurs concurrently with the classroom experience since the theory and practice components of a clinical course are viewed as a whole. The model included in this chapter illustrates the relationship of the clinical component to the overall course and demonstrates the process of planning for learning in the practice setting within the total course structure.

Table 10-3A
Model for a Unit of Clinical Course

Overview

Course:	Chronic Health Problems: A Nursing Perspective
Purpose:	This course is designed for senior students to enable them to acquire the knowledge, skills, and values necessary for care of patients with chronic health problems. The course focuses on promoting self-care within this patient population.
Prerequisites:	Senior standing. Competency in use of Orem's self-care model of nursing practice.
Course plan:	This is a six credit course with three credits for classroom instruction, three hours per week, and three credits for clinical practice, nine hours per week, over a 15-week period. A 1:3 ratio is used for determining the number of clock hours per week for each credit of clinical experience.
Units in course:	Unit I: Socioeconomic and Political Dimensions of Chronic Health Problems (2 weeks) Unit II: Nursing Management of Chronic Health Problems in Children (3 weeks) Unit III: Nursing Management of Chronic Health Problems in Adults and the Elderly (4 weeks) Unit IV: Chronic Pain Management (3 weeks) Unit V: Nursing Management of Chronic Grief and Depression (3 weeks)
Teaching personnel:	Teaching of the course is a collaborative effort of faculty with expertise in the physiological and psychosocial dimensions of care of children and adults with chronic health problems.
Teaching methods:	Lecture, discussion, media, self-paced module, computer simulation, handouts, readings, small group activities, written assignments, clinical assignments, conferences, role play, demonstrations, observation, nursing rounds.
Evaluation:	Evaluation is based on achievement of the objectives. Evaluation strategies include midterm and final examinations, term paper, observation in clinical setting, patient care conference, two nursing care plans, case study, and log. Student also will complete a self and course evaluation.

Table 10-3A

Course Objectives[a]

At the completion of the course the learner will:

C 4.2   I.   Relate Orem's self-care model to nursing management of patients with chronic health problems

C 4.2   II.   Use the nursing process in promoting self-care of patients with chronic health problems

A 4.1   III.   Formulate judgments which reflect respect for the inherent worth and dignity of patients with chronic health problems

A 4.1   IV.   Foster facilitative relationships with patients with chronic health problems, their families, colleagues, and health team members

A 4.1   V.   Assume responsibility for continued development of the knowledge base and competencies essential for promoting self-care of patients with chronic health problems

A 4.1   VI.   Affirm the accountability of nurses and the nursing profession to contribute to the development of a theory of practice for patients with chronic health problems

Unit IV: Chronic Pain Management Unit Objectives

At the completion of the unit the learner will:

C 4.2   I.   Relate Orem's self-care model to nursing management of patients with chronic pain

C 4.2   II.   Use the nursing process in promoting self-care of patients with chronic pain

A 4.1   III.   Formulate judgments which reflect respect for the inherent worth and dignity of the patient with chronic pain

A 4.1   IV.   Foster facilitative relationships with patients with chronic pain, families, and colleagues

A 4.1   V.   Assume responsibility for continued development of the knowledge base and competencies essential for promoting self-care agency in the presence of chronic pain

A 4.1   VI.   Affirm the accountability of nurses and the nursing profession to contribute to the development of a theory of practice for patients with chronic pain

Unit Objectives and Behaviors

C 4.2   I.   Relate Orem's self-care model to nursing management of patients with chronic pain

[a]The C before the behavior indicates the cognitive domain, the A indicates the affective domain, and the P indicates the psychomotor domain.

Table 10-3A *(Continued)*

C 4.2	A. Analyzes the relationship between theories of pain and Orem's model of self-care
C 4.2	B. Evaluates the biopsychosocial and cultural influences on the individual's ability to manage one's own pain
C 4.2	C. Identifies criteria for distinguishing between the use of traditional and nontraditional methods of pain management
C 4.2	D. Analyzes the various nontraditional pain management techniques in terms of the individual's and family's learning needs and self-care potential
C 4.2	E. Evaluates critically scientific rationale for implementing traditional and nontraditional methods of chronic pain management
C 4.2 II.	Use the nursing process in promoting self-care of patients with chronic pain

Assessment:

C 4.2	A. Carries out a systematic pain assessment of patient
C 4.2	B. Evaluates impact of chronic pain on patient's life style
C 4.2	C. Identifies patient's strategies for coping with pain
C 4.2	D. Appraises the impact of biopsychosocial and cultural factors on the patient's response to pain
C 4.2	E. Analyzes the influence of support systems on patient's ability to manage chronic pain
A 3.3	F. Assumes responsibility for identifying one's own values and biases that may affect the assessment
C 4.2	G. Analyzes the learning needs of patient and family in relation to chronic pain management
C 4.2	H. Formulates nursing diagnoses based on identified self-care deficits

Planning:

C 4.2	I. Develops with patient goals of care congruent with nursing diagnoses
C 4.2	J. Plans nursing management related to self-care deficits of patient and family
A 3.3	K. Supports the patient in decision making relative to options for pain management
C 4.2	L. Selects appropriate traditional and nontraditional methods of pain management
C 4.2	M. Provides for use of appropriate resources to assist patient and family

Table 10-3A *(Continued)*

Implementation:

C 4.2	N. Implements nursing interventions congruent with a scientific rationale, research, and the mutually established plan of care
P 5.0	O. Is competent in the use of traditional pain management techniques
P 3.0	P. Demonstrates skill in the use of nontraditional pain management techniques
C 4.2	Q. Initiates referrals to health care providers and/or agencies essential in assisting patient to meet optimum self-care agency
A 4.1	R. Encourages patient in use of his or her own potential and resources in addressing self-care limitations
C 4.2	S. Documents pertinent nursing observations and interventions

Evaluation:

C 4.2	T. Develops criteria for evaluating the effectiveness of the plan toward a decrease in self-care deficit and increase in self-care agency
C 4.2	U. Uses criteria in evaluating patient and family outcomes of care in terms of stated goals
C 4.2	V. Uses professional nursing standards as a framework for evaluating the process of the delivery of nursing care
C 4.2	W. Modifies plan of care as indicated by the evaluation results
A 4.1	III. Formulate judgments which reflect respect for the inherent worth and dignity of the patient with chronic pain
A 4.1	A. Defends the patient's right to be informed regarding traditional and nontraditional methods of chronic pain management relative to their expected outcomes and inherent risks
A 4.1	B. Supports the patient's choice regarding the selection of pain control methods
C 4.1	C. Provides care reflective of the patient's own sociocultural preferences, psychologic needs, health beliefs, and perception of degree of self-care deficit
A 4.1	D. Protects the patient's rights to privacy and confidentiality
A 4.1	E. Acts as advocate for patient and/or family when individuals or situations appear to impede progress toward goal attainment
A 4.1	IV. Foster facilitative relationships with patients with chronic pain, families, and colleagues
C 4.2	A. Analyzes own interactive behavior within a therapeutic or collegial relationship
A 4.1	B. Assumes a liaison role between patient and other persons who have an impact upon the health care of the individual

Table 10-3A *(Continued)*

A 4.1		C. Contributes readily to discussions and decisions that have an impact on matters concerning the patient's pain management
A 4.1		D. Maintains ongoing communication with appropriate health providers regarding the plans, implementation and evaluation of care
A 4.1	V.	Assume responsibility for continued development of the knowledge base and competencies essential for promoting self-care agency in the presence of chronic pain
A 4.1		A. Assumes responsibility for expanding one's own knowledge base regarding care of the patient with chronic pain
A 4.1		B. Maintains knowledge of current research findings which address the phenomenon of pain and its management
A 4.1		C. Is accountable for seeking out those learning experiences that enhance the development of requisite competencies
C 4.1		D. Analyzes research on chronic pain management
A 4.1	VI.	Affirm the accountability of nurses and the nursing profession to contribute to the development of a theory of practice for patients with chronic pain
A 4.1		A. Takes a position on the responsibility of nurses and nursing to protect the public against quackery and other kinds of deceptive methods purported to alleviate chronic pain
C 4.2		B. Analyzes societal, political, economic, legal, and ethical factors affecting management of the patient with chronic pain
A 4.1		C. Takes a position on issues related to care of the patient with chronic pain
C 4.2		D. Evaluates the role of the nurse as a significant health team member in the research and practice domains that address pain management
A 4.1		E. Declares a position on nursing's ethical and moral responsibilities in the various pain management methods used in practice

Table 10-3B
Model for a Unit of Clinical Course

Objectives[b]	Content	Class Teaching Method[c]
II.J,K	I. Pain: A legitimate concern of nursing	Two hours
	A. Definition	
III.B,E	1. A subjective phenomenon	Lecture/discussion
IV.B	2. Not a single entity	Transparency: Definition
VI.D	3. Perception/threshold/tolerance	of pain
	4. Chronic vs. acute	
	B. Pain: A primary reason for entry into health care system	
	C. Impact of pain	Read letter from patient
	1. Patient's perception	with chronic pain
	D. Nursing's unique contribution	Transparency: Nursing's
	1. Pain: A human response as a focus for nursing intervention	Role in Pain Management
	2. Nurse's responsibility in planning pain management	
	3. Liaison/advocate role	
	E. Patient's rights	
	1. Decision making	
	2. Mutual goal setting	
	II. Pain: Psychosocial factors	
I.B	A. Coping with pain	Film: "Coping with Pain"
	1. Factors affecting pain perception	(25 minutes)
II.B-E	B. Psychological factors affecting pain perception and response	What are some psychological factors affecting pain perception and response? Record on transparency
III.C	1. Emotionally traumatic life experiences	
	2. Personal past experience with pain	
	3. Knowledge level	
	4. Developmental level	What are the effects of developmental level on response to pain?
	a. Influence of stage of development on ability to cope	
	b. Effects of pain on developmental level	
	5. Presence, attitudes, and feelings of others	
	6. Previous coping strategies	
	C. Cultural influences affecting patient's behavioral responses and pain sensations	Transparency: Cultural influences on responses to pain
	1. Sociocultural group	How may religious beliefs influence ability to cope with pain?
	2. Age and sex	
	3. Religion	

Class	Clinical	
Learning Activity	Teaching Method	Learning Activity
Assignment: To be read prior to class 1. Unit objectives 2. Text, "Dealing with Chronic Pain," pp. 40–50		
Participate in discussion View transparency and raise questions	Plan with students for clinical assignment Explain protocol for keeping a log of activities	
Analyze message in letter		
View transparency and discuss		
View film Identify factors affecting pain perception	Clinical assignment Log	Select a patient with chronic pain in the clinical setting. Identify psychological factors affecting patient's pain perception and response and evaluate their implications. Record in log. Identify patient's developmental level and related tasks. Analyze effects of pain on development. Record in log.
View transparency and raise question	Clinical assignment (in or out of clinical setting) Log	Interview one person from a culture other than your own. Inquire regarding: —person's view of pain —how pain is handled within cultural group

Table 10-3B (Continued)

Objectives[b]	Content	Class Teaching Method[c]

	4. Body part involved in pain
	5. Meaning of pain
	6. Cultural ways of coping with pain
	D. Family factors influencing pain perception and response
	  1. Family reaction to chronic pain
	  2. Significance of role development for family member with pain
	    a. "Health leader" role
	    b. Role changes secondary to chronic illness
	E. Environmental factors influencing pain perception and response
	  1. Milieu
	  2. Time of day
	F. Other factors affecting patient's pain perception and response
		Transparency: Family Factors Influencing Pain Perception and Response
		
		Transparency: Environmental Factors Influencing Pain Perception and Response

I.A,C,E	III. Pain theories
	A. Pattern/summation
	  1. Coding of impulses at periphery
	  2. Modulation of impulses by central nervous system
	  3. Limitations of theory
	B. Specificity theory
	  1. Purely anatomical basis for pain perception
	    a. Specific peripheral pain receptors
	    b. Transported via spinothalamic tract in spinal cord
	    c. Pain center in brain
	  2. Limitations of theory
	C. Gate control theory
	  1. Melzack and Wall (1965)
	  2. Attempts to integrate physiologic and psychologic aspects of pain
	  3. Based on interaction of systems
	    a. Stimulation of large diameter fibers "closes" gate to pain
	    b. "Gate" located in substantia gelatinosa of spinal cord
	    c. Presence of a central descending control mechanism
	  4. Implications
	    a. Pharmacologic
	    b. Sensory control of pain
		One hour
		Lecture/discussion
		What is the pattern/summation theory of pain?
		Record on transparency
		
		What is the specificity theory of pain?
		Record on transparency
		
		Handout: Gate Control Theory
		
		What is the scientific rationale underlying the gate control theory of pain?
		
		What are implications of gate control theory of pain?

Class	Clinical	
Learning Activity	Teaching Method	Learning Activity
		—cultural folk remedies —when health care is elicited
View transparency and discuss one's own experiences with family when pain was present	Clinical assignment Log	Select a patient with chronic pain in the clinical setting. Assess family role in terms of health leader role and role changes.
View transparency		Identify implications for care. Record in log.
Assignment: Read chapters on pain theories and traditional pain management techniques in text prior to class		
Participate in discussion		
Read handout and raise questions		
Participate in discussion		
Discuss implications for practice	Clinical conference: Application of gate control theory in practice (one hour)	Describe patient's pain and management strategies in terms of gate control theory.

Table 10-3B *(Continued)*

Objectives[b]	Content	Class Teaching Method[c]
	5. Limitations of theory	
	6. Relationship to self-management of pain	
	D. Endogenous opiates	Transparency: Endogenous Opiates
	1. Location	
	2. Physiologic role in pain perception	
	3. Implications	Handout: Implications for Pain Management
	a. Central control mechanism for gate control theory	
	b. Rationale for hypnosis, acupuncture, and placebos	
	c. Possible use in treatment of pain	
I.C,E	IV. Traditional methods of chronic pain relief	Lecture/discussion
II.J,L,N,O	A. Surgical intervention	
III.A	B. Pain medications	Handout: Pain Medications
V.B,D	1. Utilized alone or with other treatments	
	2. Choice of medication and route dependent on many various factors	What factors influence the choice of medication and route in the treatment of chronic pain?
	3. Classifications	Self-paced module: "Medications for Pain"
	a. Narcotics	
	b. Nonnarcotics	
	c. Placebos	What is a placebo?
	(1) Use vs. misuse	
	(2) Legal and ethical considerations	
	4. Considerations in medication administration	
	a. Need for ongoing assessment and adjustments	
	b. Scheduling: ATC vs. PRN	
	c. Patient rights	
I.C,D,E	V. Nontraditional pain management techniques	Three hours Lecture/discussion

Class	Clinical	
Learning Activity	Teaching Method	Learning Activity

View transparency and raise questions

Read handout and discuss

Participate in discussion

Read handout and raise questions

	Clinical assignment Log	Choose a patient with chronic pain in the clinical setting. Review the medical record. Identify pain medications, drug classification of each, and rationale for use. Describe other methods of pain management. Record in log.
Complete module in learning laboratory		
	Clinical conference; Incident process: Issues associated with placebos (one hour)	Analyze incident in clinical conference.

Assignment: Read text and references from bibliography on nontraditional pain management techniques prior to next class

Participate in discussion

Table 10-3B (Continued)

Objectives[b]	Content	Class Teaching Method[c]

II.J,L,N,P
III.A
V.B,D
	A. Hypnosis
	  1. General effects of hypnosis
	    a. Decreased awareness of pain
	    b. Substitution of other feelings for pain
	    c. Altered meaning of pain
	  2. Advantages of hypnosis techniques
	  3. Limiting factors of hypnosis
	    a. Mechanism of action unknown
	    b. Concern about practicality
	    c. Majority of people unhypnotizable
	
	B. Distraction
	  1. Characteristics of distraction
	    a. Focus of attention on alternate stimulus
	    b. Sensory shielding effect
	    c. Use of existing objective or physical stimuli
	  2. Specific distraction techniques
	
	    a. Visual concentration and rhythmic massage
	    b. Slow rhythmic breathing
	    c. Sing and tap rhythm
	    d. Auditory stimulation via earphone
	  3. Major advantages of distraction
	
	  4. Problems related to distraction techniques
	C. Relaxation
	  1. Definition/conceptualization of relaxation
	    a. Relaxation vs. "common concepts" of relaxation
	    b. Interruption of stress-tension pain cycle
	  2. Overview of relaxation techniques
	    a. Meditation
	    b. Yoga
	    c. Progressive muscle relaxation
		What are the effects of hypnosis in relation to pain control?
		Record on transparency
		
		Transparency: Advantages of Hypnosis in Pain Management
		Transparency: Disadvantages of Hypnosis in Pain Management
		Videotape of hypnosis of client with chronic pain (10 minutes)
		Transparency: Characteristics of distraction
		
		What are examples of distraction techniques?
		Handout: Distraction Techniques
		Has anyone ever used distraction techniques?
		
		Transparency: Problems with Use of Distraction
		
		Transparency: Overview of Relaxation Techniques

Class		Clinical
Learning Activity	**Teaching Method**	**Learning Activity**

View transparency and raise questions

View transparency and discuss

View videotape and discuss

View transparency

| | Demonstration | Following demonstration of distraction techniques, choose a partner and practice techniques presented. |

Read handout and discuss

Share with class previous experiences with use of distraction techniques

Demonstrate techniques to peers.

| | Clinical assignment
Clinical conference: Use of distraction (30 minutes) | Select a patient with chronic pain in the clinical setting.
Teach patient and/or family one or several of the distraction techniques.
Discuss experience in conference. |

View transparency
Discuss problems with use of distraction

View transparency

Table 10-3B *(Continued)*

Objectives[b]	Content	Class Teaching Method[c]

	d. Biofeedback
	e. Other
	3. Effects of relaxation
	  a. Reduction of stress and anxiety
	  b. Distraction from pain
	  c. Alleviation of muscle tension or contraction
	  d. Enhancement of other pain relief measures
		What are the effects of relaxation techniques?
		List on transparency

	4. Specific relaxation techniques
	  a. Deep breath-clench fists-yawn
	  b. Heartbeat breathing
	  c. Music for relaxation
	  d. Slow, rhythmic breathing
	  e. Progressive relaxation of muscle groups
		What are some specific examples of relaxation techniques?
		Handout: Relaxation Techniques
		Tape recording of relaxation method of pain control: "Conditioned Relaxation" (10 minutes)

	5. Potential problems of relaxation techniques	What are problems and limitations associated with relaxation techniques? Record on transparency

	D. Guided imagery
	  1. Definition of guided imagery
	  2. Effects of imagery
	    a. Reduction in pain intensity
	    b. Elimination of pain
	    c. Promotion of muscle relaxation
	    d. Reduction of anxiety
	    e. Other changes
		What are the effects of guided imagery in relation to pain control?
		Record on transparency

	3. Specific imagery techniques
	    a. Images in conversation
	    b. Standardized images
	      (1) Breathing out pain
	      (2) Ball of healing energy
	      (3) Healthy body
	      (4) Beach scene
		Handout: Imagery Techniques

Class	Clinical	
Learning Activity	Teaching Method	Learning Activity

	Demonstration	Following demonstration of relaxation techniques, select a partner and practice techniques using handout as guide.
Read handout and discuss		
Listen to tape and discuss		Demonstrate techniques to peers.
	Clinical assignment Clinical conference: Use of Relaxation (30 minutes)	Select a patient with chronic pain in the clinical setting. Teach the patient and/or family one of the pain relaxation techniques. Discuss experience in conference.
Read handout and raise questions		
	Observation Log	Observe in pain clinic. Identify patients' methods for managing pain and analyze patient responses. Describe methods in terms of underlying theory. Record in log.

Table 10-3B (Continued)

Objectives[b]	Content	Class Teaching Method[c]

II.A to W	VI. Nursing process
	  A. Assessment of patient with chronic pain
	    1. Assessment categories
		Two hours
		Lecture/discussion
		What areas need to be included in the assessment of the patient with chronic pain?

III.B,C IV.A,B-D	a. Universal self-care requisites b. Developmental self-care requisites	
V.B,D	c. Health deviation self-care requisites: pain assessment (1) Impact of pain on life style (2) Patient's previous coping strategies	Record on transparency
	d. Conditioning factors 2. Self-care agency of patient with chronic pain	Transparency: Conditioning Factors
	3. Self-care deficit of patient with chronic pain	Case study: Assessment of patient with chronic pain
	4. Influence of nurse's values and biases 5. Formulation of nursing diagnosis 6. Assessment tool for client with chronic pain: McGill-Melzack (Modified)	Handout: McGill-Melzack Pain Questionnaire

	B. Planning care for patient with chronic pain
	1. Establishment of mutual goals
	2. Patient's role in decision making
	3. Design of nursing system to meet goals
	  a. Selection of pain management methods: traditional and nontraditional
	  b. Identification of appropriate resources
	4. Planning nursing system
		Interactive video (IAV)

	C. Intervention for patient with chronic pain 1. Interaction of nurse and patient 2. Comfort measures for patient with chronic pain	What actions characterize the intervention phase of the nursing process? Computer simulation: "Mrs. Shilkraut: An Uncomfortable, Terminal Patient" Learning laboratory

Class	Clinical	
Learning Activity	Teaching Method	Learning Activity
Assignment: Read text and reference from bibliography on nursing process with patient with chronic pain and issues related to pain management.		
Review McGill-Melzack assessment tool		
Participate in discussion	Nursing rounds Role play	Participate in rounds. Two students to role play and others observe. Analyze using assessment criteria presented in class.
View transparency		
Divide in groups of six Analyze case and identify nursing diagnoses	Clinical assignment Written assignment: Assessment	Select a patient with chronic pain in the clinical setting. Assess patient and identify nursing diagnoses.
Discuss handout		Complete assessment tool and submit.
Complete assigned part of IAV (on care of patient with pain)	Clinical assignment	Using same patient for assessment, establish goals to be achieved and plan to meet goals.
Discuss in terms of pain management		
Complete computer simulation in learning laboratory or home		

Table 10-3B *(Continued)*

Objectives[b]	Content	Class Teaching Method[c]

	3. Traditional and/or nontraditional interventions for patient
	4. Initiation of referrals
	5. Role as liaison and clarifier of information
	6. Documentation
	D. Evaluation of care
	  1. Evaluation criteria
	    a. Meeting of self-care deficits
	    b. Enhancement of self-care agency in relation to pain management
	  2. Evaluation of outcome
	    a. Achieved outcome vs. stated goals
	    b. Adequacy of plan
	  3. Modification of plan
		What actions characterize the evaluation process?

II.V
III.A,B,D,E
IV.C
V.A,C
VI.A,B,C,E
	VII. Personal and professional issues related to pain management
	A. Standards of care as basis of pain management
	
	B. Relation of personal philosophy to care of patients with chronic pain
	
	C. Responsibility for pain management
	  1. Patient's responsibility
	  2. Nurse's responsibility
	  3. Responsibility of other health team members
	D. Nurse's role as change agent
	
	E. Nurse's role as advocate
	F. Patient's rights
	  1. Refusal of treatment
	  2. Access to information
	  3. Privacy and confidentiality
	  4. Quality care
	  5. Termination of provider-patient relationship
	  6. Self-determination
	G. Codes for nurses: Ethical concepts
		One hour
		Lecture/discussion
		Handout: Use of Nursing Standards in Pain Management
		
		Who is responsible for managing pain?
		
		How can nurses initiate change that will result in more effective pain management for the client?

Class	Clinical	
Learning Activity	Teaching Method	Learning Activity
	Clinical assignment	Using same patient as for assessment and planning phase, implement plan including at least one nontraditional pain management technique.
	Clinical assignment Peer review conference: Evaluation of management plan (30 minutes per student)	Using same patient as assessment, planning, and implementation; evaluate effectiveness of care and suggest modifications in management plan. Present patient and management plan in conference for peer review.
Participate in discussion		
Read handout and raise questions		
Discuss responsibilities	Log	Complete self-exploration exercise on beliefs and values associated with pain and pain management. Analyze care provided to patient in terms of (a) relationship of personal philosophy to care and (b) responsibilities of patient and health care providers for care. Record in log.
	Issue conference: Patient rights in pain management (one hour)	Read vignette on patient rights. Analyze situation and discuss in conference.

Table 10-3B (Continued)

Objectives[b]	Content	Class Teaching Method[c]
	H. Ethical dilemmas in chronic pain management	Decision-making situation on ethical dilemma

	I. Accountability in chronic pain
	  1. Precautions against contributing to patient's pain
	  2. Societal, political, and economic issues
	  3. Recognition of different pain philosophies
	    a. Nursing vs. medicine
	    b. Patient's perception of own pain management
	  4. Quackery
	    a. Nurse's role in informing public
	    b. Patient's perception of own pain management
	J. Need for continued learning in relation to pain management	

V.B,D VI.D	VIII. Future directions in chronic pain management A. Transforming research into clinically useful information	Lecture/discussion

	B. Nursing research and pain management
	  1. Significance to nursing
	  2. Use of clinical nursing research in practice
	C. Future directions for nursing research
	IX. Summary of unit
		Written assignment: Critique of research

[b]Objectives are numbered according to the list of unit objectives and behaviors.

[c]Questions included with Class: Teaching Methods are to be asked by the teacher to initiate discussion of related content. (The information in this table has been adapted from course work completed by Barbara E. Banfield, Lula B. Lester, Joyce C. Miller, Judi Schneider, and Katherine M. Zimnicki in the Master's program at the College of Nursing, Wayne State University, Detroit, Michigan, with permission.)

Class	Clinical	
Learning Activity	Teaching Method	Learning Activity
Divide into groups of six. Analyze decision-making situation and discuss in small groups		
	Multidisciplinary conference	Attend multidisciplinary conference on patient with chronic pain.
	Log	Record observations in log.
Participate in discussion		
Read one article describing nursing research in area of pain management.		
Critique research and identify implications for clinical practice.		

REFERENCES

Dewey, J. (1944). *Democracy and education.* New York: Macmillan.
Orb, A., & Reilly, D. E. (1991). Changing to a conceptual base curriculum. *International Nursing Review, 38*(2), 56-60.
Reilly, D. E., & Oermann, M. H. (1990). *Behavioral objectives: Evaluation in nursing* (3rd ed.). New York: National League for Nursing.
Van Ort, S. R., & Putt, A. M. (1985). *Teaching in collegiate school of nursing.* Boston: Little, Brown.

BIBLIOGRAPHY

Bevis, E. O., & Watson, J. (1989). *Toward a caring curriculum: A new pedagogy for nursing.* New York: National League for Nursing.
Conrad, C. F., & Pratt, A. M. (1983). Making decisions about the curriculum. *Journal of Higher Education, 54,* 16-30.
Eble, K. E. (1988). *The craft of teaching* (2nd ed.). San Francisco: Jossey-Bass.
Fawcett, J. (1989). *Analyses and evaluation of conceptual models of nursing* (2nd ed.). Philadelphia: F.A. Davis.
King, I. M. (1986). *Curriculum and instruction in nursing: Concepts and processes.* East Norwalk, CT: Appleton-Century-Crofts.
Lawrence, S. A., & Lawrence, R. M. (1983). Curriculum development: Philosophy, objectives, and conceptual framework. *Nursing Outlook, 31,* 160-163.
National League for Nursing (1989). *Curriculum revolution: Reconceptualizing nursing education.* (Pub. No. 15-2280). New York: National League for Nursing.
Reilly, D. E. (1975). Why a conceptual framework? *Nursing Outlook, 23,* 566-569.
Reilly, D. E. (Ed.). (1978). *Teaching and evaluating the affective domain in nursing programs.* Thorofare, NJ: Charles B. Slack.
Scales, F. S. (1985). *Nursing curriculum development, structure, and function.* East Norwalk, CT: Appleton-Century-Crofts.
Smith, C. E. (1984). Process curriculum in nursing contrasted to product orientation. *Journal of Nursing Education, 23,* 167-169.
Torres, G., & Stanton, M. (1982). *Curriculum process in nursing: A guide to curriculum development.* Englewood Cliffs, NJ: Prentice-Hall.
Tyler, R. W. (1949). *Basic principles of curriculum and instruction.* Chicago: University of Chicago Press.

11

Clinical Evaluation

Clinical evaluation is the process of obtaining information for making judgments about the learner's performance in the clinical setting. Formative evaluation represents feedback to the learner regarding progress toward meeting the objectives for clinical practice, whereas summative evaluation provides information on the extent to which the objectives have been attained. This distinction between formative and summative evaluation is important in teaching in the clinical setting. The design must account for both formative and summative evaluation and provide direction as to when to evaluate and as to the how and what of evaluation.

The climate in which the clinical evaluation takes place is a critical determinant of the way the learner perceives the process. A supportive climate with mutual trust and respect between teacher and learner is essential for evaluation to be viewed as a means for growth and to be valued by the learner.

The nature of nursing practice and varying competencies to be achieved in the clinical setting require multiple methods for judging student learning. Evaluation methods are classified as: observation, written communication, oral communication, simulation, and self-evaluation. The teacher chooses evaluation strategies based on the objectives for clinical practice, individual learner needs, and other variables associated with the clinical experience.

CONCEPT OF EVALUATION

Evaluation is the process of obtaining information for making judgments about learners. The educational process results in changes in learners; evaluation provides the means through which these changes are assessed. Through the evaluation process, information is provided to determine student progress toward goal attainment, identify learning needs, and propose strategies for improving student learning.

Evaluation serves three major purposes: (1) selection of students for a given nursing program; (2) assessment of student learning in varied settings—classroom, learning laboratory, and clinical setting; and (3) program revision and determination of program success. The focus of this chapter is the second purpose, i.e., evaluation of student learning, although faculty teaching in any nursing program should also be knowledgeable regarding the assessment of students for entry into the program and the processes of program and curriculum evaluation.

Evaluation is a dynamic, continuous process interwoven with the teaching-learning process. This view of evaluation emphasizes its relationship to growth of the learner, for the judgments made facilitate the learner's own further development of knowledge, skills, and potential essential for professional practice. Evaluation carried out properly in an environment of trust and respect between teacher and learner aids both the teacher in the instructional process and the student in the learning process. Feedback to the learner, obtained through evaluation, is essential for improvement in learning.

There are two major types of evaluative processes: formative and summative. Formative evaluation represents feedback to the learner regarding the learner's progress in meeting the objectives. Occurring throughout the instructional process, formative evaluation is diagnostic in nature, providing information to assist in correcting learning deficiencies and promoting demonstrated abilities. Evaluation that is formative enables the teacher and student to identify areas in which further learning is needed and plan relevant learning experiences. The focus of such evaluation is on assisting the student in meeting the clinical objectives. Formative evaluation is concerned with the learner's progress during the clinical learning experience, not the end of it; it relies on feedback to guide the learner and teacher to aspects of learning which need further attention (Reilly & Oermann, 1990). With its diagnostic focus, data obtained through formative evaluation are not subjected to the grading process. Wilhite (1990) refers to formative evaluation as diagnostic evaluation in which the teacher provides learners with information on their strengths and weaknesses (p. 39).

Summative evaluation, end of instruction evaluation, provides information on the extent to which the learner has achieved the objectives. Such evaluation occurs at the end of a unit or course and is used to determine the grade for the clinical experience. Summative evaluation is "final," stating what has been accomplished rather than what can be. It is concerned with how students have changed as a result of the instruction.

Summative evaluation, while informing the teacher and student at the conclusion of an instructional period as to the degree of attainment of objectives, is not intended to identify learning deficiencies nor the appropriate experiences to assist in overcoming them. Further, with summative evaluation, objectives not mastered are often identified too late in the instructional process for students to have an opportunity to meet them.

The distinction between formative and summative evaluation is important in teaching in the clinical setting for it is formative evaluation that, as an integral part of the teaching-learning process, provides information to the learner as to knowledge and skills which have been attained and those for which further learning is needed; it also guides the teacher in planning relevant activities to assist the student in this process. Reilly and Oermann (1990) emphasize that "the concept of formative evaluation is generally accepted in principle by many teachers, but a gap exists between expressed belief and action" (p. 128). While faculty espouse the value of such evaluation, in practice it is often not an integral part of the instructional process. In a study on faculty and student perceptions of effective clinical teachers, both groups of subjects reported on the need for teachers to be fair in evaluation and provide feedback on student progress (Bergman & Gaitskill, 1990). A commitment to formative evaluation requires that a systematic approach be developed and feedback to learners be given on a continuous basis, not for use in grading but for facilitating learner growth and development. Effective clinical evaluation also requires summative evaluation that is conducted periodically.

Types of Evaluation

The distinction between norm- and criterion-referenced evaluation is important in planning for evaluation in the clinical setting. Norm-referenced evaluation is designed to compare a student's performance with that of a group of students. Such an interpretation demonstrates that a student has more or less knowledge, skill, or ability than others in the group. The learner's performance is thus *referenced* to that of the *norm* group. Rating the achievement of students in clinical practice in relation to other students in the clinical group represents an example of this approach to clinical evaluation.

In contrast, criterion-referenced evaluation compares students not in relationship to others but in terms of some performance standards. The basic intent of this type of evaluation is to measure the performance of students in relation to these standards. With criterion-referenced evaluation, the criteria to be met are established by faculty and known to learners in advance of any evaluation. The objectives of a unit or course identify the behaviors to be achieved which are based on acceptable standards. Instead of indicating that the student in clinical practice is "average," representing a normative judgment, criterion-referenced evaluation using standards indicates the learner's attainment of the clinical objectives. Criterion-referenced evaluation is the approach most relevant to clinical evaluation within a nursing program since competency in terms of specific knowledges, skills, and values is a critical outcome. Certain actions must be carried out in nursing. These actions are executed skillfully for safe and efficient practice to occur. Criterion-referenced evaluation addresses this notion. The existence of goal-free evaluation, however, must be acknowledged and recognized in the evaluation. Learning beyond the clinical objectives does occur and is significant.

NATURE OF CLINICAL EVALUATION PROCESS

Clinical evaluation is a judgmental process, reflecting the values and beliefs of the participants. Value is part of the word and since values are personally chosen, there is a subjective involvement in all aspects of the process.

E | V A L U | A T I O N

It is apparent, then, that there is no such process as "objective evaluation," which is an act of rendering judgments about performance in terms of criteria that are totally external to the evaluator. Evaluation is always subjective for it involves human beings with their own set of values that influence the process.

This value component of evaluation makes it critical for faculty to examine their values, attitudes, beliefs, biases, and prejudices about the process itself and the matter being evaluated, for these influence the judgments made of students in the field. Values affect the teacher's observations and interpretations of their meaning; the learner's values influence his or her own perception of performance in clinical practice and interpretation of the evaluative statements made by others in regard to the performance. The evaluation process can "enhance the student's personal development and learning or destroy the incentive to learn" (Reilly & Oermann, 1990, pp. 127–128). The way in which it is used depends on the teacher's beliefs about the process and role of evaluation in the clinical setting.

Quality of Fairness in Clinical Evaluation

Whereas clinical evaluation cannot be objective, it can be fair; this quality of fairness in the evaluative process should be the goal of the faculty. Fairness has two requisites: (1) clarity of the objectives identified for the clinical experience and (2) supportive climate within which the evaluation takes place. In Bergman and Gaitskill's (1990) research on clinical teaching effectiveness in nursing, students and faculty emphasized the importance of fairness in evaluating students in the clinical setting.

Clinical Objectives. The clinical objectives communicate to the learner the behaviors to be developed and, in turn, the focus of evaluation. These objectives indicate for the learner the competencies to be evaluated; the student can then direct learning toward them. The learner is thus free to learn with knowledge of the outcomes of learning to be judged. The clinical objectives also direct the teacher as to the specific behaviors to be evaluated in the clinical setting, rather than allowing the teacher's personal desires and beliefs to become the focus of the evaluation. The clinical objectives represent a contract between learner and teacher, communicating to the student the outcomes to be judged and providing structure for the teacher so that these objectives will be addressed in the evaluation.

Psychosocial Climate of Clinical Evaluation. The climate within which the evaluation takes place is a critical determinant of the way the learner perceives the evaluation process. A supportive climate denoting trust and respect between teacher and student is essential if evaluation is to be viewed by the learner as a *learning* experience, providing needed feedback for improvement in learning. Students must value feedback from the teacher and view it as an integral part of developing competence in clinical practice. A trusting relationship between teacher and learner will enable students to value feedback and seek from the teacher evaluation of performance as the learning process occurs. Hedin (1989) emphasizes the importance of faculty sharing themselves as human beings in the clinical teaching process and demonstrating a deep respect for the learner. "Concern and caring are earmarks of this relationship" (Hedin, 1989, p. 76). There is a special quality of caring in the teacher-student relationship which places evaluation within the context of promoting growth and further development of the learner.

Development of a supportive climate for clinical evaluation requires faculty clarification of one's own beliefs about evaluation. The teacher's concept of evaluation influences the way in which it is carried out. Evaluation treated as a means for control of the learner does not promote a climate in which evaluation is perceived by students as an integral part of the learning process. Instead, learners are forced to direct energies to surviving in the system rather than using the teacher as a resource for learning. A humanistic approach to clinical evaluation considers evaluation as a process for growth and development of the learner. In this context, clinical evaluation is viewed as a diagnostic process providing information to learners for their further development.

Learning in the clinical setting is a difficult process for it places students in a vulnerable position. Learning, especially that which requires a demonstrated performance, occurs as a public event in front of the teacher, clients, and sometimes even staff and peers, often resulting in the student experiencing feelings of anxiety and stress. Clinical evaluation takes place under similar circumstances, and this vulnerability of the student must be acknowledged by faculty. Much of the data obtained for clinical evaluation is through observation of the learner. The act of being observed during performance is in itself stressful. A climate based on trust, respect, and caring between teacher and learner serves to minimize some of the anxieties inherent in evaluation in the clinical setting.

Kleehammer, Hart, and Keck (1990) examined aspects of nursing students' clinical experiences which were anxiety-producing. Both junior and senior nursing students participated in the study. Areas creating stress for students in the clinical setting included communication and procedural aspects of care, interpersonal relationships with other health care providers, and interactions with faculty. When students were asked to identify the most anxiety-producing aspect of clinical, they reported, among other situations, that evaluation and observation by faculty were both stressful. Kleehammer et al. (1990) emphasize that these processes "should be done in a supportive, nonthreatening manner and be used for formative guidance" (p. 186).

Meisenhelder (1982) emphasizes the need to remain positive and supportive in the clinical evaluation process. Learners who feel threatened by the teacher will not seek feedback nor value what is given. Placed in this situation, they are deterred from their pursuit of knowledge.

RELATIONSHIP OF CLINICAL EVALUATION TO OBJECTIVES

Clinical evaluation is based on the objectives established for clinical practice which are those course objectives and behaviors for which clinical practice is required for attainment. These objectives address competencies in the cognitive, psychomotor, and affective domains at different taxonomic levels. The level of competency at which the behaviors are evaluated is determined by the taxonomic level. Strategies for evaluation need to provide data for judging learning at the particular level addressed by the taxonomy.

Cognitive Domain

Evaluation of cognitive learning relates to the learner's acquisition of the knowledge base needed for problem solving and decision making and the ability to use these skills in practice. At the lower levels of the cognitive taxonomy, evaluation is directed toward assessment of the student's knowledge and understanding of relevant concepts and theories pertinent to cognitive skill development. The student's ability to comprehend and relate data and extrapolate meaning for action is important at these lower levels. At the application level, evaluation focuses on the learner's ability to *use* abstract and factual knowledge including concepts and theories in practice. At the analysis level, evaluation addresses the ability to problem solve and make decisions through an analytic process. Evaluation reflects skill in analyzing data, comparing different alternatives and their consequences, and assessing how concepts and theories relate to one another. Strategies for evaluation at the synthesis level focus on the learner's creativity and skill in developing new products relevant to clinical practice, such as the development of one's own conceptual framework of nursing practice. It is at the evaluation level in which ability to make judgments based on internal and external criteria, such as through research, is assessed.

Affective Domain

Evaluation of affective learning in the clinical setting relates to two aspects: the experiencing behaviors of the learner which may be evidenced in practice, and the critical thinking behaviors vital to the element of choice in value development (Reilly, 1978; Reilly, 1989). It is important that evaluative data be obtained on both practice and cognition. Evaluation of the learner's behavior in clinical practice with clients and staff without cognitive evaluation does not enable the teacher to differentiate practice as value based or as a reflection of compliant or imitative behavior. Evaluation of cognitive behavior without assessment of the learner's practice only provides data on what the student *says* will be his or her own position.

The first two levels of the affective taxonomy address value indicators where beliefs are expressed and some evidence of behavior is presented. Evaluation at these levels provides data on the student's acknowledgement of the existence of a given value or a situation, condition, or phenomenon and acting on or responding to it. At the third level, valuing, patterning of behavior becomes significant; thus, evaluative data must be acquired over a period of time from more than one clinical experience. Evaluation at this taxonomic level, therefore, requires data collected over time to ascertain *consistency* of behavior with stated values. This principle of evaluating affective behavior in practice over time applies to evaluation of learning at the upper levels of the taxonomy where commitment to the underlying value is evident.

Psychomotor Domain

Evaluation of psychomotor performance competency relates to judgments of the learner's accuracy, coordination, and speed in performance. Judgment of psychomotor skill at the first two taxonomic levels reflects learner ability to perform actions with guidance, although lacking in coordination. Errors in performance and inability to carry out the skill within a reasonable time are to be anticipated at this level of development. At the precision level, performance is characterized by accuracy and ability to carry out the skill without use of a model. Critical elements of the skill are without error, although some errors may occur with other actions not requisite to effective performance of the skill. Evaluation at this level also involves collecting data on the learner's coordination in performance. It is at the articulation level that speed and timing become significant elements to be evaluated in judging skill performance. The student is able to perform the act within a reasonable time. This dimension of speed is best evaluated in the clinical setting in which it is possible to judge ability to carry out the skill with clients and adapt it as needed. Evaluation of psychomotor learning at the upper level of the taxonomy is intended to ascertain the integration of the act in nursing practice. Performance should reflect a consistently high level of coordination and competence.

Multidomain Performance

Except in instances of evaluating specifics, much evaluation entails assessment of behaviors in two or three domains of learning. This is evident in performance evaluation situations where the student is involved in administering care to a client, thus requiring an assessment of the integration of cognitive, psychomotor and affective skills. In this situation, the learner is engaged in an activity requiring a direct observation of the implementation of theory in practice. Much of performance evaluation is conducted as formative evaluation and summative data are derived from these observations.

Johnson, Lehman, and Sandoval (1988) describe use of a clinical examination for summative evaluation purposes. In this examination, several evaluation methods are used, including simulation, verbal reports, and written products. Each student is evaluated using criteria based on the course objectives. The test is based on a clinical situation and divided into six activities each with specific criteria established for evaluation. The clinical examination provides summative evaluation data about student performance. It may be used for specific nursing actions or for a holistic approach to providing care.

METHODS OF EVALUATING CLINICAL PRACTICE

Clinical practice is complex and as such cannot be evaluated by one method. Since nursing practice encompasses behaviors in the cognitive, psychomotor, and affective domains, it requires an evaluation protocol that contains multiple strategies for appraising the learner's practice competence in all three domains as appropriate.

Reilly and Oermann (1990) identify five reasons for providing diversity in evaluation strategies:

1. Complexity of human behavior
2. Individual differences in responses to learning
3. Suitability of specific evaluation approaches to specific types of learning behavior
4. Motivational factor of evaluation
5. Creative dimension to the evaluation process (pp. 133-134)

The focus of clinical evaluation is the *student* and the learner's growth and continued development. Any evaluation strategy which provides data for making judgments about the student's practice is appropriate. Evaluation methods applicable for use in the clinical setting are classified as: (1) observation, (2) written communication, (3) oral communication, (4) simulation, and (5) self-evaluation.

Observation

Observation of learner performance is a major means of evaluating students in clinical practice. Through observation, judgments may be made regarding cognitive, psychomotor, and affective performance behaviors. There are two components to any observation of learner performance; (1) the behaviors observed in the situation (data) and (2) the inference or judgment as implied by the interpretation of these behaviors. The data reflect the actual performance without the observer's interpretation. Most observations also include statements of judgments about the behavior based on specific criteria established by the teacher, learner, or both. It is important in use of observation for clinical evaluation that both teacher and learner are clear as to the data collected and the inferences made; often, different interpretations may be made of the same data.

Difficulties in the use of observation methods lie with: (1) the influence of teacher variables on the observation and the resulting judgments, (2) focus of the observation, and (3) sampling of behaviors observed which may or may not be representative of the usual level of performance of the student. Any observation of a learner in the clinical setting is influenced by the teacher's background, past experiences, values, attitudes, and biases. These teacher variables affect the actual observation, i.e., the behaviors noted in the clinical situation and the resulting interpretations.

A second problem in use of observation of learner performance relates to the focus of the observation. In any clinical situation multiple aspects of the learner's behavior may be selected for emphasis in an observation if that observation is not directed toward predetermined behaviors. For example, in observing a student changing a dressing on a client, without identification of the exact behaviors to be evaluated, the teacher could focus on any one or more of the following: (1) the dressing change procedure, (2) learner's use of nonverbal techniques, (3) relationship with the client, (4) means of preparing the client for the dressing change, and (5) other aspects of particular interest to the faculty. Faculty "see different things" in any observation. For this reason, observation should be directed toward specific clinical objectives to be evaluated which are known to both faculty and student.

Another difficulty with use of observation relates to the need for an adequate sampling of behaviors over time which often means data must be obtained from various sources before conclusions are made relative to the learner's typical performance in a particular area. Observations of performance are inevitably based on a sample of the learner's total clinical experience, so an adequate number of observations or data obtained through multiple means is necessary before drawing conclusions about the learner's achievement of specific clinical objectives.

Discussion of observations made during clinical practice with the involved learner is critical to provide for feedback, clarification, and validation of perceptions and interpretation. Litwack, Linc, and Bower (1985) emphasize the importance of providing continual feedback to students particularly in terms of observations made of their performance. Observations best fulfill a formative evaluation purpose if learners examine the data with faculty in terms of areas for further growth and development and instructional strategies for improving behavior.

Specific observations can rarely be recalled over time for a group of learners and, therefore, are generally recorded. Four methods for documenting behaviors observed in practice are: (1) anecdotal note, (2) critical incident, (3) rating scale, and (4) videotape.

Anecdotal Note. An anecdotal note is a narrative description of the behavior and activities of the learner, recorded in relation to a specified clinical objective(s). Some faculty enlarge the scope of the anecdotal note by including an interpretation of the behavior. In this case the description of the observable behavior, the data, is recorded separately from the interpretation. The anecdotal note thus represents a record of observations made in the clinical setting. Provision should be made for learners to include their own perceptions and judgments of the behavior as recorded.

Effective use of anecdotal notes can be increased by developing a systematic approach to their collection. In determining evaluation strategies, the teacher decides on methods by which each objective is to be judged. Reilly and Oermann (1990) recommend that at the time certain clinical objectives are identified for evaluation by anecdotal notes, the number of notes to be recorded for each student be specified. Such a decision, however, does not limit the total number of anecdotal notes written, for the teacher can obtain more data about student performance through this method than originally planned if the student is informed. Anecdotal notes are not the same as general notations a faculty might make after an observation.

In addition to identifying the behaviors to be evaluated with observation and anecdotal notes and specifying the number of notes to be written for each student, faculty can facilitate effective use of the note by limiting the information documented to a brief description of the incident. The observation and information recorded relate to the specific behavior being evaluated. Recording extraneous data is thus avoided. If an interpretation of behavior is also included, it is indicated as such. In documenting observations, it is important for faculty to review the manner in which the description is recorded so as not to imply only deficiencies or weaknesses as worthy of notation.

An illustration demonstrates use of anecdotal notes for evaluation in clinical practice. Anecdotal notes are most effective for formative evaluation but may also be used for summative evaluation.

Behavioral Objective

P 3.0 Demonstrates skill in administering medication using Z-track technique.

Evaluation

Two observations recorded in anecdotal notes.

Evaluation Criteria

1. Wipes skin with alcohol
2. Pulls skin laterally until taut
3. Injects needle at 90° angle
4. Aspirates
5. Injects medication slowly
6. Removes needle and immediately releases skin
7. Does *not* massage area.

Critical Incident. The critical incident technique is another means of recording information collected through observation of learner performance. In the practice area, a critical incident involving some aspect of the student's performance may be recorded and then evaluated according to specified criteria (Reilly & Oermann, 1990). Critical incident differs from anecdotal notes in that the behavior is analyzed in terms of its positive or negative influence on the outcomes of the activity. Critical implies that the behavior has a significant impact on the outcome. Critical incidents are an effective strategy for formative evaluation since they include a record of observations made regarding performance in clinical practice and allow for analysis of behavior in terms of its influence on the outcomes of the activity. Discussion of the critical incident with students provides them with information relative to their strengths and weaknesses in practice. Critical incidents are also appropriate for summative evaluation. An example of a critical incident follows.

Behavioral Objective

C 4.2 Uses nursing measures which facilitate the patient's ability to cope with pain.

Evaluation

Observation of learner's nursing actions which are recorded as critical incident.

Evaluation Criteria

Identification of measures used which were:

1. Effective in assisting patient in coping with pain.
2. Ineffective in assisting patient in coping with pain.

Rating Scale. Rating scales, used to a great extent for evaluation in the clinical setting, provide a means of recording qualitative and quantitative judgments regarding the learner's performance in practice. Reilly and Oermann (1990) suggest that rating scales have been misused in nursing education and have often been *the* method used to evaluate clinical practice to the exclusion of other strategies for evaluation. There is a continual, although impossible, search among teachers for the perfect rating scale, i.e., evaluation tool. Karns and Nowotny (1991) reported that faculty in their survey expressed the need to refine their evaluation tools and find a reliable and valid one. Similarly, Bower, Linc, and Denega (1988) suggested that faculty are always revising their evaluation tools. Rating scales have their limitations and for this reason, are best used in conjunction with other clinical evaluation strategies and for specific purposes.

The rating scale contains two major parts: (1) a set of defined clinical behaviors by which students are judged and (2) an accompanying graduated scale to rate the degree of competence with which the behavior has been performed. Rather than listing behaviors, some rating devices include a list of traits, activities, skills, or attributes to be evaluated. Generally, rating scales with behaviorally stated items are more helpful than ones with lists of traits, for the behaviors are less ambiguous and relate more clearly to the course objectives (Reilly & Oermann, 1990).

With a rating scale, the teacher makes a judgment as to the degree of the learner's performance of each behavior. Most of the rating scales used in nursing programs represent five-point scales with descriptors, such as letters, A, B, C, D, E, or numbers, 5, 4, 3, 2, 1; qualitative labels, such as excellent, very good, good, fair, and poor; normative labels like superior, above-average, average, and below-average; and frequency labels, such as always, usually, frequently, sometimes, and never (Bondy, 1983).

One of the difficulties in using rating scales is apparent with this review of typical scale descriptors. First, these descriptors are not necessarily applicable to all of the behaviors or traits evaluated. Second, many of the descriptors are vague and allow for different interpretations by faculty, contributing to problems with reliability. What is the difference between an A and a B? Is there faculty consensus as to what constitutes excellent versus very good performance? With scales that use frequency labels, what about the learner who only has an opportunity to perform a behavior a few times?

Bondy (1983) developed a criterion-referenced set of scale labels to improve the validity and reliability of rating scales for clinical evaluation in nursing. The criteria for clinical evaluation are clustered into three areas: accuracy or acceptability of the behavior according to professional standards, qualitative aspects of performance, and the type and amount of teacher assistance or cues needed to perform the behavior being judged. According to Bondy (1983), five levels of competency: independent, supervised, assisted, marginal, and dependent are applicable to each of these three areas. Bondy (1984) reported that use of these criteria to define the scale labels contributed significantly to both the accuracy and reliability of faculty scores when using the rating scale. Tower and Majewski (1987) used these scale labels for the development of their clinical evaluation tool. The authors report that clinical evaluation has been facilitated because it is based on behaviorally stated competencies and is more consistent across faculty.

If a standardized scale is used, the behaviors or other items listed may or may not be congruent with the clinical objectives for the particular unit or course upon which the clinical evaluation is to focus. Ideally, behaviors listed for evaluation should reflect those of the unit or course. Scales can be derived from the objectives/behaviors of a clinical course by designating the behaviors to be achieved in clinical practice and devising a format for judging performance of these behaviors.

If the rating scale is not developed from the clinical objectives, the teacher can review the behaviors on the scale to determine their relevancy to the objectives being evaluated in clinical practice. In this way the rating scale will contain behaviors that reflect the outcomes of the clinical experience (Reilly & Oermann, 1990). Some behaviors on the rating tool may be omitted if not relevant to the clinical objectives.

Karns and Nowotny (1991) reported from their survey of 135 NLN-accredited baccalaureate schools of nursing that 72 percent used a rating scale reflecting individual course objectives. For these programs, the clinical evaluation tool varied across courses. Twenty-five percent used a single tool throughout the curriculum for clinical evaluation.

Proper use of a rating scale requires the collection of sufficient data for judging each behavior in the scale. At times, faculty in their desire to complete the rating scale may rate behaviors without adequate evaluative data.

There also may be a lack of uniformity with which terms are interpreted by faculty, particularly in relation to the labels used to designate intervals in the continuum used in the scale. A halo effect may occur with teachers choosing a rating on the basis of prior knowledge, personal biases, or close identification with the learner (Reilly & Oermann, 1990). Scales that call for supporting data for ratings may decrease this halo effect.

Other limitations to using rating scales include difficulties with the items in the scale in that they may not represent the multidimensional nature of clinical practice nor be of equal importance. Errors of central tendency may also result in which the evaluator is hesitant to mark end categories of the scale.

Even though limitations exist with use of rating scales, they do have value in clinical evaluation. Scales provide a means of rating observed behavior over time so that a pattern emerges. This enables faculty to maintain a record of learner performance. Scales also provide a way of describing performance, suggesting areas of strength and those needing improvement, which serves an important formative evaluation purpose. Rating scales are effective strategies for compiling and presenting data regarding learner performance in terms of multiple behaviors and aspects of clinical practice, particularly when the behaviors represent the ones specified for the unit or course. Reilly and Oermann (1990) recommend they not be used as the only means of grading clinical practice because of problems associated with their use.

Videotape. One additional means of recording observation of learner performance is through videotape, followed by a session to critique the activity. Videotapes provide for visual and auditory recording of performance and have a valuable start-stop capability. Many types of performance behaviors may be videotaped in different practice settings. Videotaping is effective for formative evaluation, for the learner and the teacher or peers may then critique the performance immediately following it. Videotape also may be used for summative evaluation purposes.

The videotape may be used to present a simulated situation in which learners participate and then analyze. With videotaping, students may be asked to perform as they would in the clinical setting. Evaluation of performance can result in significant feedback to students to improve their knowledge and skills. It can also contribute to the learning of the entire clinical group. Matthews and Viens (1988) describe the use of videotaping for evaluating students' ability to complete an assessment and intervene in a simulated client situation. Students are videotaped on their performance.

Videotapes may also be used to record and then evaluate specific learner behaviors such as completing an assessment, physical examination, and interview; performing psychomotor skills; and other behaviors. The videotape provides an opportunity for the teacher and student to review the performance, provide feedback on it, and determine if further practice and learning are needed. If videotaping is done in a clinical setting, protocols of the facility related to client's privacy and other rights need to be followed (Reilly & Oermann, 1990).

Written Communication Methods

Evaluation strategies classified as written communication methods provide data on the ability of the learner to communicate in writing and on the quality of the content communicated. Through these methods, information is obtained for assessing the learner's skill in conveying ideas and thoughts on paper. Evaluation of the substance of the written material provides data relevant to the objectives. Strategies for clinical evaluation include:

1. Nursing care plan
2. Case study
3. Teaching plan
4. Process recording
5. Log
6. Nursing notes
7. Other written assignments

Nursing Care Plan. Nursing care plans are both teaching and evaluation strategies that enable the learner to analyze the client's health care problems and develop a related plan of care. The format of the care plan may represent the practice model or learning care plan developed by faculty for use as a learning strategy. Either type of care plan may be evaluated in terms of substance and clarity with which the information is communicated, use of proper terminology, conciseness of presentation, and format. An illustration of use of a nursing care plan for evaluation follows.

Behavioral Objectives

C 4.2 Derives goals of care from identified self-care deficits.

C 4.2 Develops with client and family plan of care reflective of self-care deficits.

C 4.2 Selects appropriate nursing interventions.

C 4.2 Records plan of care.

Evaluation

Two care plans.

Evaluation Criteria

1. Identifies short- and long-term goals.
2. Develops goals based on identified self-care deficits as perceived by client.
3. Involves client and family/significant others in goal setting and planning of care.
4. Selects nursing interventions which address self-care deficits and ability of client to engage in self-care.
5. Is comprehensive in planning care.
6. Uses format for recording plan of care properly.
7. Communicates information clearly, concisely, and with correct terminology.

It is advisable that a care plan devised as a learning tool be discontinued as soon as possible once the teacher assesses, on the basis of evaluative data, that the student has met the objectives. Some students may need to prepare a limited number of such plans, whereas others may need to submit a considerable number before mastery is achieved. Because nursing care plans are an integral part of nursing practice, it is advisable that the student move into the system that is operating in the setting and be evaluated accordingly. Ability to move into the practice mode is an important piece of evaluation data.

One of the major difficulties in using nursing care plans for clinical evaluation is that the written plan may or may not represent the student's own critical thinking. The care plan may reflect the existing plan for the particular client in the clinical setting or may have been developed from the literature without careful consideration of how those concepts and theories relate to this specific clinical situation. Students may use the literature and other sources for developing the care plan without understanding the particular client data base. Whether or not written care plans promote critical thinking and skill in clinical judgment has not been established through research. There is no empirical evidence to support using the care plan as the predominant teaching strategy for promoting the development of these skills nor is there evidence to eliminate it (Tanner, 1986, p. 9).

For these reasons, care plans may be more effective, particularly in terms of critical thinking and skill in clinical judgment, when presented orally and discussed with the teacher and peers. Students can then be asked to explain the data collected and differentiate relevant from irrelevant information; identify cues in the data and how they clustered them; present hypotheses generated from the data and their evaluations of each; provide a rationale why certain hypotheses were accepted and rejected; and discuss the decisions made and the *reasons* underlying those decisions. Similar discussion can occur in terms of nursing management. With this interaction between teacher and students, critical thinking and skill in diagnostic reasoning can be promoted. Discussion of care plans also promotes reflection-in-action, enabling the student to make sense of uncertain, unique, and conflicting situations of practice which may not be apparent in the written plans of care. Review and critique of nursing actions specified in the plan of care may assist the learner in recognizing that some problems do not have one correct or specific solution. This thinking about client problems and care may not necessarily be reflected in the written care plan.

Changes in the communication of nursing care plans are already underway in many agencies and will be evident in most agencies in the near future as the computer becomes entrenched in the clinical setting. The computerization of nursing care plans will alter the behaviors to be evaluated in this element of nursing. The content of the plan as it is individualized to a patient will be of significance. Evaluation will then address the skill in using the computer in planning care.

Case Study. Evaluation of a case study is particularly appropriate for judging a student's ability to present a holistic perspective of a client's care, drawing upon a related knowledge base, skill in synthesis of data, and ability to communicate this information in a logical, clear, and concise manner. A case study provides a means of evaluating a student's ability to problem solve and make decisions.

The complexity and depth of the case study is a function of the level of the behaviors to be evaluated. A study written at the comprehension level is primarily descriptive of events and relationships with a related rationale. At an analytic level, the case study would represent an analysis of a patient phenomenon, drawing upon relevant theories, and a synthesis of the elements into a creative and substantive presentation.

Case studies are often written but they can be presented orally and be subject to peer review. Case studies enable students to analyze a situation and indicate what practitioners should do in the case; they also provide an opportunity for students to indicate what they would do (Schön, 1990). Discussion of a case study in a clinical conference helps students make sense of a problematic patient care situation and perhaps one in which no known principles are involved. Students learn strategies of inquiry and become clearer as to clinical situations which are ambiguous and do not lend themselves to technical rationality. In addition, case studies assist students in making explicit "the underlying, tacit theories they bring to problem setting and problem solving" (Schön, 1990, p. 324).

Case studies that are written are effective summative evaluation strategies for they require the use of cognitive skills and the cognitive component of affective skills in an integrative format. An example of a case study for evaluation appropriate in the senior year of a nursing program is presented.

Behavioral Objectives

C 4.1 Analyzes the processes entailed in providing nursing care for a client from a theoretical perspective.

A 4.1 Includes a defense of the right of the client and family to a participatory role in decisions in all phases of the care.

C 4.2 Relates nursing decisions in all phases of the process of care to those of other disciplines involved with the client.

C 4.2 Evaluates the processes used in terms of the ANA Standards.

Evaluation

Case study of a client from practice.

Evaluation Criteria

1. Includes complete and accurate data in terms of the client's status and the theoretical framework.
2. Reflects congruency among assessment data, nursing diagnosis, plan of care, and intervention.
3. Includes nursing decisions compatible with those of other health care providers unless the reasons why these decisions are incompatible are stated and documented.
4. Provides evidence of the client's and/or family's perception of events and participation in decisions regarding management of care.
5. Addresses evaluation outcomes in terms of goals and process in relation to the integrity of the plan.
6. Presents case in a scholarly prepared document which is logically organized, clearly expressed, and substantive in content.

Teaching Plan. Evaluation of a written teaching plan provides data relative to the learner's ability to use concepts of learning and teaching to meet the educational needs of clients or staff. When used in client situations, the data for determining the learning needs of the individual are obtained during the assessment phase and the teaching plan is incorporated in the client's care plan. Similar to other written communication methods, evaluation focuses on the quality of the content and skill in communicating the information in written form. An example follows.

Behavioral Objectives

C 3.0 Relates principles of learning and teaching to patient education.

C 3.0 Develops a teaching plan consistent with patient's and family's learning needs.

A 3.1 Accepts responsibility for involving patient and family in development of teaching plan.

Evaluation
Two teaching plans.

Evaluation Criteria

1. Identifies patient's and family's learning needs in terms of knowledge, skills, and values.
2. Develops behaviorally stated objectives reflecting patient's and family's learning needs.
3. Selects appropriate content.
4. Organizes content logically.
5. Chooses appropriate teaching methods and learner activities with recognition of patient preferences and learning style.
6. Provides for patient and family involvement in development and implementation of teaching plan.
7. Selects appropriate educational materials for use in teaching.
8. Records teaching plan appropriately.

Process Recording. Process recording, when used as a teaching strategy, provides information on the learner's skill in interacting with others in the clinical setting and may be subject to evaluation. It is particularly valuable for formative evaluation, especially when used in conjunction with individual conferences with learners in which the interaction is analyzed by both teacher and student and discussed in terms of further learning experiences. It may also be used in summative evaluation as data on the student's ability to grasp the various meanings which may occur in communications. The focus of evaluation of the process recording is dependent upon the objectives. An example of the use of a process recording for clinical evaluation is included.

Behavioral Objectives

C 4.2 Identifies verbal and nonverbal cues.

C 4.2 Relates nursing actions to identified client cues.

C 4.2 Analyzes own interactive behavior within a therapeutic relationship.

Evaluation
Process recording of nurse–client interaction

Evaluation Criteria
1. Interprets accurately client verbal and nonverbal cues.
2. Identifies own verbal and nonverbal cues.
3. Selects appropriate nursing actions based on cues exhibited in communication.
4. Analyzes effect of own behavior in the relationship.
5. Identifies facilitators and blocks to communication.
6. Describes clearly own feelings during and perception of the interaction.
7. Uses format for recording interaction correctly.

Log. Learning log is another means of evaluating clinical objectives, but because of the nature of the log, it does not provide sufficient data on the learner's skill in communicating in written form. It is more of a process than an outcome evaluation strategy. Maintained concurrently with specified clinical experiences, it enables the evaluator to be a participant in the learning process through the eyes of the learner. The value of students' perceptions of experiences is often not recognized by faculty as a significant data base in the evaluation process. Use of a learning log for clinical evaluation is illustrated.

Behavioral Objectives
C 3.0 Identifies coping mechanisms used by client.
C 3.0 Assesses client system for need for planned change.

Evaluation
Log entries describing:
1. Observation of client for signs and symptoms of stress.
2. Coping mechanisms used by client.
3. Rationale for whether or not change is indicated in client system.

Evaluation Criteria
1. Identifies coping mechanisms used by client.
2. Differentiates between functional and dysfunctional adaptation.

3. Relates adaptation and change theories in determining need for planned change.
4. Assesses strengths and deficits of client system that may influence outcome of planned change.

Nursing Notes. The learner's ability to report and communicate in writing client data is an important outcome of clinical experience and another source of data for evaluation. As with other written communication methods, nursing notes may be judged in terms of their content and the learner's skill in recording. Nursing notes enable faculty to evaluate the learner's ability to collect and record relevant data about the client, identify nursing diagnoses from the data, develop and revise accordingly plans of care, and document client progress.

Criteria for evaluating the content of nursing notes include comprehensiveness and accuracy of data collected about the client, significance of interpretation of the data, and appropriateness of the plans of care and nursing interventions. Evaluation of the learner's skill in communication relates to clarity with which the information is recorded, use of proper terminology, conciseness with which presented, and order in which the information is recorded.

Evaluation of nursing notes may occur over a period of time as a longitudinal strategy or within a limited time frame for a selected number of recordings, depending on the objectives of the experience. Both approaches might be used, for the longitudinal strategy provides data about the degree of consistency with which the student documents care provided, while the incidental strategy provides the opportunity for a discrete evaluation of a particular documentation for which the student is responsible. Regardless of the structure of the evaluation, this strategy is particularly valuable for formative evaluation especially when the nursing notes are then discussed with the learner, but it may also be of value in summative evaluation.

The introduction of computers to the practice setting has altered considerably and will continue to alter the process for documenting information about clients. Nursing information systems (NIS) use computer technology to support the delivery of patient care. This includes accessing relevant data about the patient and recording patient information via a computer placed in the nurse's station or patient's bedside (Brown, 1991). With a computerized system, documentation of nursing care is computerized rather than handwritten in the patient's chart. Specific information about a client such as that included typically on a flow sheet can be entered into the computerized system. Progress notes may be edited while they are entered but cannot be changed after that time. The nurse's notes and other information collected are thus recorded in the computerized system rather than written on a variety of forms. Students' skill in using the computer system becomes another outcome of teaching in the clinical setting and area of evaluation.

McKinney (1988) reported that nurses were more organized and efficient with terminals located at the patient's bedside. It is anticipated that computerized systems will continue to be implemented and improved upon in clinical facilities. In the community setting, NIS can maintain client records and improve documentation of care (Saba, 1988). Many computer systems for both hospitals and other clinical settings provide a directory of standardized care plans that may be generated from the system. Students then require skill in modifying the standard care plan to reflect individual client needs. This may represent another area of evaluation in clinical practice.

Behavioral Objectives

C 3.0 Records pertinent client data and progress of client.

C 3.0 Revises plan of care.

Evaluation

In nursing notes, records pertinent data and revises plan of care.

Evaluation Criteria

1. Documents relevant data collected from client, family, other health care providers, and other sources.
2. Interprets data accurately.
3. Records data indicative of progress of client.
4. Presents information clearly and concisely.
5. Revises plan of care appropriately.
6. Uses proper format for nursing notes.

Other Written Assignments. Other types of assignments appropriate for clinical evaluation include reports of observations made in the clinical agency in which the student is practicing and other settings; papers reflecting an analysis of a specific clinical experience, decisions made in a particular clinical situation, and moral and ethical issues; position papers on issues encountered in clinical practice; a comparative study of different approaches to a client situation; and other written assignments related to the clinical experience.

Oral Communication Methods

Ability to convey ideas verbally is an important skill in nursing, for in most settings nursing is practiced in groups where sharing of information or the formulation of decisions for action is a frequent occurrence. This activity may involve other health disciplines.

Criteria for evaluation of oral communication skills include the ability to: (1) present ideas clearly and succinctly in group discussions, (2) assume a leadership or participant role within the group as indicated, (3) offer data and ideas or suggestions which contribute to group thinking, and (4) facilitate group process in arriving at decisions or solutions to problems. The quality of the content communicated in terms of accuracy and relevancy to the objectives of the group process are appropriate matters for evaluation.

Evaluation methods which provide data on the learner's ability to communicate verbally include:

1. Clinical conference
2. Issue conference
3. Nursing and multidisciplinary conference

Clinical Conference. Clinical conferences represent clinically focused discussions by groups in clinical practice and include such types as postconferences and peer-review conferences. Postconferences involve a group discussion or problem-solving activity in relation to experiences encountered during practice in the clinical setting. These conferences provide a means of encouraging critical thinking in that alternative perspectives may be examined and strategies proposed. In another format, the student presents a patient situation to the group for review and critical analysis. This type of conference enables students to examine decisions made and alternatives possible. Discussions of problems and solutions which are unclear may proceed during such conferences; these conferences contribute to experiences in the clinical setting which promote "thinking like a professional." Conferences such as these are effective means for evaluating the ability of the learner to present ideas, listen to the ideas of others, critique those ideas presented, and lead or participate in group action toward the goals of the conference.

Whatever the format of the conference, evaluation is concerned with the quality of the content presented, ability to communicate verbally, and skill in use of group process. Clinical conferences may be used for evaluating one or several objectives and for either formative or summative evaluation. An example of a postconference for evaluation is presented.

Behavioral Objectives

A 2.2 Discusses willingly one's own feelings about caring for patients of varied cultural and ethnic backgrounds.

C 3.0 Examines the impact of cultural stereotypes on identification of patient needs.

Evaluation

One postconference in which student presents patient of different cultural or ethnic background than own.

Evaluation Criteria

1. Describes accurately the cultural or ethnic background and behavior characteristics of the patient.
2. Identifies stereotypic attributes that she or he associates with such patients.
3. Describes own feelings about patients of this cultural or ethnic background.
4. Relates the influence of own stereotypic beliefs and feelings in assessing the patient's needs.
5. Promotes an atmosphere for sharing of ideas and feelings among individuals in the group.
6. Leads the group in exploring the significance of stereotyping of groups of patients and the care provided.

Issue Conference. Issue conferences involve group discussion of social, cultural, economic, and political as well as professional issues that are not always generated by the particular clinical experience but are relevant to that experience. Various group modalities may be used. One student or a group of students may be responsible for the presentation to the larger group. Evaluation addresses the same elements as in other oral communication methods. However, in this type of conference another dimension is added in respect to the content. These conferences are directed toward enlarging the student's perspective of the events that occur in the setting by relating them to ideas, events, or actions beyond the present boundaries. It is the ability to move from a more prescribed technical perspective of an issue to see it within the greater context that is the concern of the evaluation. An illustration of a senior issue conference is presented.

Behavioral Objectives

    C 4.2 Analyzes the impact of health insurance on quality of care.

    C 4.2 Identifies implications of being uninsured.

Evaluation

One issue conference in which learner leads discussion on health insurance and its relationship to care.

Evaluation Criteria

1. Explains the significance of health insurance in the United States.
2. Bases presentation on literature and related research.
3. Identifies the effects of being uninsured.
4. Leads group in examining implications of health insurance and selected proposals in this area for professional nursing practice.
5. Proposes strategies for improving health care to the uninsured in local and regional areas.
6. Encourages participation of group members in discussion.
7. Presents ideas clearly and in logical order.

Nursing and Multidisciplinary Conferences. Nursing team and multidisciplinary conferences provide another means of evaluating clinical objectives. The composition of the group varies from nursing practitioners only to a group of representatives from different health care disciplines, sometimes including a client. These conferences emphasize the process of collaborative decision making in which client problems are explored, plans for care are developed and revised, strategies for implementation are examined, and evaluation of care is completed. The nature of the learner's participation in these conferences varies, depending upon the objectives. In some conferences, learners may be involved primarily in sharing information about a client while in others the student may be responsible for group leadership. Criteria similar to other oral communication methods apply to evaluation of nursing and multidisciplinary conferences. An example of evaluation of a nursing team conference is included.

Behavioral Objective

C 3.0 Develops nursing diagnoses for a patient in conjunction with nursing colleagues.

Evaluation

One conference in which learner presents patient data for establishing nursing diagnoses.

Evaluation Criteria

1. Reports one's own observations of patient and data obtained through assessment.
2. Collects data from other nurses.
3. Discusses patient's resources and preferences for meeting health care needs.
4. Leads group in analyzing data and identifying priorities.
5. Leads group in identifying nursing diagnoses.
6. Provides opportunity for members to participate in discussion and group decision making.

Simulations

Another method of performance testing for the cognitive, affective, and psychomotor domains is simulations. Simulations are a valuable strategy for clinical evaluation, offering a readily available means of judging performance. The complexity of the problems simulated and related nursing actions to be performed are able to be controlled in a simulation. Evaluation may focus on cognitive, psychomotor, or affective behaviors as indicated by the clinical objectives.

Any of the types of simulations presented earlier as teaching methods may be used for clinical evaluation. In the case study method, a clinical situation is presented to the learner, requiring decisions to be made and often actions to be taken. Performance of psychomotor skills may be incorporated within the simulation. The simulation may involve a specific action or skill such as insertion of a urinary catheter or may represent a larger scope requiring a series of decisions to be made and actions taken. Evaluation may then include cognitive dimensions and skill in performing relevant technical aspects of care.

The simulation used for evaluation may be presented in paper and pencil format, through audiovisual media, and by computer. Students may observe a segment of the multimedia, then be asked to arrive at decisions or carry out some aspect of care for evaluation purposes. The focus of the evaluation depends on the objectives to be judged through this method. Matthews and Viens (1988) describe the evaluation of basic nursing skills using a simulation and then videotaping performance. The clinical group critiques the videotape during filming. Two to three faculty then view each tape and evaluate performance.

Other types of simulations appropriate for clinical evaluation include use of models, simulated patient-nurse situations, and role play. Simulations are appropriate for either formative or summative evaluation. Long and Redding (1991) describe the development and use of a clinical performance examination to evaluate psychomotor skills of baccalaureate students. The examination includes simulations in the laboratory setting and actual examinations in the patient care area. Formative evaluation is incorporated throughout the course with summative evaluation consisting of testing specific skills in the laboratory or hospital-based performance examinations. A similar system has been developed and tested for use with registered nurses enrolled in the program.

Johnson, Lehman, and Sandoval (1988) presented another view of simulation testing. In their protocol, students engage in a two-day test based on a clinical situation. There are six activities with specific criteria for evaluation of each one. Multiple evaluation methods are incorporated within the clinical examination including simulation. The clinical examination is used for summative evaluation at the completion of a nursing course. Johnson et al. (1988) also suggest that the clinical examination may be used at the end of a year of study to examine ability to transfer knowledge from one patient situation to another.

Self-Evaluation

Learner self-evaluation represents an important component of any clinical evaluation protocol. Development of this skill begins with the initial clinical nursing course and continues throughout the program. Self-evaluation "is a complex developmental skill that requires instruction and practice" (Best, Carswell, & Abbott, 1990, p. 177) and needs to be taught to students in a systematic way. It has greater value when implemented on a continuous basis for learners to examine their progress toward meeting goals. Self-evaluation should be accompanied by teacher-student discussions in which sharing of evaluation takes place and decisions are made regarding future learning experiences. For these reasons, self-evaluation is most appropriate for formative evaluation.

In a study by Abbott, Carswell, McGuire, and Best (1988), results indicated that both students and teachers perceived self-evaluation as providing direction for learning and viewed it positively. Contrary to the literature, however, students did not perceive self-evaluation as a factor in promoting their professional growth. One problem with self-evaluation of which the teacher should be cognizant is that students tend to be self-critical and underrate themselves. Abbott et al. (1988) found that although students valued participation in clinical evaluation, the process of self-evaluation generated anxiety for them and similar to the literature, resulted in underrating of performance. The authors recommend that students be given time to develop an understanding of the process of self-evaluation and become comfortable with it.

The focus of self-evaluation in clinical practice is determined by the objectives of the experience and individual learner goals. Various methods of recording evaluation data are possible, such as anecdotal notes, rating scales, logs, and reports of progress in the clinical field. Learners can also evaluate their own clinical assignments. Students have reported that personal interviews with the teacher were the most effective means of assisting them in evaluating their own performance (Abbott et al., 1988). Through this interaction, the teacher and student can share observations and perceptions, important in developing skill in self-evaluation; identify with students strengths and weaknesses; and provide direction for learning.

USE OF MULTIPLE STRATEGIES FOR CLINICAL EVALUATION

Clinical practice cannot be evaluated by one method alone. The range of behaviors to be judged in the practice setting and differences among learners require a variety of evaluation methods. An example demonstrating different evaluation strategies possible for an objective is included. The teacher can vary strategies with a group of learners or an individual learner based on needs and the clinical situation in which the evaluation takes place.

There are several significant values to the use of multiple strategies in evaluating clinical performance. In some instances, student difficulty in performance may be a function of the evaluation strategy rather than the skill implied by the objective. A written report of an interview may suggest that the student cannot perform an interview satisfactorily. A tape recording of an interview by the same student may signify that the student is indeed competent in that activity. The difficulty that the student has is in writing, not interviewing, and it is that skill which the student needs to develop. The willingness to try another method when performance is not satisfactory provides a more accurate diagnosis of the student's learning needs, whether it entails the actual skill under assessment or another skill required for data collection.

Another advantage to maintaining a multistrategy approach relates to the teacher. Repetition leads to boredom, loss of interest, and lack of creativity. The use of varied strategies with a different or even the same group of students provides the diversity the teacher needs in his or her own practice of teaching. Acceptance of this diversity leads the faculty to be challenged to the development of more creative evaluation processes and adds a sense of excitement that often accompanies change. Evaluation approaches are developed by the willingness of the faculty to be daring and comfortable with new situations.

Behavioral Objective

C 3.0 Provides for instruction of the patient and family in required measures of self care.

Possible Evaluation Methods

1. Observation in clinical setting
2. Teaching plan
3. Simulation
4. Videotape recording of teaching
5. Clinical conference
6. Nursing notes

Evaluation Criteria

1. Bases teaching on identified self-care deficits and patient's abilities to perform self care.
2. Determines priorities for teaching according to self-care deficits.
3. Involves patient and family in all phases of teaching.
4. Uses appropriate teaching strategies.
5. Evaluates effectiveness of teaching plan in terms of promoting self care.
6. Revises teaching plan based on evaluative data.

EVALUATION PROTOCOL FOR UNIT ON CHRONIC PAIN

In developing the evaluation protocol, the teacher decides on methods for collecting information on the objectives for clinical practice and plans strategies for both formative and summative evaluation. The clinical objectives specified for the unit on chronic pain management, in Table 10-2, Chapter 10, provide a means for illustrating the process

Table 11-1
Evaluation Methods for Unit on Chronic Pain Management

Clinical Behaviors	Evaluation Methods
I. Relate Orem's self-care model to nursing management of patients with chronic pain	
B. Evaluates the biopsychosocial and cultural influences on the individual's ability to manage one's own pain	Log
D. Analyzes the various nontraditional pain management techniques in terms of the individual's and family's learning needs and self-care potential	Postconference
II. Use the nursing process in promoting self-care of patients with chronic pain	
Assessment:	
A. Carries out a systematic pain assessment of patient	Written Assignment: Assessment
B. Evaluates impact of chronic pain on patient's life style	Log
C. Identifies patient's strategies for coping with pain	Case Study
D. Appraises the impact of biopsychosocial and cultural factors on the patient's response to pain	Case Study
E. Analyzes the influence of support systems on patient's ability to manage chronic pain	Case Study
F. Assumes responsibility for identifying one's own values and biases that may affect the assessment	Postconference
G. Analyzes the learning needs of patient and family in relation to chronic pain management	Videotape
H. Formulates nursing diagnoses based on identified self-care deficits	Case Study, Nursing Care Plan
Planning:	
I. Develops with patient goals of care congruent with nursing diagnoses	Nursing Care Plan
J. Plans nursing management related to self-care deficits of patient and family	Case Study, Nursing Care Plan, Peer review Conference

Table 11-1 *(Continued)*

Clinical Behaviors	Evaluation Methods
K. Supports the patient in decision making relative to options for pain management	Observation
L. Selects appropriate traditional and nontraditional methods of pain management	Case Study, Nursing Care Plan, Peer review Conference
M. Provides for use of appropriate resources to assist patient and family	Nursing Care Plan
Implementation:	
N. Implements nursing interventions congruent with a scientific rationale, research, and the mutually established plan of care	Observation
O. Is competent in the use of traditional pain management techniques	Observation
P. Demonstrates skill in the use of nontraditional pain management techniques	Simulation
Q. Initiates referrals to health care providers and/or agencies essential in assisting patient to meet optimum self-care agency	Nursing Notes
R. Encourages patient in use of his or her own potential and resources in addressing self-care limitations	Critical Incident
S. Documents pertinent nursing observations and interventions	Nursing Notes
Evaluation:	
T. Develops criteria for evaluating the effectiveness of the plan toward a decrease in self-care deficit and increase in self-care agency	Case Study, Nursing Care Plan
U. Uses criteria in evaluating patient and family outcomes of care in terms of stated goals	Peer review Conference
V. Uses professional nursing standards as a framework for evaluating the process of the delivery of nursing care	Peer review Conference
W. Modifies plan of care as indicated by the evaluation results	Nursing Notes
III. Formulate judgments which reflect respect for the inherent worth and dignity of the patient with chronic pain	

Table 11-1 (Continued)

Clinical Behaviors	Evaluation Methods
A. Defends the patient's right to be informed regarding traditional and nontraditional methods of chronic pain management relative to their expected outcomes and inherent risks	Issue Conference
B. Supports the patient's choice regarding the selection of pain control methods	Critical Incident
C. Provides care reflective of the patient's own sociocultural preferences, psychologic needs, health beliefs, perception of degree of self-care deficit	Case Study
D. Protects the patient's rights to privacy and confidentiality	Videotape
E. Acts as advocate for patient and/or situations appear to impede progress toward goal attainment	Issue Conference
IV. Foster facilitative relationships with patients with chronic pain, families, and colleagues	
A. Analyzes own interactive behavior within a therapeutic or collegial relationship	Process Recording
B. Assumes a liaison role between patient and other persons who have an impact upon the health care of the individual	Postconference
C. Contributes readily to discussions and decisions that have an impact on matters concerning the patient's pain management	Nursing Conference
D. Maintains ongoing communication with appropriate health providers regarding the plans, implementation, and evaluation of care	Written Assignment (Case Management)
V. Assumes responsibility for continued development of the knowledge base and competencies essential for promoting self-care agency in the presence of chronic pain	
A. Assumes responsibility for expanding one's own knowledge base regarding care of the patient with chronic pain	Case Study

Table 11-1 *(Continued)*

Clinical Behaviors	Evaluation Methods
B. Maintains knowledge of current research findings which address the phenomenon of pain and its management	Case Study
C. Is accountable for seeking out those learning experiences that enhance the development of requisite competencies	Log
VI. Affirm the accountability of nurses and the nursing profession to contribute to the development of a theory of practice for patients with chronic pain	
A. Takes a position on the responsibility of nurses and nursing to protect the public against quackery and other kinds of deceptive methods purported to alleviate chronic pain	Issue Conference
E. Declares a position on nursing's ethical and moral responsibilities in the various pain management methods used in practice	Issue Conference

of planning for clinical evaluation. One method, i.e., case study, may encumber more than one objective.

SUMMARY

Evaluation in the clinical setting provides data for making judgments of the learner's performance in all domains of learning. An evaluation protocol needs to include strategies for both formative and summative evaluation which are clearly differentiated. Formative evaluation represents feedback to the learner on progress in meeting the objectives for clinical practice. Evaluation that is formative enables the teacher and student to identify areas in which further learning is needed and plan relevant learning experiences. In contrast, summative evaluation, end of instruction evaluation, provides information as to the extent to which the objectives have been achieved. Summative evaluation is used to determine the grade for clinical practice.

There is no such process as objective evaluation. Evaluation is always subjective, for it is influenced by the values and beliefs of the participants. It is critical, therefore, for faculty to examine their own values, beliefs, attitudes, and biases which may affect judgments made of learners in the field. Although clinical evaluation cannot be objective, it can be fair.

Clinical practice is complex, and as such, cannot be evaluated by one method alone. Multiple strategies are needed for appraising the learner's performance in practice. These methods are classified as observation, written communication, oral communication, simulation, and self-evaluation.

Observation of learner performance is a major means of evaluating students in the field. Methods for documenting observations include anecdotal notes, critical incidents, rating scales, and videotapes.

Evaluation strategies classified as written communication methods provide data on the learner's skill in writing and quality of the content communicated. Relevant evaluation strategies are nursing care plan, case study, teaching plan, process recording, log, nursing notes, and other written assignments.

Nurses must also be skillful in conveying ideas verbally and participating in a group format. Strategies for evaluating these skills in clinical practice include clinical conference, issue conference, and nursing and multidisciplinary conferences.

Simulation, presented earlier as an instructional strategy, may also be used for evaluation of clinical objectives. Any protocol for clinical evaluation should also provide opportunity for learner self-evaluation.

A range of clinical evaluation methods is needed. Clinical practice cannot be evaluated by one method alone and instead requires a variety of methods for collecting information on the learning achieved in the clinical setting and attending to individual needs of the student. It is the faculty's responsibility to choose strategies that are appropriate for the objectives of clinical practice and carry out evaluation in an environment denoting trust and respect between teacher and learner.

REFERENCES

Abbott, S. D., Carswell, R., McGuire, M., & Best, M. (1988). Self-evaluation and its relationship to clinical evaluation. *Journal of Nursing Education, 27*(5), 219-224.

Bergman, K., & Gaitskill, T. (1990). Faculty and student perceptions of effective clinical teachers: An extension study. *Journal of Professional Nursing, 6*(1), 33-44.

Best, M., Carswell, R. J., & Abbott, S. D. (1990). Self-evaluation for nursing students. *Nursing Outlook, 38*(4), 172-177.

Bondy, K. N. (1983). Criterion-referenced definitions for rating scales in clinical evaluation. *Journal of Nursing Education, 22*, 376-382.

Bondy, K. N. (1984). Clinical evaluation of student performance: The effects of criteria on accuracy and reliability. *Research in Nursing and Health, 7*, 25-33.

Bower, D., Linc, L., & Denega, D. (1988). *Evaluation instruments in nursing*. New York: National League for Nursing.

Brown, P. A. (1991). Computers in nursing practice. In M. H. Oermann, *Professional nursing practice: A conceptual approach*. Philadelphia: J.B. Lippincott.

Hedin, B. A. (1989). Expert clinical teaching. In *Curriculum revolution: Reconceptualizing nursing education* (pp. 71-89). New York: National League for Nursing.

Johnson, G., Lehman, B. B., & Sandoval, N. B. (1988). Clinical exam: A summative evaluation tool. *Journal of Nursing Education, 27*(8), 373-374.

Karns, P., & Nowotny, M. (1991). Clinical structure and evaluation in baccalaureate schools of nursing. *Journal of Nursing Education, 30*(5), 207-210.

Kleehammer, K., Hart, A. L., & Keck, J. F. (1990). Nursing students' perceptions of anxiety-producing situations in the clinical setting. *Journal of Nursing Education, 29*(4), 183-187.

Litwack, L., Linc, L., & Bower, D. (1985). *Evaluation in nursing: Principles and practices*. New York: National League for Nursing.

Long, M. C., & Redding, B. A. (1991). Evaluating clinical skills of RN students. *Nurse Educator, 16*(3), 31-33.

Matthews, R., & Viens, D. C. (1988). Evaluating basic nursing skills through group video testing. *Journal of Nursing Education, 27*(1), 44-46.

McKinney, P. (1988). Can point of care terminals ease the threat? *Computers in Health Care, 9*(4), 62.

Meisenhelder, J. B. (1982). Clinical evaluation—An instructor's dilemma. *Nursing Outlook, 30*, 348-351.

Reilly, D. E. (1978). *Teaching and evaluating the affective domain in nursing programs.* Thorofare, NJ: Slack.
Reilly, D. E. (1989). Ethics and values in nursing: Are we opening Pandora's box? *Nursing & Health Care, 12*(2), 91-95.
Reilly, D. E., & Oermann, M. H. (1990). *Behavioral objectives: Evaluation in nursing* (3rd ed.). New York: National League for Nursing.
Saba, V. K. (1988). Taming the computer jungle of NIS. *Nursing & Health Care, 9*(9), 487-491.
Schön, D. A. (1990). *Educating the reflective practitioner.* San Francisco: Jossey-Bass.
Tanner, C. A. (1986). The nursing care plan as a teaching method: Reason or ritual? *Nurse Educator, 11*(4), 8-9.
Tower, B. L., & Majewski, T. V. (1987). Behaviorally based clinical evaluation. *Journal of Nursing Education, 26*(3), 120-123.
Wilhite, M. J. (1990). Diagnostic evaluation and grading in nursing laboratory courses. *Journal of Nursing Education, 29*(1), 39-40.

BIBLIOGRAPHY

Akers, P. A. (1991). An algorithmic approach to clinical decision making. *Oncology Nursing Forum, 18*(7), 1159-1163.
Bell, M. L. (1991). Learning a complex nursing skill: Student anxiety and the effect of preclinical skill evaluation. *Journal of Nursing Education, 30*(5), 222-226.
Burns, K. A. (1984). Experience in the use of gaming and simulation as an evaluation tool for nurses. *Journal of Continuing Education in Nursing, 15*(5), 213-217.
Grabbe, L. L. (1988). A comparison of clinical evaluation tools in hospitals and baccalaureate nursing programs. *Journal of Nursing Education, 27*(9), 394-398.
Higgins, N., & Ochsner, S. (1989). Two approaches to clinical evaluation. *Nurse Educator, 14*(2), 8-11.
Kolb, S. E., & Shugart, E. B. (1984). Evaluation: Is simulation the answer? *Journal of Nursing Education, 23,* 84-86.
Larson, C. E. (1987). Use of the microcomputer as a tool for subjective grading. *Computers in Nursing, 5*(5), 186-191.
Leino-Kilpi, H. (1989). Learning to care—A qualitative perspective of student evaluation. *Journal of Nursing Education, 28*(2), 61-66.

Lenburg, C. B., & Mitchell, C. A. (1991). Assessment of outcomes: The design and use of real simulation of nursing performance examination. *Nursing & Health Care, 12*(2), 68-75.

Malek, C. J. (1988). Clinical evaluation: Challenging tradition. *Nurse Educator, 13*(6), 34-37.

McDowell, B. J., Nardini, D. L., Negley, S. A., & White, J. E. (1984). Evaluation clinical performance using simulated patients. *Journal of Nursing Education, 23*, 37-39.

McNight, J., Rideout, E., Brown, B., Ciliska, D., Patton, D., Rankin, J., & Woodward, C. (1987). The objective structured clinical examination: An alternative approach to assessing student clinical performance. *Journal of Nursing Education, 26*(1), 39-41.

Novak, S. (1988). An effective clinical evaluation tool. *Journal of Nursing Education, 27*(2), 83-84.

Plunkett, E. J., & Olivieri, R. J. (1989). A strategy for introducing diagnostic reasoning: Hypothesis testing using a simulation approach. *Nurse Educator, 14*(6), 27-31.

Shellenbarger, T. (1991). Use of a database for clinical assignments and student evaluation. *Nurse Educator, 16*(2), 39-41.

Wakim, J. H. (1986). Developing evaluation tools. *Nurse Educator, 11*(4), 26-30.

Waltz, C. F., & Miller, C. H. (Eds.). (1988). *Educational outcomes: Assessment of quality—A compendium of measurement tools for baccalaureate nursing programs*. New York: National League for Nursing.

12

Grading of Clinical Experience

Summative evaluation often leads to some type of system by which the results are "readily interpreted" and communicated. In American education, that system is usually referred to as *grading*, the process by which some symbol is designated to represent the sum total of achievement for an educational experience. Evaluation and grading are two distinct processes, although some persons use the terms interchangeably. Evaluation can occur without grading; grading should not occur without evaluation. The use of a grading symbol, whether a letter or number, to convey a complex and diverse array of competencies and attributes is reflective of a need for simple answers or responses. The meaning conveyed by the symbol is generally instantly "understood" by the viewer.

MEANING OF GRADES

What do grades mean? It is interesting that grades are identified as quantitative symbols of qualitative dimensions of behavior, even though no absolute standard is available for interpretation. As one ponders the meaning of the term *grade*, Boulding's (1971) postulation about the differentiation between the image and the message comes to mind. He postulates that a highly learned process of interpretation and acceptance influences how one receives a message. He states, ". . . What this means is that for any individual or group or organization, there are no such things as *facts*. There are only messages filtered through a changeable value system" (p. 14). Grades may well reflect the values, past experiences, and beliefs of the interpreter.

Grades are a context dependent phenomenon with the broadest frame of reference provided by social-historical era in which the grade is assigned (Milton, Pollio, and Eison, 1986). They are human, contextual judgments which have a temporal dimension. Milton et al. identify five factors which influence the meaning of grades; (a) socio-historical era (including grade inflation and deflation), (b) educational institutions, (c) academic discipline, (d) instructor policies, and (e) student characteristics (p. 25). They further describe grades as unidimensional symbols into which complex and multi-dimensional judgments are compressed. Jedrey (1984) perceives that a "grade conveys a relatively unambiguous message about a student's progress in universally understood system of academic notation" (p. 104).

Although educational institutions may have protocols for ascribing meaning to grades, there is generally little consistency in their use. There can be marked differences among graders in any given institution as to the dimensions of the educational process that relate to the grading practice. This differentiation can be not only institution-wide, but found within departments and among faculty involved in the same course.

Grading as currently perceived is a system for ranking or rating an individual; i.e., categorizing the person in relation to a phenomenon called academic achievement. Academic achievement is a nebulous concept. Warren (1971) notes that academic achievement is itself defined only in terms of composites of course grades. "It has no independent definition against which the validity of course grades can be checked" (p. 2). The symbol used denotes unidimensional information and keeps concealed data about many different kinds of performances which may have been used to arrive at the grade. Thus the concept of academic achievement projects a single entity that is global in nature, when in reality it represents many interrelated components.

The meaning behind the ranking, therefore, lacks consistency among users whether the symbols used are letters of the alphabet, numbers, or descriptive words. Is an "A" an "A"? No standard exists for supporting such a contention; there are certain variables which mitigate against standardization in the meaning of a grade.

Perceptions of Participants

The meaning of a grade is not the same for the person awarding the grade, the recipient of the grade, and the user of grades such as admission officers, or employers. Meanings are derived from values, experiences, motivations and knowledges within the life-space of each individual.

Faculty attitudes toward and perceptions of grades are particularly relevant since they are charged with the responsibility for awarding grades. Studies of faculty grading practices evidence considerable variance in the data base used for assigning a grade, the notion of the role that grades play in the total educational endeavor, and the standards used in assessing performance, i.e., the perfection or the growth model. Faculty behavior patterns which tend toward flexibility or rigidity, and reflect these beliefs about individuals as learners, influence the grading process. In the study of faculty behavior regarding accommodating grades to particular circumstances, Milton et al. (1986) found that the majority of faculty followed the rules and made no exception. The few who did adjust grades identified two major reasons; progressive improvement from an exceptionally poor start and personal crises.

Faculty and students have significant disagreements regarding grading as noted in the Milton et al. (1986) national study. Both agree that the student is the primary audience for the grade, but faculty, more than students perceived grades as relevant to success in life. Faculty felt that there was too much emphasis on grades, while students felt that more was needed. Faculty view grading as evidence of fairness and high standards whereas students see grades as fostering a faculty reputation of unfairness. Grading was perceived by both parties as having an influence on the student-teacher relationship, but students were more sensitive to the power disparity between students and faculty. Although faculty tend to downplay the power aspect and seek to empower students, in reality, the person who makes the final judgment of performance does have more power. This power can also create conflicts for faculty when the final grade is a determinant for other demands in society, such as affirming draft status of a student in time of war, or influencing career choices. Milton et al. (1986) note that the variance in views between students and faculty indicate that the desired partnership within the total learning experience is not being achieved.

Business leaders are users of grades of potential employees. Grades are used as criteria, even though business leaders have not done any studies to ascertain their reliability and validity. They place considerable emphasis on the reputation of the institution awarding the grade when interpreting its significance. The appropriateness of using grades for this purpose is discussed later.

Grades and Student Learning

What is the relation of the pursuit of grades to the student's motivation for learning in academic programs? Faculty in their ideal posture would suggest that the pursuit of learning, not pursuit of grades is the force behind student's educational endeavors. In reality, however, pursuit of grades is the motivational force for many students, especially in American society where "acceptable grades" are the entry into further study, professional careers, or the job market. Although faculty often profess the value of learning rather than grades as a motivation, in practice many tacitly or overtly refer to grades within their course as a reminder to improving performance or as a means of controlling student behavior. Indeed, some take pride in announcing the vagaries of their grading practice and the value of the grades they assign. The utilitarian value of grades is presently demanding more notice about grading process in each course with specific information as to the quantitative value of each learning task. The legalistic orientation of present society is seeing grade challenges in the courts, although the prerogative of faculty to assign grades has generally been respected. All of these activities increase the pressure of grades on the faculty and students and cannot be ignored.

Grade orientation and learning orientation are two separate entities, yet both may be present in the same student. Milton et al. (1986), in their study of educational orientation, derived a four-fold typology.

1. High Learning-Orientation/High Grade-Orientation
   (High LO/High GO)
2. High Learning-Orientation/Low Grade-Orientation
   (High LO/Low GO)
3. Low Learning-Orientation/High Grade-Orientation
   (Low LO/High GO)
4. Low Learning-Orientation/Low Grade-Orientation
   (Low LO/Low GO) (pp. 130–131)

Particular personality characteristics of students in each group were identified in the study and a profile of each group was compiled. Students in the HighLO/Low GO group are inner directed, self-motivated, possesses high levels of abstract thinking and sensitivity, are challenged by new ideas and intellectual matters and are less anxious in testing situations. In contrast, the students in Low LO/High GO group are not inner-directed, approach learning experiences with tension to do the "right thing," are more comfortable with concrete than abstract thinking, believe in luck and fate as powerful influences in their lives and exhibit a high level of test anxiety. Students in the Low LO/Low GO group have similar characteristics as the Low LO/High GO group with a greater degree of frustration and tension with marked introversion. Students in the High LO/High GO group are relaxed learners, less able than the High LO/Low GO students and seek concrete information regarding grades as a determinant of how well they are doing and evidence a high level of test anxiety.

The profile of the groups derived from the study of Milton et al. (1986) provides a framework for faculty to consider in teaching and testing students. The authors also make apparent to teachers that grades assume a significant role in student learning and call for teaching strategies that assist the learner in obtaining an enriching educational experience. Too often the grade oriented student relies on memorization in testing situations and develops a mechanical posturing in life pursuits often resulting in cheating or withdrawal from the experience when success is threatened. Creativity is often lost and the full potential of the learner is not realized.

Variation in Data Base

A second variable is the inconsistency in the quantity and quality of the evaluative data base; i.e., the summative evaluation used by the person assigning the grade. Data may measure only one type of performance, such as writing a paper or answering questions on an examination, regardless of whether or not the performances are the appropriate ones. On the other hand, a grade may represent data from a composite of numerous evaluation strategies that deal with many dimensions of the learning experience. A grade may represent the student's skill in handling the evaluative procedure rather than the attainment of the learning inherent in the objectives of the experience. Thus, a grade may reflect relevant competencies or may reflect the attempt to use one symbol to depict accomplishment as to varied and unrelated abilities.

Another dimension of quality relates to the consistency with which the data base really reflects the objectives. Does the grade have enough support to convey the student's progress, or have the evaluation strategies been irrelevant to the goals of the experience? As an example, do the objectives relate to skills in problem solving and decision making while the data upon which a grade is based relate to skills in information recall? Is it possible that a grade may reflect learner behavior unrelated to the objective such as, tardiness, appearance, or some personal attribute? Use of these latter criteria connotes a punitive dimension to the grading process when reflecting negative attributes. The practice of integrating scholarship and conduct within a single grade was addressed in 1870 at Harvard University with the following statement:

> *Voted, that the deductions from the scale of scholarship for absence, tardiness, and misconduct, as well as those which accompany the various admonitions shall be discontinued; but the numbers representing such deductions and other similar numerical marks of censure shall be regularly entered in the Dean's office, and shall form a separate scale of demerit. (Smallwood, p. 74)*

Over 100 years later, the practice of incorporating scholarship and conduct within one grade continues within the educational system in many institutions of higher learning. The inconsistency in endorsing this practice among graders adds to the lack of congruency in interpreting meanings of grades. One hopes that eventually, grades will refer to scholarship attainment of the students without further distractors.

Base Standard

A third variable is concerned with the basis for the standard in determining grades. In some instances, the standard is based on evidence of growth throughout the learning experience, the *process*; whereas in other instances, the standard is based on the degree of learner attainment of the objectives at the conclusion of the experience, the *outcome*.

In general, grading is directed toward the outcome pattern, the degree of learner attainment of the objectives. There are discrepancies in the approach used by various graders. Some teachers rely only on summative evaluation strategy results, whereas others incorporate formative evaluation results leading to the objective attainment.

As the concept of mastery of learning increasingly influences the educational process, the focus of evaluation is on learner attainment of the objectives. A system of formative and summative evaluation operates to assure the student's mastery of the task to be learned. Standards for grading are then criterion-referenced standards. These standards, usually ascertained from empirical evidence, derive from the performance desired for a given task. In the criterion-referenced approach, the teaching-learning process is closely interwoven with formative evaluation, with summative evaluation indicating if the learner has mastered the task.

Computation Method

The method of computing grades is a fourth variable which is highly individualized and mitigates against grade standardization. How are grades determined? In some situations, the normal curve is used as the basis for determining grades. The underlying assumption of the normal curve, however, is incompatible with an educational process, for it is based on a random sample. Do learners in nursing represent a random sample? A negative response is generally in order, especially in light of the selection procedures employed in many nursing programs. What is the random element? Teaching itself cannot meet this criterion, for it is a purposeful activity. Bloom, Hastings, and Madaus (1971) in their statement on mastery learning state: "We may even insist that our educational efforts have been *unsuccessful* to the extent that the distribution of achievement approximates the normal distribution" (p. 46).

Milton et al. (1986) concur with the above statement that the results of the use of a normal curve represent failure rather than achievement, especially in a college population where students are selected and do not reflect a normal distribution in society. When a normal distribution of grades occur, they see this fact as a "symbol of failure, failure to teach well, failure to test well, and failure to have any influence at all in the intellectual lives of students" (p. 225). Geisinger, Wilson, and Naumann (1980) report in their study of grading practices that university faculty favored norm-reference grading which involves use of the normal curve more than did any other faculty group. Community college faculty prefer self-referenced grading which is based on actual student performance. When the norm-referenced grading system is used, the grade received by each student is in essence a symbol of rank order, not a symbol of learning progress in accord with goals.

Grades derived from the normal curve show a small percentage of students with an "A," an equal percentage with a failure. The failure may be more representative of the student's rank order in a group than the student's failure to grasp the essential learning in the course of study. A skewed curve would be the expected outcome in a professional program.

The expectation of learner performance in the mastery of learning system is markedly different. Using a criterion-referenced approach, this theory posits the notion that 95 percent of the learners for any given task have the potential for mastery, meaning a grade of "A," if that symbol is used. The other 5 percent may have a special disability for the particular learning task and, thus, are not able to achieve mastery. Although the theory recognizes the potential for most students to achieve mastery, such an outcome is not guaranteed, for much of the mastery of any learning rests with the intent, commitment, and persevered effort on the part of the learner.

Another aspect of computing grades to be considered is the procedure for the weighting of different sources of data for arriving at the ultimate grade. Much variation exists in the way faculty allocate weight for items such as tests, especially final examinations; papers; nursing care studies; and conference presentations. Weighting is a function of any particular course, but the basis for such a decision even lacks a rationale that could be used as a standard.

In response to an earlier question, one can say that "an A is not an A." A possible definition of a grade as presently used could be that it is a symbol representing the learner's degree of academic achievement as defined by an individual teacher in light of competencies and attributes deemed appropriate and as arrived at by that teacher's choice of the data base to be used and the computation strategy to be followed. In spite of the poor fidelity the grade symbol has in encoding evaluative data and the lack of reliability and validity of the grade, the grading system is highly institutionalized in our society and thus is to be used in educational programs, especially those that carry some kind of credit.

USES FOR GRADES

The grade is a ubiquitous symbol, but it prevails in the American educational system and is used as a basis for decisions critical to the life of the individual. Administratively, grades are used as a basis for determining admission to and continuance in programs of study and for awarding honors, scholarships, or other special means of recognition. The use of grades as a predictive variable occurs in spite of data to the contrary. Warren (1971) confirms this question of predictability when he states: "For most students previous grades do predict later grades moderately well over relatively short time periods. Undergraduate grades predict first year grades in graduate and professional schools moderately well, but they predict advanced grades poorly, particularly in clinically oriented programs" (p. 10). This conclusion is based on studies by Bartlett (1967), Gough (1967), Gohn (1968), and Hanlon (1964). Erickson and Bluestone (1971) address the predictive value of grades: "Regardless of in-house controls and refinements, the accumulated grade record fails as a useful indicator of post graduation success" (p. 4). Milton et al. (1986) in their recent study found that the assumption that grades are predictors of future success in life still prevails. Faculty, more than any other groups studied, accepted this premise while students were less convinced.

Educationally, grades may be perceived as stimuli for learner motivation; although the motivation may be to meet academic demands, not to develop the competencies inherent in the learning task. Erickson and Bluestone remind faculty of the "distinction between study effort and learning benefit; between time spent at the books and material absorbed for productive application beyond the exam" (p. 2). In general, the effort a student extends is more a function of the value the student places on the course than the grade to be received. An additional consideration is the timing of the awarding of the grade, often at the conclusion of the experience or course. At this time it is too late for a student to become motivated to effect behavior change in the experience.

A current use of grades is social; to certify individuals to perform certain functions in society. The use of grades as an admission feature fosters the "gatekeeper" role of an educational program, the means by which it selects who may enter certain fields of endeavor, thus in essence, maintaining class structure and controlling access to high social and economic levels (Warren, 1971). Employers also use grades in selecting from applicants, a practice challenged by Erickson and Bluestone (1971) by the question: "Do colleges have either the responsibility or the right to provide encapsulated evaluation of student achievement to sources beyond the classroom?" (p. 6). A suggestion is made that the employing agency determine its own criteria for evaluation to which the college could respond.

The national survey conducted by Milton et al. (1986) explored the issue of use of grades. There was a marked discrepancy between the preferred use of grades and the actual use. Preference for use of grades was expressed as a means of communicating data to students as to the actual learning achieved. However, about 80 percent of the respondents felt that in the current period, the primary purpose is to provide information to other educational institutions for their decision-making. Faculty also viewed grades as useful to industry's selection of employees. About 84 percent of the companies said that grades were moderately to very important for hiring an individual, but once the person was employed, grades had no significance for future decisions (pp. 86-87). The authors in accord with the position of Erickson and Bluestone (1971) raised questions about the colleges and universities becoming personnel selection agencies rather than agencies responsible for promoting the learning potential of students. Concerned about the impact of this role on the faculty, they state, "In our view, serving as personnel selection agents for society is a distortion of the faculty role in the first place; the job should require them to focus on promoting learning in the classroom and not classifying students for industry" (p. 84).

TYPES OF GRADING SYSTEMS

The most frequently used system is the multidimensional system, usually representing a five-point scale of symbols from "A" to "D" and "F." Its long-time usage and accepted respectability by administrators, faculty, and some students make it the most common form in use.

A second pattern that became fairly popular in the seventies is the two-dimensional system with only two symbols. This dichotomous system could include such combinations as: (1) pass (P)-no pass (NP); (2) satisfactory (S)-Unsatisfactory (U); (3) credit (C)-noncredit (NC). The S-U system is usually an administrative decision and pertains to all students in the course; whereas, the P-NP is an individual student option. The premises underlying this pattern are: (1) students can take difficult courses without fear of lowering their grade point average, (2) students have more option to experiment with courses outside their major, (3) emphasis is on the learning process, (4) anxiety about grades is reduced, (5) students can be self-directing, and (6) less time is wasted by students and teachers in playing the "game of grades."

Responses to this approach vary among students and faculty. There is no doubt that articulation from undergraduate to graduate school is impeded because of administrative preference for the five-dimensional system. Students wishing to pursue advanced study may be jeopardized, especially if the system is used for courses in the major. Students who require structure and the five-dimensional grading system as a frame of reference for guiding their own learning may increase their anxiety with this less structured format. Others find that with the release from competition and "grade getting" learning is less of an anxiety-producing process. An interesting phenomenon has occurred. Students and many faculty do not perceive this two-dimensional system as a grading system, which it is, nor do they perceive that the letter symbols students receive are actually grades.

Some faculty find that they cannot change their grading practices. They keep two sets of records, one in five-dimensional grades and the other in two-dimensional grades. The change to the new system is in reality a translation of symbols from one system to another. There seems little question that an ethical issue exists when a system of records of grades not chosen by the student is maintained.

When dual grading systems are used by students; i.e., selecting five-dimensional grading for some courses and two-dimensional for others, there is a tendency for students to place priority of learning on those subjects requiring the more discriminating five-dimensional system.

A study was conducted by faculty in the College of Nursing, Wayne State University to determine faculty and student responses to the use of a two-dimensional grading pattern (Reilly, 1973). Student responses were generally favorable to the two-dimensional system, while faculty, particularly graduate faculty, were less supportive. Results were similar to those found in the literature with some student polarity evident on such issues as the impact of the system on anxiety, motivation, and competition. Faculty were less supportive of the belief that in this system there is more emphasis on learning than on obtaining a grade. Many respondents expressed concern about the evaluation process that underlies the two-dimensional grading system, suggesting that poor evaluation processes could therein be hidden.

An often voiced objection to this system is the inability to distinguish between academic excellence and barely satisfactory performance. As a result, descriptive terms are added or the use of a plus (+) or minus (−) with the letter is instituted so that in reality a four- or five-dimensional grading system results.

A third grading system has had limited use. It is the descriptive grading system which uses no letters, but rather provides for a written evaluation of student performance. At Santa Cruz University, where this system was used with a pass-no pass system, comments ranged from one word euphemisms for letter grades to several paragraphs of expressive prose (Andrews, 1970). Although there is no agreement on terminology or criteria, there is a possibility that a computer could select from stored descriptions of student performance relevant aspects of a particular performance and merge them into a standardized summary. This descriptive approach presents difficulty to decision-making groups, such as admission officers. Descriptive grading is effective if used in conjunction with the other systems.

Very few educational programs today use the number system which denotes a specific quantitative value to the achievement rather than a range of measures as in systems using letters as symbols. The inexactness of the measurement component of many evaluation strategies mitigates against the use of such a specific quantitative symbol and makes the grader vulnerable to challenge. It is difficult to defend the choice of a grade of 89 over 90.

Contract grading is another system, which in reality uses the five- or two-dimensional system with clarification of the basis for determining the grade. Mind set is a significant dimension in approaching any learning situation. Contract grading fosters such a mind set in the student as the decision for the grade to be achieved is made by the student. The decision, however, may or may not be to the advantage of the student. An agreement to engage in learning experiences in accord with a "B" grade may not be the wisest use of the experience when selected by a student with potential for greater achievement. Likewise, a student may desire to achieve an "A" level but lack the resources to meet such a goal. Student counseling is essential in using this system so that the decision is congruent with student resources, potentials, and ultimate goals.

Findings in the national study by Milton et al. (1986) suggest that a grade scale with the greatest number of categories is desired by many of the participants. The more numerous the categories, the more precision in differentiating individuals and the more individualized is the grading. The authors suggest that such quantified precision may be delusional, for the basis used is not necessarily sound and may reflect "measurement myopia." They recommend a grading system based on a reduced number of categories.

It is evident that there are deficiencies in all grading systems. In too many instances of change there has been a manipulation of the symbols and as Silberman (1970) states:

This kind of tinkering fails to come to grips with the real problem; how to make evaluations serve the ends of education instead of being an end in itself. . . . What is wrong with the present system is not the use of grades, per se, but the fact that the awarding of grades has been divorced from the large function of evaluation (p. 347).

Erickson and Bluestone (1971) concur with Silberman: "The crux of any system of grading is to establish criteria relevant in learning to reduce the disparity between evaluation and grading" (p. 5).

ISSUES ON GRADING CLINICAL PERFORMANCE

Clinical performance is a form of academic achievement in a professional program, and therefore the allocation of a grade on the basis of appropriate evaluation data is in order. The use of grades for denoting achievement in a clinical practice experience is often fraught with apprehension, uncertainty, and diverse beliefs as to its applicability. The solution selected to address this matter usually entails a shift from a five-dimensional grading system to a two-dimensional system. Faculty tend to perceive this action as the discontinuance of a grading system; the awarding of a symbol, a letter such as P, NP, and so on, is not acknowledged as a grading process.

Rationale for discontinuing the traditional approach is based on the premises previously stated for the two-dimensional system. Even more so, it often reflects the insecurity of faculty as the search for the impossible, *objective* evaluation and grading, is pursued. As previously indicated, grading is not *objective*, (no human judgment can be objective), but it can be *fair* if the data on which it is based address the objectives through judicious selection of evaluation strategies. In the clinical component of a course of study, there tends to be a greater reliance on one evaluative tool as a basis for grading than is true for the classroom component. The tool is usually some form of rating scale which is translated quantitatively for a grade. The scale may or may not reflect the objectives of the learning experience. The tool is often too limited to provide the data necessary, for the diversity of competencies at any point in time requires a variety of data-gathering methods.

Grading for classroom activities is perceived to be more accurate because the methods lend themselves more easily to quantification.

Perhaps this notion is more myth than reality, for it is primarily the objective format tests that are readily quantifiable. Performance testing that employs such methods as problem-solving situations, papers, essay questions, and group activity generates as much uncertainty for the evaluator as do the clinical performance activities in the clinical area such as nursing care plans, process recordings, and performance of nursing actions. Strategies removed from the one-answer format depend upon the application of pre-determined criteria and judgment on the part of the teacher if they are to be used widely and fairly in determining the grades whether for class or clinical experiences. They also require the openness to hear and see the "different," which signifies the creative approach from the learner. A touch of humility when evaluating leaves the teacher in a position to acknowledge the "new" from the learner.

Concern is often expressed about the inability of grades to differentiate among students who have competency in achieving classroom objectives but are unable to master the necessary clinical performance, or vice versa. It is acknowledged that a grade represents complex, diversified abilities and is unable to encode the values attached to specific abilities which are in essence a part of the grade. However, the inability to denote the differences in performance in either of the major components may be a function of the grading system used in arriving at a grade. If a policy exists which states that failure to achieve in either of the two components, regardless of the performance in one of the components, results in failure of the total course and that policy is explicit in public announcements of the school, then no further grade computation is necessary if the failure occurs in one component. Note that it is the computation that is stopped, not the evaluation. This policy has particular meaning if clinical practice is not passed because of the practice nature of the nursing discipline. When there is passing performance but marked discrepancy between that in the classroom or clinical field, the system of grade computation should make this fact evident. Perhaps one of the systems later proposed will address this matter for some individuals.

The trend toward using a two-dimensional grading system for clinical practice experience while maintaining the five-dimensional system for the classroom experience raises some critical concerns. When a two course system is used, one for classroom (theory) and one for clinical (practice), it becomes evident that the theory component represents more discriminating evaluation. What messages are conveyed to the learner? Theory may be perceived to be more valuable because its grading is more discriminating; therefore, time for studying and preparation is allocated in that direction. Clinical practice, on the other hand, may be perceived to be less valuable and only an activity experience with little cognitive input necessary.

If both class and clinical components are combined in one course, then the final grade in this type of grading system, represents only performance in regard to the classroom objectives. It is not possible to transfer a grade from a two-dimensional system to one in the five-dimensional system. A "P" is just that; it has no further meaning. In this instance is the grade that appears on the transcript for the clinical courses misleading since in reality it only represents the classroom experiences?

Regardless of the pattern of courses, in a mix of the two grading systems, it is the classroom grade that is perceived to be significant and the one that is used in determining the grade point average. The clinical performance is assumed to be satisfactory but carries no weight in the student's average for the total program. A less confusing approach would be for faculty to decide on one grading system for both components of the course. Any system will have its strengths and its limitations, requiring faculty to make the choice with full knowledge of the implications in the use of the selected system.

GRADING SYSTEMS FOR CLINICAL PRACTICE EXPERIENCE

With recognition of the significant place that the grading system occupies in the American educational system and the lack of standardization for whatever system is chosen, several systems for grading the clinical experience are proposed. Whatever system is ultimately developed by a faculty, it must be acknowledged that the field of grading is an inexact one and the professional judgment of faculty is the key factor in making decisions. Fairness is obtained in adhering to the use of evaluative data that address the objective and the weighting of items in relation to their significance in contributing to the goal of the course and to the ultimate goal of the program. Weighting must be justified and each faculty member is held responsible to peers for such a decision.

Whether one uses a two-dimensional or five-dimensional grading system, two criteria are essential:

1. Evaluation data-gathering strategies must be congruent with the stated objectives and behaviors.
2. The data base to be used must be identified and declared.

Because clinical practice requires certain specific competencies for safe and effective execution, a criterion-referenced system of evaluation and therefore a criterion-referenced system of grading are in order.

Objectives as Framework for Computation of Grades

As previously demonstrated, clinical course objectives include behaviors most appropriately achieved in the clinical field. The extrapolation of the clinical behaviors from those of the overall course provides the evaluation form for use in clinical evaluation. It is this list of objectives and behaviors that constitute the basis for a grading system. Since these objectives and behaviors are in essence a contract with the learners by which they are assured that the teaching and learning experiences will be directed toward the attainment of the objectives and that evaluation will be so directed, grading also must be in accord with the contractual statements. There is no assurance that students will indeed attain the designated behaviors, for student choice continues to be a major factor in making the required effort to achieve.

For each objective, specific behaviors are expressed that must be attained if the objective is to be met. Achievement in certain behaviors is essential while others are significant, but their full attainment may not be reached within the time allocated to a particular course or unit of study.

Faculty judgment is the basis for determining which behaviors are essential in a criterion-referenced system. Some persons call these behaviors critical elements; others refer to them as non-negotiable behaviors. The latter signifies a very definitive approach—these behaviors *must be achieved.* No bargaining is possible. Achievement of other behaviors is not a substitute. In other words, *all* of the non-negotiable behaviors must be attained if the objective is to be considered to be passed. Alterations in decisions about behaviors must be agreed upon by all faculty concerned. One faculty member cannot modify the decision to meet individual expectations. The objectives and behaviors with the non-negotiable behaviors so noted are provided to all faculty and students concerned. This action fosters fairness in grading as it communicates specifically the expectations for an acceptable performance.

Table 12-1 depicts the designation of non-negotiable behaviors for the unit Chronic Pain Management, which was previously presented in Table 11-1, Chapter 11. Since this unit is developed for senior students, it can be expected that many of the behaviors would be classified as non-negotiable for they have been in development throughout much of the program. It is their interpretation within the context of the topic under discussion that is new.

Table 12-1
Clinical Behaviors—Unit of Chronic Pain Management

C 4.2   I. Relate Orem's self-care model to nursing management of patients with chronic pain

*   C 4.2 B. Evaluates the biopsychosocial and cultural influences on the individual's ability to manage one's own pain

     C 4.2 D. Analyzes the various nontraditional pain management techniques in terms of the individual's and family's learning needs and self-care potential

C 4.2   II. Use the nursing process in promoting self-care of patients with chronic pain

Assessment:

*   C 4.2 A. Carries out a systematic pain assessment of patient
*   C 4.2 B. Evaluates impact of chronic pain on patient's life style
*   C 4.2 C. Identifies patient's strategies for coping with pain
*   C 4.2 D. Appraises the impact of biopsychosocial and cultural factors on the patient's response to pain
*   C 4.2 E. Analyzes the influence of support systems on patient's ability to manage chronic pain
     A 3.3 F. Assumes responsibility for identifying one's own values and biases that may affect the assessment

* Denotes a non-negotiable behavior.

Table 12-1 (Continued)

*	C	4.2 G.	Analyzes the learning needs of patient and family in relation to chronic pain management
*	C	4.2 H.	Formulates nursing diagnoses based on identified self-care deficits

Planning:

*	C	4.2 I.	Develops with patient goals of care congruent with nursing diagnoses
*	C	4.2 J.	Plans nursing management related to self-care deficits of patient and family
	A	3.3 K.	Supports the patient in decision making relative to options for pain management
	C	4.2 L.	Selects appropriate traditional and nontraditional methods of pain management
*	C	4.2 M.	Provides for use of appropriate resources to assist patient and family

Implementation:

*	C	4.2 N.	Implements nursing interventions congruent with a scientific rationale, research, and the mutually established plan of care
*	P	5.0 O.	Is competent in the use of traditional pain management techniques
*	P	3.0 P.	Demonstrates skill in the use of nontraditional pain management techniques
	C	4.2 Q.	Initiates referrals to health care providers and/or agencies essential in assisting patient to meet optimum self-care agency
	A	4.1 R.	Encourages patient in use of his or her own potential and resources in addressing self-care limitations
*	C	4.2 S.	Documents pertinent nursing observations and interventions

Evaluation:

*	C.	4.2 T.	Develops criteria for evaluating the effectiveness of the plan toward a decrease in self-care deficit and increase in self-care agency
*	C	4.2 U.	Uses criteria in evaluating patient and family outcomes of care in terms of stated goals
	C	4.2 V.	Uses professional nursing standards as a framework for evaluating the process of the delivery of nursing care
*	C	4.2 W.	Modifies plan of care as indicated by the evaluation results
A 4.1		III.	Formulate judgments which reflect respect for the inherent worth and dignity of the patient with chronic pain
*	A	4.1 A.	Defends the patient's right to be informed regarding traditional and nontraditional methods of chronic pain management relative to their expected outcomes and inherent risks

Table 12-1 *(Continued)*

*	A	4.1	B.	Supports the patient's choice regarding the selection of pain control methods
*	C	4.1	C.	Provides care reflective of the patient's own sociocultural preferences, psychologic needs, health beliefs, and perception of degree of self-care deficit
*	A	4.1	D.	Protects the patient's rights to privacy and confidentiality
	A	4.1	E.	Acts as advocate for patient and/or family when individuals or situations appear to impede progress toward goal attainment
A 4.1			IV.	Foster facilitative relationships with patients with chronic pain, families, and colleagues
*	C	4.2	A.	Analyzes own interactive behavior within a therapeutic or colleagial relationship
	A	4.1	B.	Assumes a liaison role between patient and other person who have an impact upon the health care of the individual
*	A	4.1	C.	Contributes readily to discussions and decisions that have an impact on matters concerning the patient's pain management
*	A	4.1	D.	Maintains ongoing communication with appropriate health providers regarding the plans, implementation, and evaluation of care
A 4.1			V.	Assume responsibility for continued development of the knowledge base and competencies essential for promoting self-care agency in the presence of chronic pain
*	A	4.1	A.	Assumes responsibility for expanding one's own knowledge base regarding the care of the patient with chronic pain
			B.	Maintains knowledge of current research findings which address the phenomenon of pain and its management
*	A	4.1	C.	Is accountable for seeking out those learning experiences that enhance the development of requisite competencies
A 4.1			VI.	Affirm the accountability of nurses and the nursing profession to contribute to the development of a theory of practice for patients with chronic pain
	A	4.1	A.	Takes position on the responsibility of nurses and nursing to protect the public against quackery and other kinds of deceptive methods purported to alleviate chronic pain
*	A	4.1	E.	Declares a position on nursing's ethical and moral responsibilities in the various pain management methods used in practice.

Since achievement of non-negotiable behaviors is considered to be passing, the two-dimensional system uses the data as a basis for a passing grade. The five-dimensional system for grading involves further interpretation. In an undergraduate program using the five-dimensional grading system, a grade of "C" is considered passing in most professional schools; a grade of "B" is passing in a graduate program. Quantitative allocation of criteria in this system is presented in Table 12-2.

In institutions where there is use of plus (+) or minus (−) signs, the numbers of behaviors can be discriminated more finely. One other quantitative datum must be in place before the grading process can proceed. The weighting of the value of each objective is indicated on the basis of faculty judgment in terms of the purpose of the course or unit. Although categories of objectives are consistent in all courses, the value of each may vary according to the major emphasis of the course. Because nursing process is the methodology of practice, it can be assumed that the nursing process objective would receive the highest weighting in a clinical practice course.

Table 12-2
Quantitative Allocation for Grading

Undergraduate			Graduate		
Letter Grade	Numerical Equivalent	Criteria	Letter Grade	Numerical Equivalent	Criteria
A	4	All behaviors met	A	4	All behaviors met
B	3	All non-negotiable behaviors and at least half of the others met	B	3	All non-negotiable behaviors and at least half of the others met
C	2	All non-negotiable behaviors met	C	2	One half or more non-negotiable behaviors met
D	1	One half or more non-negotiable behaviors met			
F	0	All or most non-negotiable behaviors not met	F	0	All or most non-negotiable behaviors not met

As an illustration, a possible weighting of the objectives for the unit on Chronic Pain Management is noted:

Weight	Objective
20%	1. Relate Orem's self-care model to nursing management of patients with chronic pain.
40%	2. Use the nursing process in promoting self-care of patients with chronic pain.
15%	3. Formulate judgments which reflect respect for the inherent worth and dignity of the patient with chronic pain.
10%	4. Foster facilitative relationships with patients with chronic pain, families, and colleagues.
10%	5. Assume responsibility for continued development of the knowledge base and competencies essential for promoting self-care agency in the presence of chronic pain.
5%	6. Affirm the accountability of nurses and the nursing profession to contribute to the development of a theory of practice for patients with chronic pain.

When the evaluation process has been completed, data are ready to be translated into the symbol designated by the grading process which the faculty selected. Each objective is accorded the grade symbol allocated to the behaviors that have been attained as specified in the system for quantifying the behaviors. An illustration of this process with the unit Chronic Pain Management is in Table 12-3. Because the five-dimensional grading system is most often used for classroom grading, it is the one used in the illustration.

After the grade and numerical value are determined for each objective, these data are used in accordance with the weighted value for each objective to obtain the grade for the clinical component for the unit. In this illustration, the computation generates the grade as depicted in Table 12-4.

A further step is indicated in instances when one course grade representing both clinical and classroom components is the practice. Grading in this manner has the advantage of communicating to students and others that a clinical nursing course is a total entity which entails a synthesis of theory and practice. When these two

Table 12-3
Grading of Clinical Practice

Objective	Total No. Behaviors	Total No. Non-Negotiable Behaviors	No. of Behaviors Achieved Non-negotiable	Others	Grade	Numerical Value
I	2	1	1	1	A	4
II	23	17	17	3	B	3
III	5	4	4	1	A	4
IV	4	3	3	0	B	3
V	3	2	2	0	C	2
VI	2	1	0	1	F	0

components are separated into two courses, their interrelationship is often not as apparent.

In order to combine the classroom and clinical grade, one must know the credit allocation for each component within the course. The grading process for the clinical achievement using the objectives and behavior has been developed so as to result in one grade. The same process could be used for computing the classroom grade. The weight attached to each cumulative grade is a function of the credit allocation. In the current illustration, each component represents three credits, thus the course grade is the result of averaging the cumulative grade for

Table 12-4
Computation of the Clinical Grade

Objective	Numerical Grade	Value	Weight	Numerical Weight
I	A	4	20	4 × 20 = 80
II	B	3	40	3 × 40 = 120
III	A	4	15	4 × 15 = 60
IV	B	3	10	3 × 10 = 30
V	C	2	10	2 × 10 = 20
VI	F	0	5	0 × 5 = 0
				Total 310
				Numbered Value 3.10
				Grade B

each component. In the instance where the distribution is not equal, the grade for the course is comprised of the averaging of the two cumulative grades as prescribed. As an example, where the unit credit allocation is designated as two credits for classroom activities and four credits for clinical activities, the course grade computation would be:

Classroom grade   × 1
Clinical grade   × 2

Designated Evaluation Strategies as a Basis for Grading

The grading process presented uses the objectives and behaviors directly as the data source in determining the grade to be awarded. It is noted that the word *awarded* is used instead of the word *given*. The teacher does not *give* a grade; the student earns it and the teacher awards it.

Another approach is to use the objectives and behaviors indirectly through the use of selected evaluation strategies as the major source of data. One evaluation strategy may provide data on one behavior or numerous behaviors. If the source of data for each behavior is so designated and all behaviors are included in the evaluation process, the results on the various evaluation strategies can become the data base. It is still possible to highlight the non-negotiable behaviors for special consideration. The evaluation strategies selected and the weighted value of each are functions of faculty judgment based on the purpose of the course or unit. An illustration of this pattern of grading is presented in Table 12-5.

The cumulative clinical grade is then subjected to the same computation procedure for determining a course grade when it comprises both classroom and clinical components as was described for the previous grading system.

Several approaches to arriving at a clinical grade when the five-dimensional grading system is used have been described. They are not meant to be inclusive, but rather they suggest means of addressing the grading of clinical practice that are congruent with that generally found in grading the classroom performance. The systems are

Table 12-5
Computation of Clinical Grade II

Evaluation Strategy	Grade	Numerical Value	Weight	Numerical Value
Process Recording	C	2	15	2 × 15 = 30
Care Conference Presentation	A	4	30	4 × 30 = 120
Performance Rating	A	4	35	4 × 35 = 140
Analysis of Log	B	3	20	3 × 20 = 60
			Total	350
			Numbered Value	3.50
			Grade	B

criterion referenced using the stated objectives and behaviors as the framework. Criterion-referenced grading is the method of choice because nursing is a practice discipline which calls for certain competencies that must be mastered. The standard used as a basis for criterion-referenced grading must be selected with care in terms of the purpose of the grading and must not be too narrow and rigidly fixed. This approach does not suggest an objective system, but it does foster a fair system.

Reliability of grades is a function of internal consistency of individual instructors. Internal consistency of a grade measures the degree to which the various observations made by a teacher to arrive at judgment about grades of students in a course reflect a common form of academic performance (Warren, 1971). Reliability of grades is a function of their dimensionability with a decrement in reliability occurring as attributes used increase unless there is a strong relationship among attributes. Warren suggests that: "The high reliability of grades across courses and instructors, for example, in spite of differences in course emphasis and methods of evaluation is probably due to the common element of verbal ability in most academic evaluation" (p. 21).

One of the significant limitations of the computation patterns presented is the tendency to foster rigidity with no room for flexibility and recognition of a transcendent quality in the student, which portends success or failure in future endeavors. Just as intuition is an important element in nursing, so too is it meaningful in teaching. The demand in present society for specific documentation for each computation precludes decisions which arise from faculty's own perceptions and judgment. There is a phenomenon known as goal-free learning which can often get lost in the measurement process.

Faculty who acknowledge this nonmeasureable attribute in grading often place themselves at risk. Students have the right to know the basis used for grading for any learning experience, but when a trusting relationship exists between the student and the teacher, the teacher is more free to interpose his or her own professional judgment in the final interpretation of the data used in grading. As an illustration, if a "C" is equal to 2.0, the teacher might feel that a particular student with a grade point average of 1.8 will succeed in the program more readily than a particular student with a 2.2 average. Could the former student receive the grade "C," while the latter student did not receive a passing grade? An analysis of the data for the grade may provide the rationale for such a decision. The latter student may have received the 2.2 average on the basis of a high grade in a group activity, sufficient to compensate for a poorer performance in self-directed activities. Likewise, the former student may evidence satisfactory performance in most activities, but the skill required for one type of activity may be deficient.

Grading is a fact of life in the American educational system and evokes many ambivalent feelings among all involved. Westland (1969) speaks of grades thusly: "Grades probably do represent something useful; we just don't know what it is" (p. 358). Warren (1971) raises the issue of our lack of knowledge as to what grades represent as indices of academic performance. He states: "When the components and structure of grades are better described, we will be able to attack not only the current, rather limited issues, but the more substantial ones that bear heavily on the entire educational enterprise" (p. 26).

SUMMARY

Grading is a process by which some symbol is used to designate some degree of academic achievement. Various systems are selected by faculty, such as the two-dimensional or five-dimensional. The symbol is arrived at through a computation system for interpreting evaluation data. Grades have different meanings and lack a universal standard due to various individual perceptions of grading and grades, variations in data base used, differences in base standard, and types of computation methods.

Many issues accompany the concept of grading the clinical practice experience, often arising out of faculty uncertainty, insecurity with the process, and the search for an "objective" grading system. Fairness, not objectivity, is the goal. When a two-dimensional grading system is used for clinical practice and a five-dimensional grading system is used for classroom activities, confusion results and it is only the five-dimensional grading system that is ultimately used in determining the grade point average of the total program of study for a student. The five-dimensional system is often perceived to be more discriminating, thus suggesting greater value for the activities involved than is noted with the two-dimensional system.

The grading processes that are criterion referenced are: (1) the use of objectives and behaviors of a course which are to be achieved in the clinical field with certain ones designated as non-negotiable, and (2) the use of evaluation strategies which imply indirectly the objectives and behaviors. Both of these approaches lend themselves to either the two- or five-dimensional system of grading.

Grading is an integral part of the American system of education and thus cannot be dismissed. The selection of a system must reflect thoughtful consideration on the part of the faculty involved as to its strengths, limitations, and consequences.

REFERENCES

Andrews, F. C. (Ed.). (1970). *Report on grading at the University of California, Santa Cruz*, Committee on Educational Policy.

Bartlett, J. (1967). Medical school and career performance of medical students with low medical college admission test scores. *Journal of Medical Education, 42*, 231–237.

Bloom, B. S., Hastings, J. T., & Madaus, G. F. (1971). *Handbook on formative and summative evaluation of student learning.* New York: McGraw-Hill.

Boulding, K. E. (1971). *The image.* Ann Arbor, MI: The University of Michigan Press.

Erickson, S. C., & Bluestone, Z. (1971). *Grading and evaluation: Memo to faculty, No. 46*. Ann Arbor, MI: Center for Research in Learning and Teaching, University of Michigan.

Geisinger, K., Wilson, A., & Naumann, J. (1980). A construct validation of faculty orientations toward grading comparative data from three institutions. *Educational and Psychological Measurement, 40,* 413–417.

Gohn, L. A. (1968). An investigation of the selection techniques of veterinary science and medical students at Purdue. *University Abstracts 28A,* 446.

Gough, H. C. (1967). Non-intellective factors in the selection and evaluation of medical students. *Journal of Medical Education, 42,* 642–650.

Hanlon, L. (1964). College grades and admission to medical schools. *Journal of Higher Education, 35,* 93–96.

Jedrey, C. (1984). Grading and evaluation. In M. Gullette (Ed.), *The art and craft of teaching.* Cambridge: Harvard University Press.

Milton, O., Pollio, H., & Eison, J. (1986). *Making sense of college grades.* San Francisco: Jossey-Bass.

Reilly, D. E. (Ed.). (1973). *Report of ad hoc committee to study grading.* Unpublished manuscript. Wayne State University, College of Nursing, Detroit, MI.

Silberman, C. E. (1970). *Crisis in the classroom: The remaking of American education.* New York: Random House.

Smallwood, M. (1935). *An historical study of examinations and grading in early American Universities.* Cambridge: Harvard University Press.

Warren, J. R. (1971). *College grading practices: An overview, Report 7.* Washington, DC: ERIC Clearinghouse on Higher Education.

Westland, G. (1969). The philosophy of student assessment. *Universities Quarterly, 23,* 350–60.

BIBLIOGRAPHY

Beyer, F. J. (1983). Setting passing scores. *Nursing & Health Care, 4,* 518–22.

Brazziel, W. (1985). Waiting for the older student. *AAHE Bulletin, 37*(6), 8–9.

Chickering, A. (1983). Grades: One more tilt at the windmill. *AAHE Bulletin, 35*(8), 10–13.

Cureton, L. (1971). The history of grading practices. *Measurement in Education, 2*(4), 1–9.

Duke, J. (1983). Disparities in grading practice. Some resulting inequities and a proposed new index of academic achievement. *Psychological Reports, 53,* 1023–1080.

Eizler, C. (1983). The meaning of college grades in three grading systems. *Educational Research Quarterly, 8*, 12–20.

Geisinger, K., Rabinowitz, W. (1982). Individual differences among college faculty in grading. *Journal of Instructional Psychology, 1*(1), 20–27.

Geisinger, K. (1982)b, Marking Systems. *Encyclopedia of Educational Research, 3*, 1139–1149.

Hales, L. W., Bain, P. T., & Rand, L. P. (1973). The pass-fail option: The congruence between the rationale for and student reasons in electing. *Journal of Educational Research, 66*, 295–298.

Hills, J. R., & Gladney, M. B. (1968). Factors influencing college grading standards. *Journal of Educational Measurement, 5*, 31–39.

Huckabay, L. M. (1979). Cognitive-effective consequences of grading versus nongrading of formative evaluations. *Nursing Research, 28*, 173–178.

Lenburg, C. B. (1979). *The clinical performance examination.* New York: Appleton-Century-Crofts.

McFarland, M. B. (1983). Contract grading. *Nurse Educator, 8*(4), 3–6.

Morgan, M. K., & Irby, D. M. (Eds.). (1978). *Evaluating clinical competence in the health professions.* St. Louis: C. V. Mosby.

Perry, L. B. (1968). College grading: A case study and its aftermath. *Educational Record, 49*(4), 78–84.

Reilly, D. E., & Oermann, M. H. (1990). *Behavioral objectives: Evaluation in nursing* (3rd ed.). New York: National League for Nursing.

Rezler, A. G., & Stevens, B. J. (Eds.). (1978). *The nurse evaluator in education and service.* New York: McGraw-Hill.

Sgan, M. R. (1970). Letter grade achievement in pass-fail courses. *Journal of Higher Education, 40*, 638–644.

Stallings, W. M., Smock, H. R., & Leslie, E. K. (1968). The pass-fail grading option. *School and Society, 96*, 179–180.

Stancato, F., & Eizler, C. (1983). When a "C" is not a "C". The psychological meaning of grades in educational psychology. *Journal of Instructional Psychology, 10*, 158–162.

13

A Future Perspective: The Clinical Setting

A familiar adage cites the need for nurse educators in preparatory programs to prepare nurses not only for today, but also for tomorrow. Likewise, staff educators are charged not only with keeping practicing nurses up to date with current knowledge and practice, but they must prepare them for tomorrow. But tomorrow is today. The seeds of tomorrow are already evidenced today. What does today suggest tomorrow will be like in nursing practice, and therefore what will teaching in the clinical field be like at that time?

Loye (1984) makes note of the fragile nature of future forecasts.

All forecasts for the future upon which we rely for personal and national survival . . . are warped and distorted by the personality and ideology of the forecaster and because these personal differences are hidden, from us and indeed generally from the forecaster themselves, we walk on quicksand in viewing the future. (p. 66)

With some risk, the future of nursing practice is forecasted and the resultant implications for teaching this practice are examined and addressed. It is essential that faculty explore the potential directions of the future and search for their meanings, for the way nursing practice responds to these directions, the roles and responsibilities attributed to nurses, and the very actions the nurses undertake are all part of the substance of today's nursing education.

Caution in examining the future is suggested by Bolles (1983) when he states that the future has two parts: *change* and *constancy*. He sees both parts as essential, with change representing "challenge risk taking, adventure and at its height, a kind of magic and enhancement lent to our life while constancy represents familiarity, safety, comfort and security" (p. 7). A view of the future that stresses only change provokes a state of anxiety, fear, uncertainty, and powerlessness. Likewise, a future perceived as constant with an aura of nostalgia provokes a state of boredom and inertia, as well as emotional, mental, and spiritual stagnation. It is both elements, the constant and the change, which must be incorporated in the faculty's perception of the future as it pertains to teaching in the clinical field.

Nursing practice is not an island unto itself. It has its own microworld with its own boundaries and delineated actions, but it is part of the macroworld, which constantly moves, threatens, and even permeates the boundaries. It functions within an ever-expanding knowledge generation and within a rapidly evolving information society characterized by high technology and marked demands on all resources. As with other disciplines, nursing's rapidly developing knowledge base is demanding efficient means of organizing that knowledge so that it can be readily available for use. This new knowledge is altering for the better the capabilities of nursing in intervening both qualitatively and quantitatively in health matters, while modifying its roles, responsibilities, and activities. Its constancy rests in the certain goal of assisting clients in meeting their health care needs toward fulfilling their maximum potential.

The information society with its concomitant high technology provides for intervention in physiologic or anatomic aberrations to a remarkable degree but at such cost that it threatens financial resources for all health care in the society and poses moral and ethical questions relative to the "rightness" of the intervention and the eligibility of the recipient. In an effort to address the dislocation of health care dollars, regulation of the health care delivery system through cost effective measures is undertaken in the public and private sector. One effect of these measures is a marked change in both of these settings. Changes in clinical practice for the future are concerned both with the practice settings and the characteristics of the activities within those settings, while constancy is maintained through the affirmation of the caring role with the client as the primary focus. Many nursing functions will be basically constant, but they may seem different because of the changes in their execution.

THE INFORMATION SOCIETY

Naisbitt (1982) states that our society is ". . . drowning in information, but starved for knowledge" (p. 17). Information is perceived to be high in quantity but low in usability in its present disorganized and uncontrollable state. Nurses are only too aware of Naisbitt's observation as they seek to deal with the extraordinary influx of information generated not only by their own discipline, but also by disciplines whose knowledge bears directly or indirectly on nursing practice. Knowledge will continue to evolve with increased momentum and must be harnessed so that it can be a directed force used to improve the health care in the society. Ownership of knowledge cannot be a private preserve for the health professional; knowledge must be used for the benefit of others within the context of professional practice.

Technology

The fact that technology permeates the lives of all, at least in the western world, is well acknowledged. The fact that its intrusion is occurring at such a rapid rate so that in many instances there is not enough time to react to its presence is not as readily realized until it threatens some way of life. Some technology improves life for individuals; some causes disequilibrium in the balance of an individual's life, while some may threaten the very existence of life.

The health care field is in the center of much new technology: some of it has been proven essential for forward movement; some of it has yet to attest to its value; and some of it may address one problem but create new ones. The use of technology in health care has occurred in two major areas; the instrumentation of care and cure and the computerization of data into information systems.

Instrumentation. Technology is a significant part of the cure component of health care. Assessment instrumentation has moved far beyond the glass thermometer and the stethoscope and in time these tools will become obsolete as newer devices are developed to monitor vital signs more efficiently and accurately. Monitoring can now occur even when geographic distances separate the client from the health care provider. Technology provides for continuous observation of many body functions as is evidenced in intensive care units. New technology, such as scanners, imagery, and their successors, permit more accurate assessment of body structures and functions not easily accessible with the usual assessment techniques.

Technology has altered significantly the instrumentation aspect of intervention so that many aberrations in body structure or function previously unperceived or untreatable are now addressed with reasonable assurance of improvement in the quality of life for the individual. Some technology is making older intervention strategies obsolete. The advent of laser surgery portends the obsolescence of some currently used surgical procedures. Technology has permitted life processes to be maintained when the body's own mechanism fails; an action which may be important for a prescribed period of time, but which possesses the potential of extending beyond the need, resulting in feelings of anxiety and guilt on the part of the families and care givers when the purpose is no longer relevant and cessation of the process should be undertaken.

It is beyond the purview of this book to identify the various types of instrumentation currently used in practice or on the drawing board for future implementation. Suffice it to say, the assessment of an intervention in body dysfunction is becoming increasingly technologic. This is a significant factor in preparation of practitioners.

Computerization. The reference to "information society" causes an immediate association with the word computer. The computer is one means for bringing order to the vast array of available information and making it more accessible. Naisbitt (1982) sees the computer developing information systems which incorporate the essential data relative to their purposes and functions, and provide for demonstration of their interrelationships as needed. This communication network organizes the multitude of data pertinent to agency functioning and yields data necessary for meeting a designated problem or situation. It is obvious that employees in these agencies who have decision-making responsibility will be required to be functional in the use of a computer.

The role of computers in concert with technology is presently in use for monitoring the many physiologic processes of vital functions of clients. The addition of the computer provides an important dimension, for it lessens the demand for the nurse to "monitor the machine." The computer also interprets the findings and provides the protocol for action when any findings suggest body system dysfunction.

Computer technology is already integrated in the health care field, with each discipline developing its own information system, i.e., Nursing Information System (NIS). Saba (1988) states that the most common use of NIS presently is in managing nursing services and patient care in hospitals and nursing homes (p. 487). For management of services that include staffing patterns, four acuity-based systems are being used in classifying needs: (1) self-care deficits of the patients, (2) time required to carry various nursing activities, (3) patient care requirements, and (4) nursing dependency as defined in a nursing diagnosis by a primary care nurse (Saba, 1988, p. 488). Some hospital systems (HIS) incorporate nursing care planning in the main frame, using one of two models, medical model or nursing diagnosis model.

Halloran (1988) conducted a study to determine if the HIS plans which are based on the DRG system address nursing. Originally designed for cost-effectiveness data, the present DRG systems combine medicine and business. Halloran (1988), using a nursing dependency construct including physical, social, and psychological incapacities, found that the DRG system did not provide for nursing care and that the care provided was determined by the nurses' judgment as to the level of care needed (p. 199).

The favorable impact of computer technology on nursing in the practice setting is expressed by many in the field, Brown (1991), Gross (1988), Saba (1988), Millholland, K. (1988), Graves and Corcoran (1989), Blum (1986) and others. Brown (1991) comments on the effect of computer systems on nursing:

> Computers are helping to improve the quality and efficiency of nursing care delivery through the use of information systems that facilitate

the input, processing and retrieval of patient information and nursing care planning programs that assist the nurse with decision-making. (p. 197)

Gross (1988) notes the value of HIS in the improvement of the quality of discharge planning and follow up through its ability to compare the actual care given with accepted standards of care.

A new dimension of nursing knowledge is developing which is referred to as nursing informatics. Graves and Corcoran (1989) define this term:

Nursing informatics is a combination of computer science, information science, and nursing science designed to assist in the management and processing of nursing data, information, and knowledge to support the practice of nursing and the delivery of nursing care. (p. 227)

The developing of nursing informatics is proceeding through the analytic processes of research and is providing a system for using nursing knowledge, developing new knowledge, and expediting nursing decision making. The contribution that nursing informatics makes to research and development of nursing knowledge is particularly significant. Werley (1985), one of the leaders in knowledge development in the area of nursing data sets states "through computerized information systems, nurses can collect, manipulate and retrieve nursing data in systematic ways to advance nursing knowledge" (p. 2). As new knowledge is generated from data sets, Graves and Corcoran (1989) note that nursing informatics is an integral part of nursing science, not a branch of computer or information science applied to nursing (p. 228).

Influence of Technology on Hospital Care

Donley (1984) refers to hospitals as "temples of technology" (p. 4). Technology is well integrated into all systems of hospitals with evidence that this trend will continue in the future. High technology is associated primarily with acuity of illness. This factor accounts for hospitals becoming centers of acute care requiring sophisticated technologic instrumentation used by highly trained technical practitioners. McClure and Nelson (1982) note that the acuity issue has fostered an increased specialization phenomenon relative to medical and nursing care and concomitantly to specialization or segregation of particular areas of the hospital. Although this costly technologic specialization occurs predominantly in medical centers, even small community hospitals are required to have intensive care units to provide for immediate service to their communities.

A significant factor about high technology in health care to consider is the difference of its impact on the health care system from what one finds in industry. In the latter, technology often reduces the cost for labor, causing a shift of the cost to capital which can be spread out over a period of time. Curtin (1984) notes that in the health care system, the introduction of cybernetics increases capital costs without the concomitant decrease in labor costs, for in practice it actually increases the need for employment. Two results of using high technology in the delivery of health services are cited by Curtin:

1. Sicker people now can survive, but their care consumes more human and material services.
2. The resultant increase in population ultimately increases demand for services. (p. 70)

She concludes, "In short, mortality rates still come one to a person, only now people tend to die of long-term, chronic or debilitating diseases that require increasingly sophisticated interventions over longer periods of time" (p. 70).

Technology, rather than contributing to a reduction in costs of health care, in essence accounts for much of its increase. Its effect is found in its ability to prolong life, with or without improvement in its quality. Value questions arise in addressing cost in relation to life. Health care dollars are not finite, hard choices lie ahead in their control and allocation.

Because of the high cost of technology, patient days in the hospital are restricted to the time necessary for the use of the technology, not to the time necessary for the patient to be prepared to manage self-care outside the hospital. This means that hospital stays for patients will be shorter, patient turnover will be more rapid, and hospitals will be centers of intensity and complexity with high stress for all a complicating factor. Naisbitt (1982) refers to the effects of technology in changing the care aspect in the hospital: "The more high technology we put into our hospitals, the less we are being born there, dying there . . . and avoiding them in between" (p. 38).

Hospital care as previously known is in transition, if not in revolution. Birthing centers for new life, hospices for the dying, chronic hospitals as step-down centers for persons discharged from high-tech centers, ambulatory centers for general surgery and medical therapies, managed care systems including nursing centers, and organized home care services will be the pattern for delivery of health care in those matters previously tended to within the hospital domain. The decrease in the dependence on hospitals will foster the self-care movement in which individuals will place more emphasis on staying well and learning how to meet their own health needs except in acute situations or those which impede their usual activities.

Changes in Role and Responsibilities of Nursing

The technology diffusion in health care settings has altered the responsibilities of nursing. Donley (1984), using Toffler's notion of societal waves, considers the mechanical technologic nursing seen today as reflective of a second-wave society with some evidence of a third-wave society in the use of some sophisticated technology. To a lesser degree, hands-on care, characteristic of the first wave continues. In a mechanical technologic setting, nursing responsibilities entail clinical knowledge for rapid decision making and technologic expertise. Naisbitt (1982), however, sees high technology creating dissonance in life patterns of many persons resulting in resistance to the dehumanizing effects of such mechanisms.

Nurses' knowledge of technology as an integral part of patient care and their responsibility to clients whose care involves technology are critical factors in assuring humanistic care. Technology is rapidly advancing in the health care field and mandates nurses' attention to the implications which it brings. Zwolski (1989) provides a framework for enabling nurses to examine issues related to the extensive use of technology. He cites four principles which describe a technological health care system:

1. Technique is distinguishable from technology. Zwolski uses Barrett (1978) to provide the definition of these two entities. A technique is simply a standard method that can be taught, a recipe that can be duplicated, and that if followed, will always lead to the end desired. Technology is the embodiment of technique and/or the material products of technique.
2. A technique cannot produce the philosophy that directs it. A danger exists that the means (technique) and the ends (technology) will become blurred so that the means becomes the end. A question to be raised by the nurse, "What is the good of this technique for the client and under what circumstances should it be used?" (p. 240)
3. Technology in its incomplete and imperfect stages creates new problems. The possibility of iarthogenesis problems arises as well as problems of autonomy and control for individuals in the system.
4. Technology produces fragmentation. Fragmentation often results in competition among groups for scarce resources and personalization of care. (pp. 238-241)

Recognizing that technology is also permeating the care in the community and even patient homes, nurses who profess holistic, humanistic care need to be in tune with the rationale for use of the technique and the patient's vision of its meaning. To assist nurses to examine technology and the techniques it represents, Zwolski (1989) suggests use of the four principles cited while pondering some professional themes; the use of alternate techniques, the allocation of resources, ethical concerns and issues of control and autonomy, advocacy, education and creativity (p. 242).

Nurses working in high-tech hospital settings, although challenged by the "wonder machine," must develop skills in "high touch"; a process of sensitivity to the humanity of the client and to those who share love and concern for the client. High-touch skills are most vulnerable in a highly charged environment where client stay is short, negating a long-term relationship and where client response level is diminished by the nature of the pathologic processes and the therapies being used to ameliorate these processes.

Nurses need to participate in decisions as to what advances in technology are acceptable in the setting. Questions as to technology's value, its effect on the value system of individuals and the society, and its effect on the health care delivery system are in order.

The high-tech environment in hospitals includes computerization of the data relative to assessment of patient physiologic responses and protocols for patient management or treatment for deviations in response. Many clinical judgments are thus preprogrammed, with the major decisions related to the selection of the appropriate protocols for the particular problem involved.

There is some concern in the minds of some nursing leaders relative to the possibility of nursing autonomy, legitimate control over nurses' own work, becoming reality in hospital settings (Donley, 1984; Jacox, 1982; Rosenow, 1983). Although nurses have the ability to make clinical judgments, their actions are limited by role definition in a bureaucratic system. Rosenow notes: ". . . the authority for nursing actions comes from physicians through orders or from the hospital through rule and specified routines" (p. 35). In describing the intensive care situation with its high technology, she identifies the activities of the triad: administration, physician, and nurse; the administration assures the availability of essential resources, the doctor determines the services to be offered and the nurse executes and monitors the delivery of services. The nurse in this setting does not have professional autonomy; rather, the nurse functions in a supportive role carrying out tasks delegated by a member of another profession. To have professional autonomy, Freidson (1971) cites two significant criteria: ". . . (a) the professional must have control over an area of work separate from that of a dominant profession; (b) the practice must occur without routine contact or dependence on the dominant profession" (p. 79).

Maraldo (1990) sees nursing gaining greater preeminence in health care delivery as the shift from in-patient delivery system to a community-based system occurs where "managed care nursing is best suited for patient advocacy, patient education and practitioner in the care of the chronically ill" (p. 12). Nursing entrepreneurs have already established nurse managed care centers and in many instances are receiving fees from third party payers.

Within the work place, the bureaucratic fiat or order is being replaced by participatory style. Maraldo (1990) sees a different relationship between employer and employee in a knowledge society where employees are independent, mobile, and colleagual in their relationships (p. 9). The identity of nurses in the "knowledge society" is with their profession, its philosophy, goals and practices, not with any institution. As nurses become more autonomous and career oriented, their power in the work place will increase, an occurrence which will be threatening to others who previously dominated policy and decision making.

Feminist theory which emphasizes the caring component, sharing, and equality in relationships is contributing to the knowledge of nursing empowerment in decision making. Mason, Backer, and George (1991) identify three dimensions in which nursing needs to develop for empowerment in political action; raising the consciousness of social-political realities, developing positive esteem with emphasis on group consciousness, and political skills (p. 72). Nursing's cultural history is a deterrent, but not a barrier to nursing becoming a major force in the political area where health concerns are argued and decided. The dimensions cited above provide direction for education of nurses and nursing students for this critical role.

A significant action was the decentralization of decision making nearer the locus of action. In the study of magnet hospitals (American Academy of Nursing, 1983) the decentralization of decision making was a major factor in attracting and maintaining nurses because it enabled nurses at the unit level to have a sense of control over the immediate work environment. The decentralization of decision making is an essential concept of the networking system which affords authority to those who know, not to those who hold a designated position in a hierarchy. Networking as an organizational framework has not appeared at this time in hospitals to any significant degree in the mid-eighties, but its acceptance in other major organizations will influence the processes in hospitals. Three reasons are cited by Naisbitt (1982), for the emergence of a network system:

1. Dearth of traditional structures.
2. Din of information overload.
3. Past failures of hierarchies. (p. 220)

Differences between a networking system and a hierarchical system are identified by McInnes (1984):

1. Authority tends to be decentralized, residing in individuals with pertinent information rather than in those who occupy an assigned position.
2. Policies and boundaries tend to be fluid rather than fixed.
3. Personnel tend to relate among themselves and with others as equals rather than as subordinate or superior.
4. Procedures tend to be people centered.
5. Style tends to be sociable rather than officious.
6. Structure tends to be polycentric rather than monocentric. (p. 9)

Present trends in some nursing departments suggest that in the future, nursing will move into a networking system which provides for information linkages horizontally, vertically, and multidirectionally. This system change will result as more highly educated and prepared nurses enter the practice setting with professional knowledge and the expectation to be active participants in the decision-making process with control over their own practice. Because of nurses' need to manage large quantities of information in a short space of time, nurses will see validity to Naisbitt's concept of networking as a "structure for transmitting information in an organization that is quick, more high touch and more energy efficient" (p. 215).

Alterations in locus of decision making relative to patient care have potential for fostering a networking organizational system in hospitals. Jacox (1982) notes the internal authority conflict occurring in hospitals as outside forces exert control over patient care decisions, formerly the primary responsibility of the physician. The cost-effective measure, prospective payment for health care provided for Medicare patients, places the administration with the support of government in a decision-making position relative to patient discharge, a practice rarely occurring in the past. The change in power of the physicians in the hospital and their movement toward becoming salaried employees of hospitals, and the development of nurse managed care as well as the affirmation of nursing's knowledge domain, provide an opportunity for nursing to consolidate its domain of practice over which it has autonomy. With the recognition and acceptance of the expertise of each group working within the hospital and the allocation of responsibility and authority accordingly, a networking, rather than a power-oriented management system is a real potential for the hospital of tomorrow. The increasing complexity of decisions is no longer the domain of any one group; decisions require the synthesis of expertise of all involved.

HEALTH CARE DELIVERY COSTS

The 1990s is a crisis period in the health care of America. How this crisis is resolved influences significantly the nature of nursing practice, its roles within the health care system, and the types of the settings where practice occurs; all of which have direct bearing on the future of nursing education. The impending arrival of a new century raises serious questions for all health care professionals, for present decisions will influence the pattern of health care in the next century. Samuel Johnson stated, "The future is purchased from the present" (Evans, 1978). What will nursing be purchasing? What will be nursing's agenda in this new century? What will be its relationship to a world-wide schema of health care? For what and how will its new members be prepared? The future of nursing is purchased from the beliefs, values, commitments, and practices of today.

Nursing visionaries such as, Maraldo (1990), Maraldo and Solomon (1987), Lynaugh and Fagin (1988), Donley (1984), and Barnum (1989) have presented their views of nursing's future with marked implications for the present. Their future suggests that the time is ripe for nursing to move to control its own destiny. Maraldo and Solomon (1987) even title their article to denote this premise, "Nursing's Window of Opportunity."

At this time when American society is demanding, as a national priority, health care at a reasonable cost for all its citizens, nursing is being provided with the opportunity to demonstrate its expertise, its cost-saving potential, and its readiness to enter the health care market as a competitor.

The future, as perceived by these visionaries, will see nursing with a stronger voice in health care policy decisions, empowered to have a definitive role in influencing the direction of and declaration of the basic philosophical assumptions underlying a health care system. Participation in the provision of health care services will reflect the autonomy of the profession as it acts colleagually with other health care providers. Through a strengthening of its caring dimension of practice, it will promote the values of human rights, self worth and human dignity, often lost in a health care world of technology, and will provide an ethical and moral voice in decisions relative to the goal of a health care system, the expenditure of health care dollars, and the role of the consumer's voice in health matters affecting them. Nursing's long time association with the community as a health care provider places it in a unique position for advocacy of a humanistic health care system, emphasizing allocation of funds for preventive as well as curative care with consideration of the affordability, availability, and accessibility of health care resources to the varied population in the community to be served.

Health Care Issues

Nursing's future as a viable force in shaping the delivery of health care services is closely related to the directions the society takes in meeting the peoples' demand that a cost-effective health care system be instituted for all the citizens. The United States has one of the most sophisticated and advanced health care practices in the world, yet access to that advanced care is denied to 18 percent of its population (35 million) who have no health insurance. Over half of these individuals are employed and about two-thirds have incomes above poverty levels (Harrington, 1990). Payment for health care in the country is through government programs, primarily in the form of Medicare, designed for the elderly and selected categories of disabled, and Medicaid, a state allocation for the poor, and private funding programs from insurance plans. Grace (1990, p. 127) reports on the allocation of health care financing in 1985 as:

Public (government)	40%
Private	31%
Direct–out of pocket	27%

Most insurance plans are the result of a link of the insurance companies and business so that insurance for health care is tied into employment. Although this plan worked well for a long time, the high cost of health care is forcing industry to review this practice and many are now requiring that employees pay part of the health insurance cost. This model of health insurance has many serious deficits and accounts for the large number of uninsured individuals. The high cost of health insurance prevents small companies and businesses, who pay minimum wage to their employees, from offering health insurance as a benefit. In companies where health insurance is a benefit, laid off or fired employees lose their health insurance when they leave their job, while other workers feel compelled to remain in a job, even though it is not to their liking, because they cannot afford to pay the high cost of health insurance as independent subscribers. The present situation leaves many individuals without access to health care, health needs unmet, and with preventive practices so essential to family development nonexistent. These individuals enter the health care system primarily through emergency services often the result of neglect.

High Costs of Health Care

The issue of insurance affordability and accessibility is a critical one, for health costs in America are extremely high and basically out of control. Lack of money for health care is not the issue, for the United States spends more money for health care than any other country, about 500 billion, 11 percent of the gross national product (Freudenheim, 1988). There are numerous reasons for high cost health care, with a major one being the role afforded to doctors, hospitals, and insurance companies as arbitrators of what health care is and how it is to be delivered and administered. Emphasis on the bio-medical model results in high-cost curative care requiring expensive technology and the use of highly priced medical specialists rather than preventive care whose long term results decrease the need for such expensive intervention.

Grace (1990) identifies four major reasons why health care costs have become so high: overcapacity of hospitals, surplus of highly specialized care providers, inequitable financing of health care services, and passive role of the consumers (p. 124). Other causes include the opportunistic behavior of groups, such as, pharmaceutical companies who price drugs way beyond their generic value, hospital system of charging patients for many items beyond their inherent worth, and doctors, health care delivery agencies, and others who misappropriate health care dollars to satisfy their own greed. Reports of misuse of funds are frequent occurrences in the media such as the one which appeared in *The New York Times* on November 24, 1991 labeled, "Mental Hospital Chains Accused of Much Cheating" (Kerr, 1991, p. 1).

Califano (1986) addresses the present situation thusly, "The American way of health has been voracious in its pursuit of more and more money, too often unrelated to better care. Unless we change its course, our health care system will break the bank, set off the nastiest generational and political conflict our nation has ever experienced, provide increasingly extravagant first-rate health care to fewer and fewer Americans, and put life-and-death power in the hands of government, which no free people can tolerate" (p. 7).

Efforts to Control Costs

Cost control of health care needs to be approached from many fronts, financial, social, ethical, geographic, psychological and therapeutic. Since hospitals absorb the highest use of health care dollars, efforts to control costs have been undertaken in several ways.

Prospective Payment System. Following efforts since 1960 to control costs by determining a realistic cost basis for patients in hospitals, the government-sponsored reimbursement for hospitalized patients receiving Medicare became prospective rather than retrospective.

In a retrospective reimbursement system the hospital was paid at the conclusion of services rendered including a per diem for routine and special care as well as ancillary services such as diagnostic and therapeutic tests at a cost specified by the hospital. With few restrictions on costs to health care providers, individuals, and agencies, there was no sense of urgency to provide cost-efficient care. The inflation of health care costs at a higher rate than was evident for other aspects of society prompted the government to develop a system of payment with built-in cost controls, which are in effect expenditure controls.

On April 20, 1983, the Social Security Amendments of 1983, law H.R. 1900 (P1 98-21), passed by Congress, was signed by President Reagan. This law authorized the use of a prospective payment system based on DRG (diagnostic-related groups) for all hospitals serving Medicare. The primary objective of the system is to define types of cases that would be expected to be similar in the amount of usage of hospital services, with the length of stay as a measure of hospital services (Plomann & Schaffer, 1983). The length of stay is a significant factor, for experience suggests that ancillary services, such as diagnostic tests and treatments, increase proportionally to the time the patient stays in the hospital.

The categories selected are based on patient diagnosis, age, treatment procedures (inclusive of surgery), discharge status, and sex. This classification system reinforces the already established disease orientation of the hospital, in contrast to nursing's health orientation. Rates are set in advance according to a formula which takes into account regional and national rates and for each hospital, the cost experience updated for inflation.

The model has now also been adopted in states for their Medicaid system and is a factor in some private insurance programs. Results of studies of the effect of the system are now being reported. There has been a notable shift in the demand for health care from the hospital to community services. Haddon (1990) notes that the prospective payment system has resulted in increased efficiency spending, but costs have not been substantially reduced because of the costly hospitalization needs of the elderly and individuals with AIDS (p. 27). Bull (1988) suggests that the Diagnostic-Related Group system (DRG) has facilitated discharge planning and communication and collaboration among health care providers. Since the community is receiving much of the impact of the new system, studies by Phillips, Fisher, MacMillan-Scattergood and Baglioni (1989) note greater demands on nursing. The need to see patients soon after discharge from the hospital, the increase in the number of visits, and the greater number and more complex services required for each visit have greatly increased the nursing care needs for community nurses. Oermann (1991) notes the increased acuity of the illness factor in patients returning to their home under the DRG system; so that nurses skilled in acute care need to be employed by these community agencies. It is also noted that the community health nurse is the primary care-giver in the community where a disparity in payment for services exists. Medicare reimbursement for these services is based only on the visit regardless of the services required, while in the hospital, reimbursement is based on a array of services.

Utilization Review Cost Control Program. Another approach to controlling hospital costs is the utilization review method where authorization for patient admission to a hospital is required. This method is limited to addressing two elements, inpatient care and diagnostics. Studies have generally shown about a 12 percent decrease in hospital admissions and a 9 percent decrease in inpatient expenditures (Robert W. Johnson, p. 6). A study by Wickizer, Wheeler, and Feldstein (1991) examined the relationship between the decreased costs in hospitalization and the costs for outpatient services. The finding indicated a 20 percent increase in outpatient costs in institutions using utilization review cost control program. With the most notable increase in outpatient surgery, questions could be raised as to a possible practice whereby this service was used by doctors to circumvent the need for prior review.

Other Measures. Some movement is now underway to decrease the expenditure in another high cost area, doctors' fees. Medicare has made some alterations in this area, decreasing the remuneration for specialists' fees and increasing the remuneration for general practitioners and primary care providers. Some doctors have withdrawn from the Medicare and Medicaid programs in protest of the decreased fees.

At this time the political leaders have heard the consumers' demand that the health care system be put in order so that care is within the reach of all peoples in the country. Discussions within political bodies are suggesting three possible approaches to health care funding: (1) repair the present system by addressing the weak areas, (2) remodel the present system to make it more responsive, and (3) scrap present plans and develop a new plan for a national health insurance similar to the one in Canada and other western countries. The eventual model will probably entail both government and private funding. Although its form is uncertain, it is *certain* that some type of plan will be forthcoming.

Nursing and Health Care Issues

Nursing's future direction may well be determined by the commitment and intensity with which it becomes involved in the development of a health care plan for American society. Nursing leadership is already involved in developing strategies for assuring that the nursing voice is a recognized part of these deliberations. Maraldo and Solomon (1987) see nursing's need to gain economic and political power and to relate the health needs of society to the goals of nursing. Weisfield and Amor (1991) believe that nursing will have the greatest impact on health policy by demonstrating the positive effect of nurses' ideas on care and health care policy concerns, i.e., access, quality, and cost containment. Lynaugh and Fagin (1988) suggest that nursing needs to acknowledge the advancement that nursing is making in the health field, i.e., the 20,000 nurses, as reported by the American Nurses Association, who have started independent ventures such as family primary care, clinics, birthing centers, home health agencies, and in 25 states nurses are receiving third party payment from insurance companies (*Perspectives*, 1987, p. 186). The immediate challenge is to have the Medicare restrictions rescinded so that nurses have the right to bill the agency for services to clients. Within the practice area and legally, nurse midwives, nurse anesthetists, and clinical specialists are recognized as expert practitioners. Nursing research and researchers are acknowledged on the national and international scene for their scholarship and relevancy to the health care needs of individuals and society and their potential for directing solutions to the health problems. Nursing's developing knowledge in nursing ethics theory facilitates nurses in providing the humanistic health care service which the consumer is requesting. Nursing's emphasis on primary care, prevention, and restoration as critical components of a health care system promotes a more realistic and cost efficient model.

Nursing has the knowledge, the expertise, and the fundamental philosophical basis for an active role in the evolution of an American health care system. Nursing leaders completed in 1991, a proposal for a health care system, called *Nursing's Agenda for Health Care Reform*, (National League for Nursing, 1991) which has been adopted by 42 nursing organizations. A thoughtful, relevant and comprehensive proposal, it mandates intensive examination by all nurses and students in nursing, for it speaks for nursing. In citing the need for this agenda, the authors state, "Our (nursing) constant presence in a variety of settings places us in contact with individuals who reap the benefits of the system's most sophisticated services, as well as those individuals seriously compromised by the system's inefficiencies" (p. 4). The plan reflects the basic values and assumptions to which nursing subscribes; cost effective universal access to health care; consumer involvement as primary focus of the care, responsible for own self care and health care, and entitled to a full range of quality services; emphasis on primary as well as secondary and tertiary care; efficient use of financial and other resources; and accommodation for catastrophic illness or impoverishment. The funding incorporates private and public money within the present system of deductibles and copayments which can be altered if they become a barrier to any individual's care.

Managed care and case management systems through which consumers have access to quality care on a cost-effective basis are advocated in the plan. These systems incorporate nurses as primary care givers as well as being involved in secondary and tertiary care. Some managed care services are already developed and in operation by nurse entrepreneurs.

The *Nursing Agenda for Health Care Reform* has received considerable attention and recognition in the professional communities and the political areas of government. It is less known in the general nursing community, yet these members of the profession are needed to bring the document to the attention of all levels of government in the community. Political persuasion is in order as well as dialogue with consumers to show the positive relationship of the proposal to their desire for universal cost-effective quality health care.

One significant component of society has not or chooses not to recognize the potential role of nursing in ameliorating the inequities and high cost of health care. That is the press. Burest, Gordon, and Bell

(1991) conducted a study of the major publications and found that there is a dearth of material in which nursing is a source of information on health care and their expertise is ignored in any such discussion. A recent issue of *Time Magazine,* November 25, 1991, contained a lead article by Castro, entitled, *10 Ways to Cure the Health Care Mess.* The word, nursing, was not even mentioned. Burest et al. (1991) state that nursing as a group "has no influence in development of public policy and allocation of resources unless it can be seen and heard as part of public discussion" (p. 108).

The culture of nursing and society explain in part the failure to cite nursing as a significant force in the politics of health. Lynaugh and Fagin (1988) identify five paradoxes of the nursing profession which serve as barriers to nursing's involvement in society beyond the caregiver role.

1. Nursing's mission to care is undervalued by society.

2. Nursing's limited involvement in the economic system has affected nursing to the point that the price of nursing service is still unknown.

3. Nursing is primarily a woman's profession. (97 percent) is dominated by male values of American society which accepts these values.

4. Nursing's history as an oppressed group, i.e., one controlled from outside itself, leads to low self-esteem, intragroup conflict, and self hatred.

5. Nursing's preoccupation with professional status as an ideology has led to division in nursing. (pp. 185–188)

These paradoxes do not represent insurmountable obstacles to nursing's movement into health care policy-making, but they need to be understood so that corrective actions can be instituted. They are appropriate areas of study in the educational programs with opportunities for students to turn them from barriers to opportunities.

It is in the clinical setting where much of the impact of the health care system issues can be experienced by the students as they view the inequities in care offered and plan with patients to meet their health needs. Case analysis which also includes the financial component is in order. When clinical practice is in the various community settings, health care access, affordability, and availability take on a reality which can challenge students to take a stand on some of the issues and move into action in the political sphere.

The Shift Toward Health Care in the Community

The movement of more health care into the community signifies a different client-health care provider relationship than one encounters in the hospital. In the latter, the client is "captive" with relatively little say about services provided. Tests are done, routines are followed, standard meals are served, and each group's territory is specified. In the community, however, the health caregiver is on the client's turf and the client is more free to decide whether or not to follow the prescribed regime of care, or indeed to accept any care. Some of the decisions will be based on clients' priority for expenditure of their own money, for there is less reimbursement money for diagnostic and therapeutic measures when carried out outside the hospital domain. Care of clients within their own cultural milieu represents a different source of power in health care decisions than when caring for a client within the hospital culture.

The cultural milieu of the client in the community represents several elements, ethnic, socio-economic, gender, family composition, and geography, all of which influence the life-style and patterns of the individual. Knowledge of and respect for various cultural groups, their values, their beliefs, and their patterns of behavior is essential for nurses in the community centers, especially when facilities are located in particular ethnic communities. Humanistic nursing care requires the nurse's sensitivity to these ethnic patterns and their meanings so that the nursing measures which are used will be in concert with the ethos of the individual not in violation of it.

The early discharge of patients means a change in the nature and amount of nursing that will be required in the home. Some patients will move into chronic hospitals as a transition from the acute care hospital to home. Others, however, will be discharged directly to their homes, often needing care and the use of technical equipment, once thought to be available only in the hospitals. Teaching of patients, families, and even volunteers will become a major focus of nursing action in the maintenance of a therapeutic regimen within the community settings. Because the early discharged patient still needs monitoring and care, Schraff (1984) recognizes that the planning for these patients involves more than the types of professional services needed; planning will need to consider client needs over a 24-hour period. Interagency planning, flexibility of community agencies with time schedules determined by need for services, and a networking system designed so that client and family have access to whatever care is needed are essential if continuity of care is to be provided.

Other activities, formerly conducted in the hospital, will be incorporated into community health care. The high cost of acute hospital care means that the time as a patient in that setting must be maximized and focused directly on the resolution of the health problem. The practice of admitting patients for preoperative preparation, both diagnostically and educationally, can become obsolete as practice increasingly occurs in the community prior to hospital admission.

All of these changes in practice occur with a shift in population groups needing care. The increasing age level of the public is documented in the literature and brings with it increased demand for use of health care resources and dollars; for illness, especially chronic, is more frequent in the older age group. Care emphasis will shift from custodial to the maximizing of the social potential of these elderly individuals so that they can assume greater responsibility for self-care. Another goal of this change is to minimize the cost of their care.

Fries (1986) has developed a theory, *Compression of Morbidity*, which proposes means by which health care costs for the elderly are minimized and their quality of life maximized. Three eras of illness since entering this century are identified: (1) the era of infectious disease, (2) the era of chronic noninfectious illness which is beginning to fade, and (3) the era which we are now entering and in which we will be involved for the next 25 years, major health burdens associated with aging population per se rather than specific diseases. In this era, the frailty of the organism becomes the immediate cause of death and major cause of dependence on others.

Fries sees the medical model appropriate for a simple world where "diseases have causes (germs) and the task of the bio-scientific enterprise is to identify the cause and to devise an appropriate and specific cure" (1985, p. 10). Current medical problems are not responsive to the medical model, for they require multiple disciplinary approaches inclusive of those from the social and behavioral sciences.

The *Compression of Morbidity* concept is based on acknowledgment of limits of Human Life expectancy—i.e., the relative stability of a natural life span—approximately 85 years with 90 percent of death occurring between ages of 70 and 100. Aging, a universal, incremental phenomenon begins early in life with first symptoms beginning later in life. The concept of compression of morbidity is addressed to decreasing the total life spent infirm through two goals: (1) postponement of onset of chronic illness and (2) preservation of maximum functional ability. These goals are targeted at developing a society of healthy and independent persons who maintain physical and cognitive functions until very close to the end of the natural life span. Emphasis stresses identification and control of high risk factors, development of personal responsibility and support for independent living. The compression of morbidity phenomenon is compatible with the concept of nursing we have articulated for a long time—wellness, prevention, health promotion, fostering of self-help, etc.

Milo (1989) concurs with Fries when she states, "The fundamental health problem today is premature aging–having people enter their late decades disabled from early onset of chronic and other damaging conditions" (p. 315).

At the opposite end of the age spectrum are the very young who need the essential care to assure a healthful life. Neglect at this age often dooms the individual to a life of health problems which puts increased demand on health care resources. Prevention, early correction of deviations, and health promotion and teaching are the foci of health care dollar expenditure for this young group. Although these two groups of the population place the highest demands on health dollars and resources, other age groups have specific health needs which must also be addressed.

Very serious health problems are evident in the community which require considerable expenditure of health dollars and services of varied health care providers. AIDS, now occurring at an increased pace, is a progressively deteriorating disease process with limited intervention modalities to stop its progress. Emergency services in communities are seeing an alarming number of victims of violence, a major public health problem in American society. The saturation of some communities with drugs has led to much violence, often involving young children. Spouse and child abuse appear too often at health care facilities and are destructive to the persons involved as well as the very fiber of the community.

New systems of health care delivery services are appearing in communities, many of which provide for prevention services to minimize the high cost of medical care. These models are in accord with nursing's belief about the importance of primary health care for our society. The new systems represent various forms of managed care with the goal of offering quality care at minimum cost.

One of the earliest recognized prepaid group practice models was the health care maintenance organization (HMO) resulting from the Health Maintenance Act of 1973 which specified that any HMO must be both the insurer and provider of health care. Drew (1990) reports that in 1988 there were 30.3 million people enrolled in 653 HMOs of various types with numbers expected to increase in the 1990s (p. 146). Emphasis on prevention and decreasing the need for hospitalization accounts for cost containment. The increasing number of elderly and indigent is placing great stress on these organizations in terms of cost expenditure and maintenance of quality care. Other types of prepaid group health care systems resembling the HMO model have been developed, many by private groups, and have met with varied success.

Nursing managed care centers have been developed in communities using a similar model. In 1987, a task force on nursing centers published a document which describes centers. The definition in the publication, *Nursing Center: Concept and Design* (Aydelotte, 1987) offers this definition, "Nursing Centers, sometimes referred to as community organizations, nurse managed centers, nursing clinics, and community nursing centers–are organizations that give the client direct access to professional nursing services" (p. 2). Barber (1991) identifies the key elements stated in the total definition as, complete nursing control and responsibility for the centers and the services they provide, patient-centered care which encompasses diagnosis and treatment and promotion of health and optimum functioning, and reimbursement for all services (p. 191). Reimbursement by third party payers is still not acceptable in some states. Warner (1988) found that even in South Dakota where third party funding has been approved legislatively, insurance companies do not notify their customers of the available nursing option nor are insurance personnel told that nurses are legitimate care providers.

Nursing centers may be free standing organizations, associated academic centers, home health care agencies or associated with hospitals. Some of the nurse managed care facilities are primarily for primary care, others address specific groups such as mothers and children, but all are guided by the goal to meet health care needs of the community. Rural areas are particularly responsive to nursing centers because of their limited access to health care services and the large number of people with chronic illness (Barber, 1991). Since these nursing centers are business operations, nursing executives requiring knowledge of business practices for the centers must ultimately demonstrate cost effectiveness of their services.

The concept of community will expand in the new century as worldwide concerns for health care are articulated and approached multilaterally by various countries. The implications of international nursing are the concern of American nurses (Maraldo, 1990). Milo (1989), Maglacas (1989), Gosnell (1985), De Santis (1988). Maraldo (1990) sees globalization of international economy which will open new markets for nursing services and literature (p. 13). Milo (1989) notes that "the new world is one of interdependence among nations, communities and groups; between environments and individuals; between policies and patterns of action" (p. 315). Maglacas (1989) notes the Alma-Ata Declaration of Primary Health Care of 1978.

Nations of the world join together in expressing the need for urgent action by all governments; all health and development workers and the world community at large to protect and promote the health of all people of the world. (p. 304)

Maglacas (1989) expresses the opinion that community health nurses are supporters of the document advocating health care for all, but nurses working in hospitals are not truly informed nor do they care about the international call for equity of health care for all peoples. At this time the will of nurses to respond to the new realities is missing among nurses in most countries (p. 312).

Nursing practice will change. Nursing knowledge will change. Nursing administration will change with more involvement of nurses in decision making. Donley (1984) sees dimensions of knowledge needed as a "gestalt of technical, humanistic and ethical knowledge" (p. 6). She elaborates on each of these dimensions. Super-technical knowledge refers to the professional who has established parameters of assessment and use of information to make clinical decisions. Humanistic knowledge enables nurses to address the philosophical meaning of health, illness, life, and death. Ethical knowledge enables the nurse to ascertain the goodness or badness of both clinical decisions and social policies which influence public decisions about resource allocation.

Harriman (1984) believes that in any rapidly changing world, ". . . innovative skills will be increasingly sought and implemented as more and more competing new challenges appear because it will be practical to do so" (p. 104). The ability to move within a changing system requires problem-solving skills that do not rely on past solutions but rather call upon the formulation of new ideas. This requires the ability to connect seemingly irrelevant data to a problem without the demand for assurance of fit but with the willingness to risk to think differently. Change is not linear; neither is problem solving. Nurses will need skills far removed from a routine, principled, or procedural approach to respond to obstacles or novel problems which will characterize the future of health care.

THE USE OF THE CLINICAL SETTING IN THE FUTURE

Change in the present presages the directions that will be found in the future. Health care, delivery of health care, and nursing practice are all enmeshed in a radical change that alters the foreseeable future. Nursing education, likewise, is an integral part of this change. The current directions influence nursing practice in the future and thus will influence the character of learning knowledge and skills in the clinical setting. Two significant changes in the use of the clinical field are apparent: change in the settings and change in the types of learning in these settings.

Change in Setting

Cost-containment measures in the system do not include educational costs for students using hospitals as a practice field. Although in some instances, nursing service is charging a fee for use of the setting as a student affiliation, this practice was not supported by four nursing directors discussing the future of nursing (Nursing & Health Care, 1984). Walker, responded to this trend thusly: "I think it is absolutely ridiculous for nursing directors to get into this mentality, because then we are cutting off our nose to spite our face" (p. 314). Another director, Sr. M. Flaherty, noted a disadvantage to interfering with the system of clinical affiliation, especially in chronic care hospitals. Positive experience as a student is an important factor in the recruitment of graduate nurses. It is also recognized that the presence of students in a practice setting positively influences the quality of care provided, for they serve as an incentive to the staff to improve care and reevaluate the care they are providing. The future possibility of charging for clinical affiliation remains to be decided, but such a decision is critical relative to its possible impact on both nursing service and nursing education.

Although the nursing literature in recent years has referred to the emphasis on wellness through prevention and health promotion as a primary focus in professional nursing preparation, there has been limited evidence of this fact in many nursing curriculums. In most instances, the majority of clinical experiences, indeed even the first such experience for a student, occur in the hospital, where emphasis is on cure. The pattern continues in spite of the increasing complexity of patient needs while hospitalized. If the development of professional competencies proceeds from simple to complex, practice fields must be selected that provide for the orderly process to occur. Movements to the community and its agencies, other than acute hospitals, for learning experiences is in the future, with hospitals providing experience in acute nursing care at an appropriate time in the program when students have the requisite entry competencies for practicing in such a setting.

Community as a Practice Setting

The reference to the community as a practice field must recognize its diversity in purpose, clientele, and services within the system of health care delivery. Its chronic care hospitals, long-term facilities, and nursing homes provide experience which is generally continuous, not subject to radical changes in patient health status, and is opportune for learning to establish a nurse-patient relationship and to use the nursing process in practice. Emphasis can be on prevention, health promotion, and cure, which brings persons to optimum health status. The experience is available for such learning but may need to be selective with the arrival of more acutely ill patients coming from an early discharge from the hospital.

Ambulatory care facilities will increase and provide experience in monitoring health status, participation with diagnostic and therapeutic measures, and fostering self-help capacities of clients and their families. The facilities are often the locus for preparation of people for hospital admission, which includes preoperative and pretherapeutic teaching, thus enabling the student to gain experience in addressing the informational and emotional needs of clients prior to hospitalization. The nurse-patient relationship is episodic and may or may not recur. In this field, the student learns to maximize time with the client and develop precision with assessment and intervention skills, particularly teaching and counseling competencies. Nursing care centers provide experiences in primary nursing where a continuing relationship with clients is a factor. Students also learn to accommodate their own notions of health care to the culture of clients in terms of their practices, life styles, values, and priorities.

Home care as a field of practice brings the student in direct contact with the client's culture where client acceptance or rejection of care and counsel may be related to the nurse's sensitivity to the multiple forces that affect health care decisions. Nursing experience in a home care setting ranges from simple to complex and often entails a continuing nurse-patient relationship. Experiences are selected on the basis of the student's readiness to participate. In some situations monitoring and teaching are the primary activities. In situations where the patient is discharged from the hospital early and requires considerable technologic intervention, students must be reasonably competent in their own practice to become involved. Whereas many of these interventions are carried out in a regular regime in the hospital and in the home, the patient, family, or others must be prepared to follow the regime beyond the nurse's professional visit. A network for patients' use summoning for assistance whenever needed is a critical component of care. The high nursing intensity required by these patients is the proper concern of the more advanced student.

The illustrations of different types of community agencies and some of the learning experiences available have been identified. The illustrations are not inclusive but suggestive of the experiences which faculty can choose as the curriculum is developed. Knowledge of and skill in computer usage within an information system is required for all students in community settings, for linkages are being established and data from patients will be computerized.

Greater use of the community as a field of practice demands that students be more informed about various community resources to assist client health needs. Often the nurse serves as the coordinator of care and needs to have a functioning knowledge of appropriate resources to which the client must be referred as well as the systems by which they operate, the procedures for entry, and costs and financial arrangements required.

As nursing education responds to the need to address the geographical inequities in nursing education programs, the notion of community takes on a broader meaning. The need to prepare many nurses in professional programs at the undergraduate and graduate level has forced faculty to examine the geographical barriers which prevent students from fulfilling the profession's goal of providing professional nursing services to all communities. Universities and colleges are beginning to recognize their responsibilities and are bringing their degree programs to students in outreach sites. One of the major concerns of faculty relates to the perception that practice can occur only in centers documented as "models" in terms of some selected criteria. There is hesitancy to use health care delivery agencies in rural or smaller communities. Yet since the goal of an outreach program is to provide access for students to achieve their degrees, an outreach program must use health care agencies in the local community. Reilly (1990a) states that "the faculty's ability to move within new practice environments to view their potentials from a less rigid set of criteria and to sense the challenge and excitement in moving from the "tried and true" greatly influences the success of the endeavor" (p. 98). Students in non-urban areas are generally knowledgeable about the types of practice resources available, their quality and their potentials for accommodating the demands of a new type of educational program. Since many of these communities do not have a highly structured system of health care agencies with territorial claims, nurses themselves are often more creative in planning for care. Faculty in outreach programs have considerable opportunity to be creative in planning and teaching in practice settings new to them while still maintaining the objectives and integrity of the program as stated on campus.

Hospital as a Practice Setting

The role of the hospital in preparing nurses is being altered as the result of the system of health care which is evolving. The acuity of patient needs and problems and the intensity of nursing demands in a high-stress environment create a practice field for more experienced students who have mastered skill in making clinical judgments, using the nursing process and using technical skills, and who are comfortable with themselves in a patient care milieu. The experiences provided include opportunity to participate in care where decisions are apt to be made rapidly and where patient-nurse-family relationships occur under highly stressful situations. The use of information systems by which care data and therapeutic prescriptions are computerized gives significant meaning to "Hi-Tech-Hi-Touch" care. Sharing in the decision-making process not only with nurses, but with members of other disciplines provides a broad perspective of the various perceptions of individuals involved in patient care. Skills in moral reasoning become particularly developed when decisions as to who receives care, who pays for the care, and what care is appropriate become of concern.

Discharge planning skills of the student are fostered as patients are sent from the hospital with a lesser degree of recovery than previously. Many institutions will develop a computerized discharge planning model which assures a systematic approach to providing continuity of care. A multidisciplinary discharge planning model using the Computerized Medical Information System (MIS) has been developed at the Clinical Center, National Institute of Health and is reported in the literature (Romano, 1984). New knowledge is needed relative to discharge planning which addresses the needs of early discharged patients and the use of community resources, often limited, to meet these needs.

Implications of Setting Change for Faculty

The change in emphasis on setting and the inherent nursing activities place new demands on the preparation of faculty so as to use effectively the various fields available for experience. Most faculty preparation dichotomizes nursing faculty roles into those prepared to teach within hospitals and those prepared to teach in the community. Another type of faculty is required: one who has the competencies to function in both settings and can facilitate involvement of students in the patient's transition from home to hospital and then to another community agency or home. The essence of continuity will become a critical factor in teaching, for the transfer of patients to various health care settings poses a real danger of the patient becoming "lost" in the process.

Many faculty teaching in hospitals today will not have the high technological knowledge and expertise necessary for patient care and for teaching that care to students. This factor will require these faculty to further their education in the competencies required or to be retrained to function within a community setting. It is in the latter where the need for faculty will be greatest in the future and where there is the greatest deficit currently. These faculty must be expert in home or long-term care and in coordination of health care resources, and comfortable with the values, practices, and life styles of various cultural groups. There will also be a need for coordination between faculty associated with acute episodic care in the hospital and those involved with long-term needs in the community so that the student experience provides for a holistic perspective of the client's needs for health care. Changes in health care patterns and delivery affect markedly the preparation of nursing faculty and support the need for faculty to maintain practice competencies. Increasingly, faculty practice plans will become commonplace in nursing education institutions.

Research in nursing education is a critical need in the future, especially as it explores the new knowledge and skill demands and their incorporation in a teaching modality which is most cost effective. Cost factors in educating future students relative to the new patterns of care must be identified through research for they are critical variables in determining programs. A teacher-student ratio appropriate for a geographical field reasonably circumscribed may not be sufficient for one with more diffuse boundaries as characteristic of nursing in the community.

New uses of information processing teaching modalities, preceptors in practice settings as models, and new knowledges derived from research in the learning process must be explored and instituted into the teaching program. Delineation of the *essential* knowledges and skills which are within the purview of any particular preparatory program is needed. Trivial pursuits and vested interests of faculty or others cannot with impunity dominate program decisions. Quality and quantity of the substance of learning, cost-effective teaching strategies, and the most expeditious use of faculty and clinical experts in the field are all matters for specific renewed exploration and research. The future demands precision in nursing education with quality of experience provided by those with expertise in their domain of nursing practice and teaching practice.

Research in all domains of nursing education is in progress at this time. The Council of Research in Nursing Education, now located within the National League for Nursing, was started in 1982 and has been a critical force in reestablishing such research as an essential component within the research movement in nursing. The Council provides for a forum where dialogue, dissemination of ideas, and critique of research endeavors occurs. Reilly (1990b) notes that nursing's introduction into the research area was primarily through studies in nursing education. This entry was related to nursing's entry into institutions of higher learning through educational schools, the first being Teachers College in Columbia University from which most of the early advanced degrees earned by nurses were awarded. As nurses earned degrees in the science fields and eventually in nursing itself, research interests were directed toward clinical practice and the development of nursing knowledge. Educational research in nursing became less favored, even to the point of questioning its legitimacy, as an appropriate research domain for nurses. Although nursing educators continued to conduct their own research on a limited basis, it was the forum of the Council meetings that brought renewal to the efforts.

Reilly (1990b) expressed the need for research in nursing education when she states, "New ways of thinking, new strategies and new standards are essential if we are to prepare practitioners possessing skills of analysis and problem solving for addressing the real problems in an increasingly complex society" (p. 143). It is important that as research in nursing proceeds, Mahdi's (1987) concern is addressed. He feels that the emphasis in much of education has been on *maintenance learning* rather than *innovative learning*. He further states that we need "the development of new criteria and parameters, as well as statistical norms and standards to monitor achievements in the field of education and learning" (p. 60). Research in nursing education will continue to evolve and provide the knowledge essential for facilitating teaching and student learning of nursing's body of knowledge expeditiously and effectively within a realistic cost-effective framework so that nursing's goals in the health care field can be achieved. Nursing education does have a body of knowledge.

EFFECT OF CHANGE ON USE OF CLINICAL SETTING FOR PREPARATION OF PRACTITIONERS

The caution that any view of the future must incorporate both change and constancy was stipulated by Bolles (1983). The change component has received the bulk of the attention in this chapter, but some explicit and implicit references were made to the constancy in the goal of nursing which is providing health services to clients in such a way as to contribute to the quality of their lives. Does any other constancy exist for the future which is significant for faculty?

This book began with suggestions for use of the clinical area in professional education as proposed by Argyris and Schön, which are: learning how to learn, handling ambiguity, thinking like professionals, and developing personal causation. Although the general notion of the goal of applying theory to practice is acknowledged, the other purposes denote a broader concept of this application more fitting for a professional so that the *how to do* does not become an end in itself.

Is there evidence of constancy in these four purposes, in spite of all the changes that are affecting nursing and nursing education? A review of their intent suggests that they are even more relevant today and for the future. They are most important outcomes in a field whose students will enter a society dominated by change.

The first outcome stated is *learning how to learn*. Facts and "how to do" are not sufficient subject matters for the clinical field experience, for both are consistently subject to questioning and are often altered as new knowledge is developed. Students must learn the facts and the *how to do* acceptable at any point in time, but they must equally be prepared to accept the probability of their transiency. Ever alert to the advent of new knowledge, the student will need to acquire the cognitive skills of rational and creative thinking, problem solving that provides for innovation as indicated, and decision making within a humanistic context. These skills enable the student to adopt the present state of knowledge, yet maintain the flexibility to accommodate to the new. Learning how to learn means the rigidity of knowledge ownership is inappropriate. It means the development of the posture of a continuous learner, the maintenance of a scholarly approach to developing knowledge, and a readiness to examine decisions and actions critically. The projection of the future of nursing includes the potential instability of much of its current knowledge and practices and affirms that *learning how to learn* is still an important purpose for clinical experience.

The second purpose stated is *handling ambiguity*. Nursing, like other health disciplines has many ambiguities in its practice. In particular, the delivery of health care services lacks a rationale which assures the delivery of the right care to the right client at the right time with the right intensity. The ambiguity of many actions in the entire health field becomes even more evident with the introduction of cost effectiveness as a major priority in the delivery of services. The health care provider who is a dualist thinker needing the *right and only answer* will be at a great disadvantage in the world of future nursing. Studies cited earlier showing that nursing programs are remiss in moving students from dualistic to relativistic thinking and ultimately to commitment is a cause of great concern. The future of nursing requires practitioners who can handle ambiguity and not rely on absolutism, but are self-confident in making decisions with use of the best of present knowledge, even when the outcome is not certain. Uncertainty, not certainty, will characterize nursing in the future, thus supporting the purpose, *dealing with* ambiguity as a legitimate one for use of the clinical field in nursing education.

The third purpose stated is *thinking like professionals*. The evolution of a theory of nursing practice is ongoing and will become increasingly obvious. Professional nurses base their practice not from a task orientation, but rather from a questioning and exploratory posture which seeks answers to the *why* and *what if* of nursing actions. Each professional practitioner is expected to develop an individual theory of practice that includes a systematic self-examination of decisions and actions. An action is not a *fait accompli*—it demands an analysis based on theories of nursing and other relevant disciplines in terms of its potential contribution to nursing practice knowledge.

Professionals also examine their own practice, beliefs, and modalities as they interface with the sociopolitical and economic forces of the larger society. Practice is not perceived from the position of personal territory; it is recognized as a part of a larger system which is influenced by that system but must also contribute to the system. Nursing in the future will be involved intimately with that larger system of health care, which in turn will be involved with the greater society—locally, regionally, nationally, and internationally.

Thinking like a professional means that the students in the future have a large view of their practice, develop as a scholar and contributor to nursing knowledge, and assume an active role in helping nursing to meet health needs of individuals in a complex socio-economic, political world. If nursing is to take its rightful place in that endeavor, practice experience needs to move the student from a self-interest posture to one that is enlightened by the values and behaviors of the professional in a world society. The purpose of the clinical experience to help students learn to *think like professionals* is basic for the attainable future for the profession.

The fourth purpose is *developing personal causation*. Accountability for one's actions is an essential criterion for any member of a society, but is required of those who are licensed by society to practice nursing. Development of information systems in health care settings will monitor the actions of nurses and others in the delivery of their services and more specifically identify the issues of accountability. The complexity of health care and the varied settings in which it occurs place demands on the nurses, not only for what they do, but also for the possession of requisite knowledge and skills for engaging in these actions. Accountability for knowing and doing in a future world of rapid knowledge generation will be a particular charge to the nurse.

Students can develop this quality of personal causation early in their clinical experience as it pertains to their accountability for their own knowledge and skills for the actions in which they participate. The emphasis, however, accommodates the expectation that learners make mistakes in the process of learning and can learn from their mistakes.

Accountability for preparation for clinical assignments, recognizing areas of knowledge and knowledge deficits as they pertain to the involved activities, and careful documentation of actions help students to recognize professional accountability as a legitimate value of a professional. The purpose, *personal causation* development, will become a critical outcome of nursing education as the student prepares to enter a field characterized by ambiguity with some uncertainty of its areas of autonomy, and involved in a society capable of declaring its expectations and issuing sanctions if its expectations are not realized.

A constancy in the future of nursing education's use of the clinical setting has been identified. Although the substance of the practice and settings where it occurs will be subject to alteration, its purposes remain constant. The charge to nursing educators is to accept the constancy of the purposes while interpreting them within the context of change, a characteristic of the future.

SUMMARY

The future of nursing and thus the future of nursing education is already evident today. The current developing practices need to be examined in relation to their predictive value for the future.

The change is resulting from many strong movements in society which are altering patterns for delivery of health care. The entrenchment of technology into the health field is evident in many diagnostic and therapeutic modalities and in the computerization of data which are retrieved for use in practice and for discovery of new nursing knowledge. Each of the parties involved in the health care field are developing information systems. Nursing information systems (NIS) are in use in some settings for management of nursing and patient care. Nursing systems relevant to patient care are developed with nursing diagnosis as the focus. Technology in the health field has brought about marked increase in health care costs.

The crisis of the 1990s is in relation to quality health care, its affordability, accessibility, and availability for all citizens in the country. The consumer demand for humanistic quality health care is forcing government bodies to develop some type of funded national health care program so that basic health needs can be met for all. Nursing is prepared, having developed its own agenda for health care, to enter into the critical dialogue at the policy making level to stress its position that primary care services are a vital element of any plan for national health care to avoid the high cost entailed in managing degenerative diseases or other illnesses which are the product of neglect. Primary care contributes remarkably to the health care and well being of the people in society.

Increases in health care costs occurring within a limited financial resource has resulted in the federal government's initiation of the prospective case mix reimbursement system as a basis for payment of services provided for hospitalized Medicare patients. The issue of cost containment will be paramount in all health care services for the future. Patterns of health care delivery are already being altered, so that hospital care which is the most costly, will be reserved for the acutely ill requiring high technology intervention. Hospitals will foster early discharge of patients, thus placing a much greater burden of health care on the community agencies.

The changes influence the delivery of nursing care by making the hospital the setting for high intensity acute care requiring nursing competencies reflected in a well-developed knowledge base, skill in technology with a high-touch component, and the requisite knowledge and skills for making clinical judgments in a rapidly changing, high-stress environment. The community agencies will require many more nurses equipped not only with the requisite knowledge of a professional practitioner, but also the knowledge and skills essential for coordination of patient care over a 24-hour period with use of multiple community resources. Nurses will be carrying out many activities of care previously carried out only by nurses practicing in the hospital, such as preparation of patient for hospital admission, assisting with surgical procedures in ambulatory centers, and carrying out many more complex technical interventions in client's homes, clinics, or other settings.

A third major force in the change process is the increasing age of the population which will put greater demand on the use of health care resources. Technology is now permitting life to many individuals who in earlier days would have died. Now with lengthening life spans, the need for continuous monitoring of health status requires increased health care dollars.

The clinical area for nursing experience of students will be more prominent in the community with the hospital designated as the setting for the more experienced student who is able to cope with and learn in a highly technical, stressful environment. The shift to more use of practice fields in the community will raise questions as to the appropriateness of the present preparation of faculty, costs entailed in using the fields which are less geographically circumscribed, and the identification of the knowledge and skills essential for a professional practitioner.

Change in the future relates to where students will have their practice experience and the knowledge and competencies they will need to practice in the future. Constancy in the future rests with the intent of the preparation—to provide humanistic nursing care to clients in order to facilitate optimum health. For the educators, the source of constancy remains in the purposes for the use of the clinical field in preparation of tomorrow's nurses; learning how to learn, dealing with ambiguity, thinking like professionals, and developing personal causation. Both constancy and change are in the future of nursing education.

The past is recollected in the present. The future is anticipated in the present. In a sense, the "past" is gone; the "future" never comes. Now is the time to move with the future.

REFERENCES

American Academy of Nursing. (1983). *Magnet hospitals: Attractions and retention of professional nurses.* Kansas City, MO: American Academy of Nursing.

Aydelotte, M. et al. (1987). *The nursing center: Concept and design.* Kansas City: American Nurses Association.

Barber, S. (1991). The nursing center: A model for rural practice. *Nursing & Health Care, 12*(6), 295-296.

Barnum, B. (1989). Nursing's image and the future. *Nursing & Health Care, 10*(1), 19-21.

Barrett, W. (1978). *The illusion of technique.* New York: Anchor Press/Doubleday & Co.

Blum, B. (Ed.). (1986). *Clinical information systems.* New York: Springer-Verlag.

Bolles, P. (1983). Life/work planning: Change and consistency in the world of work. *The Futurist, 12*(60), 7-11.

Brown, P. (1991). Computers in nursing. In M. Oermann, *Professional nursing practice: A conceptual approach* (pp. 197-215). Philadelphia: J. B. Lippincott.

Bull, M. (1988). Influence of diagnosis-related groups on discharge planning, professional practice, and patient care. *Journal of Professional Nursing, 4*(6), 415-421.

Burest, B., Gordon, S., & Bell, N. (1991). Who counts in news coverage of health care? *Nursing Outlook, 39*(5), 204-208.

Califano, J. (1986). *America's health revolution: Who lives? Who dies? Who pays?* New York: Random House.

Castro, J. (1991). Condition: Critical. *Time Magazine,* (21), 34-38, 39-40, 42.

Curtin, L. L. (1984). Prospective payment: Winners and losers. In American Academy of Nursing, *Nursing research and policy formation: The case of prospective payment.* Kansas City, MO: American Nurses Association.

De Santis, L. (1988). The relevance of transcultural to international nursing. *International Nursing Review, 35,* 107-108.

Donley, Sr. R. (1984). Nursing: 2,000, an essay. *Image: Journal of Nursing Scholarship, 16*(1), 4-6.

Drew, J. (1990). Health maintenance organization: History, evolution. *Nursing & Health Care, 11*(3), 145-149.

Evans, B. (Ed.). (1978). *Dictionary of quotations,* p. 262. New York: Avenel Books.

Freidson, E. (1971). *The profession of medicine: A study of the sociology of applied knowledge.* New York: Dodd, Mead.

Fries, J. (1986). The future of disease and treatment: Changing health conditions, changing behaviors, and new medical technology. *Journal of Professional Nursing, 2*(1), 10-19.

Freudenheim, M. (1988, Nov. 19). U.S. health care spending continues sharp rise. *The New York Times.*

Gosnell, D. (1985). The international implications of nursing education and practice. *International Nursing Review, 32,* 108.

Grace, H. (1990). Can health care costs be contained? *Nursing & Health Care, 11*(3), 124-131.

Graves, J., & Corcoran, S. (1989). The study of nursing informatics. *Image: Journal of Nursing Scholarship, 21*(4), 227-231.

Gross, M. (1988). The potential of information systems in nursing. *Nursing & Health Care, 9*(9), 477-479.

Haddon, R. (1990). An economic agenda for health care. *Nursing & Health Care, 11*(1), 21-26.

Halloran, E. (1988). Computerized nurse assessments. *Nursing & Health Care, 9*(9), 497-499.

Harriman, R. (1984). Creativity: Moving beyond creativity. *The Futurist, 18*(4), 17-20.
Harrington, C. (1990). Policy options for a national health care plan. *Nursing Outlook, 38*(5), 223-238.
Jacox, A. J. (1982). Role restructuring in hospital nursing. In L. H. Aiken (Ed.), *Nursing in the 1980s: Crises, opportunities, challenges*. Philadelphia: J. B. Lippincott.
Kerr, P. (1991, Nov. 24). Mental health chains accused of much cheating. *The New York Times*.
Loye, D. (1984). The forecasting brain: How we see the future. *The Futurist, 18*(1), 63-68.
Lynaugh, J., & Fagin, C. (1988). Nursing comes of age. *Image: Journal of Nursing Scholarship, 20*(4), 184-190.
Maglacas, A. (1989). Close encounters in international nursing: Impact on health policy and research. *Journal of Professional Nursing, 5*(6), 304-314.
Mahdi, E. (1989). Learning needs in a changing world. *The Futurist, 21*, 60.
Maraldo, P. (1990). The nineties: A decade in search of meaning. *Nursing & Health Care, 11*(1), 10-15.
Maraldo, P., & Solomon, S. (1987). Nursing's window of opportunity. *Image: Journal of Nursing Scholarship, 19*(2), 83-86.
Mason, D., Backer, B., & George, C. (1991). Toward a feminist model for the political empowerment of nurses. *Image: Journal of Nursing Scholarship, 13*(2), 72-77.
McClure, M. L., & Nelson, M. J. (1982). Trends in hospital nursing. In L. H. Aiken (Ed.), *Nursing in the 1980s: Crises, opportunities, challenges*. Philadelphia: J. B. Lippincott.
McInnes, N. (1984). Networking: A way to manage our changing world? *The Futurist, 18*(3), 9-10.
Millholland, K. (1988). Patient data management systems. *Computers in Nursing, 6*(6), 237-241.
Milo, N. (1989). Developing nursing leadership in health policy. *Journal of Professional Nursing, 5*(6), 315-321.
Naisbitt, J. (1982). *Megatrends*. New York: Warner Books.
National League for Nursing. (1991). *Nursing's agenda for health care*. New York: National League for Nursing.
Oermann, M. (1991). *Professional nursing practice: A conceptual approach*. Philadelphia: J. B. Lippincott.
Perspectives. (1987, May 11). Medicine and health, 3.
Phillips, E., Fisher, M., MacMillan-Scattergood, D., & Baglioni, A. (1989). DRG ripple and the shifting burden of care to home health. *Nursing & Health Care, 10*(6), 325-327.

Plomann, M., & Shaffer, F. (1983). DRGs as one of nine approaches to case-mix in transition. *Nursing & Health Care, 4*(8), 438-443.

Reilly, D. (1990a). *Graduate professional education through outreach: A nursing case study.* New York: National League for Nursing.

Reilly, D. (1990b). Research in nursing education: Yesterday-today-tomorrow. *Nursing & Health Care, 11*(1), 138-144.

Robert Wood Johnson Foundation. (1991). Hospital cost control through utilization review. *Advance Newsletter, 4*(3). Princeton, NJ: Robert Wood Johnson Foundation.

Romano, C. (1984). A computerized multidisciplinary discharge care planning model: NIH model. *Computer Technology, 2nd National Conference.* Monograph of National Institute of Health.

Rosenow, A. (1983). Professional nursing practice in the bureaucratic hospital revisited. *Nursing Outlook, 31*(1), 34-39.

Saba, V. (1988). Taming the computer jungle of nursing systems. *Nursing & Health Care, 9*(9), 487-491.

Schraff, S. (1984). As quoted in nursing in transition: Four perspectives. *Nursing & Health Care, 5,* 312-316.

Walker, D. (1984). As quoted in nursing service in transition: Four perspectives. *Nursing & Health Care, 5,* 312-316.

Warner, S. (1988). Third party payments for nurses: Untangling the web. *Nursing & Health Care, 9*(4), 181-185.

Weisfield, N., & Amor, G. (1991). Toward a national policy for nursing. *Nursing Outlook, 39*(2), 73-76.

Werley, H. (1985). School hosts international conference to develop nursing minimum data sets. *Input/Output, 1*(3), 1-4.

Wickizer, T., Wheeler, J., & Feldstein, P. (1991). Have hospital cost containment programs contributed to the growth in outpatient expenditures? *Medical Care, 29*(5), 442-451.

Zwolski, K. (1989). Professional nursing in a technical system. *Image: Journal of Nursing Scholarship, 21*(4), 238-242.

BIBLIOGRAPHY

Aaronson, L. (1989). A challenge for nursing: Reviewing a historic competition. *Nursing Outlook, 37*(6), 274-279.

Aiken, L. (1982). *Nursing in the 1980s: Crises, opportunities, challenges.* Philadelphia: J. B. Lippincott.

Aiken, L. (1989). The hospital nursing shortage: A paradox of increasing supply and increasing vacancy rates. *Western Journal of Medicine, 151,* 87-92.

Aiken, L. (1990). Charting the future of hospital nursing. *Image: Journal of Nursing Scholarship, 22*(2), 72-78.

Bailey, D. (1988). Computer application in nursing. *Computer in Nursing, 6*(5), 199-203.

Ball, M., Hannah, K., Gordon-Jelger, U. & Peterson, H. (Eds.). (1988). *Computers in health care: Nursing informatics. Where caring and technology meet.* New York: Springer-Verlag.

Barger, S., & Bridges, W. (1990). An assessment of academic nursing centers. *Nurse Educator, 15*(2), 31-36.

Barker, A. (1991). An emerging leadership pattern: Transformational leadership. *Nursing & Health Care, 12*(4), 204-207.

Blair, E., & O'Brien, R. (1990). Deliberations on nursing practice. *Nursing & Health Care, 11*(10), 514-517.

Carter, M. (1989). The beat goes on. *Journal of Professional Nursing, 5*(6), 299.

Carolyn Davis speaks out. (1988). *Nursing & Health Care, 9*(7), 355-359.

Chibuye, P. (1989). Nursing in action: Nurses influence in research and health policy development. *Journal of Professional Nursing, 5*(6), 326-329.

Chinn, P. (Ed.). (1991). *Health Policy: Who Cares?* Kansas City, MO: American Academy of Nursing.

Cohen, S. (1990). The politics of medicaid, 1980-1989. *Nursing Outlook, 38*(5), 229-253.

Donley, Sr. R., & Flaherty, Sr. M. (1989). Analysis of the market-driven nursing shortage. *Nursing & Health Care, 10*(4), 182-187.

Fagin, C. (1986). Opening the door in nursing's cost advantage. *Nursing & Health Care, 7,* 356-358.

Goertzen, I. E. (Ed.). (1991). *Differentiating nursing practice: Into the twenty-first century.* Kansas City, MO: American Academy of Nursing.

Grayson, C. (1984). Networking by computer. *The Futurist, 18*(3), 14-17.

Griffith, H. (1987). Direct 3rd party reimbursement for nursing services: A review of legislation and implementation. *Nursing Administration Quarterly, 12*(1), 19-23.

Haddon, R. (1989). Tri-care: A new concept in health care. *Nursing & Health Care, 10*(4), 196-201.

Harrington, C. (1990). Policy options for a national health care plan. *Nursing Outlook, 38*(5), 223-228.

Harrington, C., & Culbertson, R. (1990). Nursing left out of health care reimbursement reform. *Nursing Outlook, 38*(4), 156-158.

Hassanein, S. (1991). On the shortage of registered nurses: An economic analysis of the RN market. *Nursing & Health Care, 12*(3), 152-156.

Heller, B., & Romano, C. (1988). Nursing informatics: The pathway to knowledge. *Nursing & Health Care, 9*(9), 483-484.

Hawken, P., & Hillestad, A. (1990). Promoting nursing's health care agenda through collaboration. *Nursing & Health Care, 11*(1), 17-19.

Kaler, S., Levy, D., & Schall, M. (1989). Stereotypes of professional roles. *Image: Journal of Nursing Scholarship, 21*(2), 85-89.

Kent, V., & Hanley, B. (1990). Home health care: Policy evolution, cost effectiveness, and trends. *Nursing & Health Care, 11*(5), 234-241.

Krugman, M. (1990). Nurse executive role socialization. *Nursing & Health Care, 11*(1), 526-531.

Kippenbrock, T. (1991). I wish I'd been there: A sense of nursing history. *Nursing & Health Care, 12*(4), 208-212.

Lindquist, G. (1990). Integration of international and transcultural content in nursing curricula; A process for change. *Journal of Professional Nursing, 6*(5), 272-279.

McCarron, L. (1991). Equal access to health care: Ethical issues in determining public policy. *Journal of Professional Nursing, 7*(2), 10.

McCormick, K. (1991). Future data needs for quality of care monitoring DRG considerations, reimbursement, outcome and measurement. *Image: Journal of Professional Nursing, 23*(1), 29-38.

Mc Kay, S. (1989). Nursing education in nuclear age. *Journal of Professional Nursing, 5*(3), 152-158.

Mc Kinney, P. (1989). Can patient care terminals ease the threat? *Computers in Nursing, 9*(4), 348-351.

Mitchell, C. (1988). One view of the future: Non-traditional education as the norm. *Nursing & Health Care, 9*(4), 187-190.

Mitchell, P., Kruger, J., & Moody, I. (1990). The crisis of the health care non-system. *Nursing Outlook, 38*(5), 214-217.

Newman, M., Lamb, G., & Michaels, C. (1991). Nurse case management: The coming together of theory and practice. *Nursing Outlook, 12*(8), 404-409.

Moccia, P. (1989). Shaping a human agenda for the nineties. Trends that demand our attention as managed care prevails. *Nursing & Health Care, 10*(1), 14-17.

Nursing and Nursing Education: Public policies and private actions. (1983). Washington, DC: Institute of Medicine.

Nursing research and policy formation: The case for prospective payment. (1984). Monograph of the American Academy of Nursing. Kansas City, MO: American Academy of Nursing.

Polk-Walker, G. (1989). Aerospace nursing. *Journal of Professional Nursing, 5*(4), 224-230.

Rantz, M. (1990). Inadequate reimbursement for long term care: The impact since hospital DRG. *Nursing & Health Care, 11*(9), 470-473.

Raudonis, B., & Griffith, H. (1991). Model for integrating health services research and health care policy formation. *Nursing & Health Care, 12*(1), 32-36.

Robert, S. (1983). Oppressed behavior: Implications for nursing. *Advances in Nursing Science, 5*(1), 21-22.

Saba, V., & McCormick, K. (Eds.). (1986). *Essentials of computers for nursing.* Philadelphia: J. B. Lippincott.

Schramm, C., & Gabel, J. (1988). Prospective payment: Some therapeutic observations. *New England Journal of Medicine, 318*(25), 1682.

Sinclair, V. (1988). Data base management: Solving information overload. *Nursing & Health Care, 9*(9), 493-495.

Sharp, N., Biggs, S., & Wakefield, M. (1991). Public policy: New opportunities for nurses. *Nursing & Health Care, 12*(1), 16-18.

Stark, P. (1991). Health care under siege: Challenge for change. *Nursing & Health Care, 12*(1), 26-31.

Stimpson, M., & Hanley, B. (1991). Nurse policy analyst: Advanced practice role. *Nursing & Health Care, 12*(1), 10-15.

The impact of changing resources on health policy. (1981). Monograph, American Academy of Nursing. Kansas City, MO: American Academy of Nursing.

Toffler, A. (1980). *The third wave.* New York: Bantam Books.

Trice, L. (1990). Meaningful life experiences to the elderly. *Image: Journal of Nursing Scholarship, 22*(4), 248-251.

Werley, H. (1987). The nursing minimum data set. In K. Hannah & N. Reimer (Eds.), *Clinical judgment and decision making; The future with nursing diagnosis* (pp. 540-555). New York: John Wiley and Sons.

Werley, H., Devine, E., & Zorn, C. (1989). Nursing needs its own minimum data set. *American Journal of Nursing, 88*(12), 1651-1653.

Wheeler, C., & Chinn, P. (1989). *Peace and power: A handbook of feminist process* (2nd ed.). New York: National League for Nursing.

Zerwekh, J. (1991). At the expense of their soul. *Nursing Outlook, 39*(2), 58-61.

Index

Ability, 36, 249
Accountability:
  faculty and, 282-284
  significance of, 12-13
Affective domain:
  attitudes, 301-302, 332
  behavior and, 291
  beliefs, 299-300, 332
  care phenomenon and, 297-299
  choice making, 306-307
  clinical setting and, 320-321
  community influence on, 294-295
  conflict, 296. See also Conflict
  ethics, 305, 332
  evaluation and, 386-387
  goals, 331-332
  morality, 305-306, 332
  moral reasoning, 302-305, 319, 332
  need for, 293
  objectives preparation, 321-325
  political influence on, 295
  skills development, 299-307
  society and, 293-296
  taxonomy of, 321-322
  teaching-learning process and, 292
  teaching approaches, 313-320
  teaching methods regarding, 326-331
  values, 300-302, 312-318, 332
Age increase, clients, 473-474
Agency personnel, relationships with, 120-123. See also Clinical setting
Alavi, C., 274-275

Ambiguity, management of, 7-8, 19, 485
Ambulatory care facilities, future of, 479, 488
American Academy of Nursing, 461
American Nurses Association:
  Nursing, A Social Policy Statement, 76-77, 316-317, 332
  Standards of Nursing Care, 78, 315-316, 332
  studies by, 316-317, 322, 469
Analysis, as teaching tool, 326
Anecdotal notes, as evaluation tool, 390-392
Argyris, C., 4, 9, 13, 15, 484
Articulation level, psychomotor skill development, 270-272, 278
Aspy, D. N., 147-148
Assessment of learner in instructional process, see Learner, assessment of
Assessment of learner needs, 150, 152-154
Assessment process:
  data gathering/analysis, 61-63
  defined, 59
  diagnosis, see Diagnosis
  operations of, 61
  patterning, 69, 70
  problem recognition, 61-62
  theory frameworks, 79, 94-95
Associate/diploma programs, 12, 274
Attitudes, defined, 301-302
Augmented feedback, 266-267

Baccalaureate degree programs, 12
Baldwin, D., 187, 263
Barber, S., 475-476

497

Barger, S. E., 111-112
Barnum, B., 58, 463
Bayesian decision model, 224
Behaviorist theory of learning, 25
Beliefs, defined, 299-300
Bell, N., 470-471
Benner, P., 3, 5, 15, 33, 215, 225-226, 297-298
Bergman, K., 140, 142-143, 145, 150, 381, 383
Biases of health care workers, 308-310
Bill of Rights, Constitution, 313
Bill of Rights for Patients, 314
Bloom, B. S., 41, 43-44, 50, 153, 234, 428
Bolles, P., 452, 484
Bondy, K. N., 393-394
Bower, D., 390, 393
Bower, F., 72, 74
Boyer, E. L., 141, 145
Brown, I. D., 267-268
Brown, P., 60, 168, 403, 455
Bruner, J. S., 32-34, 44, 50, 96, 98, 209, 219
Burest, B., 470-471

Caring component:
   development of, 3
   design for, *see* Planning operation
   phenomenon of, 297-299
   process of, 78
   significance of, 48
Carnegie Commission on Higher Education, 308-309
Carnevali, D., 55, 72, 223
Carpenito, L., 55, 63, 86
Carroll-Johnson, R., 64
Case study:
   cognitive skills development and, 239
   as evaluation tool, 399-400, 417
   as teaching tool, 169, 211
Characteristics of different cognitive styles, *see* Cognitive styles
Characterization level, affective domain, 324
Chickering, A. W., 27
Choice making, development of, 306-307
Chronic pain management model:
   evaluation protocol for, 412-416
   grading system for, 438-440
   objectives classification and unit for, 349-352, 357-377
Churchill, L., 305, 326, 331

Clayton, G. M., 44, 143, 197
Clinical agencies, *see* Clinical settings
Clinical assignment:
   cognitive skills development and, 238-239
   as teaching tool, 165-167, 327
Clinical conferences:
   as evaluation tool, 405-406, 417
   as teaching method, 181-183
Clinical experience, 115-117, 149-151
   grading of, *see* Grading
   historical, 15-16
   nature of, 60-61
   objectives of, *see* Clinical objectives
   planning for, 353-355
   program objectives, 344-345
   purposes of, 5, 58-60, 484-487
Clinical evaluation, *see* Evaluation, clinical
Clinical evaluation methods, *see* Evaluation, clinical, methods of
Clinical judgment process:
   development of, 240
   teaching of, 232-233
   theories of:
      decision theory, 224-225
      information processing theory, 222-224
      phenomenologic theory, 225-227
Clinical objectives, 152, 156, 348-356, 384-388
Clinical performance grading systems:
   course objectives and, 437-444, 447
   criteria, 437
   evaluation strategies and, 444-446
   fairness, 436, 447
   See also Grading systems
Clinical practice:
   historical perspective, 15-19
   holistic approach to, 95-100
   professional practice, 1-3
   purposes of, 5-10
   theories of, 3-5
Clinical setting:
   benefits of, 115-117
   community as, 478-481
   contract with, 124-125
   evaluation of, 132-133, 154-156
   faculty responsibilities, 117-120
   future changes in, 477-484
   hospital as, 481
   instructional process, 151-152, 154, 156

learning experience selection, 149-151
nature of, 113-115
objectives, 152, 156, 348-356, 384-388
purposes of, 113
relations with agency, 120-123
selection of:
  assessment instrument, 128-131
  clients, 127
  criteria, 126-128
  importance of, 123, 134
  instrument for, 128-131
setting and faculty, 126-127
staff, 127
student/faculty resources, 128
types of, 110-113
Code for Nurses, 314-315, 332
Cognitive development, 219-221
Cognitive domain:
  evaluation and, 386
  psychomotor skill development and, see Psychomotor skill taxonomy of, 233-237
  skills development, 98-100
  taxonomy of, 235-236
  teaching framework and, 227-237, 241
  teaching methods, 237-240
  theories regarding, 219-221
Cognitive field theory, 29-31
Cognitive skills, 207-227
  teaching of, 228-240
Cognitive style:
  field-dependent, 36-38, 42, 48, 118
  field-independent, 36-38, 48, 118
  recognition of, 48-49
  types of, 35-38
Collaboration, see Diagnosis, collaborative
Communication skills:
  significance of, 76
  verbal expression examination, 329-330
Competency:
  faculty and, 141-142, 156
  five levels of, 225-226
Compression of Morbidity, 473-474
Computation of clinical grades, see Grading
Computer-assisted instruction:
  cognitive skills development and, 239
  psychomotor skills development, 283
  purpose of, 190-191, 211
  See also Simulation

Computer technology:
  instruction and, see Computer-assisted instruction
  introduction of, 60, 403, 454-456
  patient privacy issue and, 296
  systems, see Nursing information systems (NIS)
Computerized Medical Information System (MIS), development of, 481
Concept-Based Learning Activity (CBLA), 211
Concept learning:
  attainment, 210-211
  defined, 208-210
  role of, 208-210, 240
  teaching and, 227-228
Concepts, see Concept learning
Conference(s):
  as evaluation tool, 407, 417
  peer review and, 102
  as teaching tool, 181-183, 201, 238, 327, 332-333, 405-407
  See also specific types of conferences
Conflict:
  consequence of, 296
  response to, 332
  sources of, 308-312
Confrontation, as teaching tool, 326-327
Contract(s):
  with clinical agency, 123-125
  learning, 192-195
Convergent thinking, defined, 33
Cooper, S. S., 180, 185-186
Cooperative education/work study programs, 199-200
Cost containment, effect on nursing education, 488
Cost of nursing care, 478-488. *See also* Health care costs
  technology's effect on, 457-458
Crick, M., 39-40
Critical thinking:
  cognitive development, 219-221
  development of, 217-221
  teaching of, 231-232
Cross, K. P., 145, 320
Culture, 39-40, 50
Curriculum:
  components of, 342-348
  course model, 355-377

Curriculum (Continued)
  courses, 346, 348
  definitions of, 342
  expansion of, 3
  nursing conceptual framework and, 342–343
  objectives, 348–349, 353, 356
  planning of clinical components, 353–356
  program objectives and, 344–345
  purpose of, 344
  school philosophy, 343
  student level and, 345–347
  themes of, 3

Davis, A. J., 300, 302, 319
de Tornyay, R., 187, 191
Decision-making:
  decentralization of, 461
  development of, 240–241
  intuition and, 33
  models of, 224
  process of, 215–217
  student knowledge level and, 230–231
Demonstration, as teaching tool, 186–187
Dewey, J., 28, 35, 50, 295
Diagnosis:
  classification systems, 64–69, 210
  clinical judgment and, 64, 226–227
  collaborative, 71, 121
  definitions, 63–64
  issues, 70–72
  labeling, see Labeling
  taxonomy, 71
  validation of, 66
Diary/learning log, as teaching tool, 169
Diekelmann, N., 47, 143, 145
Divergent thinking:
  cognitive field theory and, 50
  defined, 33
Donaldson, S., 1, 333
Donley, Sr. R., 456, 458, 460, 463, 477
DRG system, 455, 467–468
Dualism, 219, 221
Dubos, R., 26, 306–307

Early discharge from hospital, 472
  impact on community health agencies, 472–477
Eble, K. E., 44, 46, 142, 144

Education, future perspective, 451–489
Elstein, A. S., 222–224
Erickson, S. C., 429–430, 434
Ethics:
  decision-making and, see Ethical decision making
  defined, 305
  See also Affective domain; Moral reasoning; Values
Ethical decision making, see Affective domain; Ethics
Evaluation, clinical:
  affective domain and, 386–387
  anecdotal notes, 390–392
  clinical objectives and, 384–388
  cognitive domain and, 386
  concepts of, 380–385
  conferences, 405–408
  criterion-referenced, 382
  critical incidents and, 392
  defined, 379–380
  fairness, 383–385
  formative, 101, 154–156, 380–382, 390, 416, 427
  methods of, 411
  model of, 412–416
  multidomain performance, 388
  multistrategy approach to, 411–412, 417
  norm-referenced, 382
  nursing process and, 78
  objectives, relationship to, 385–388
  observation and, 389–390
  oral communication, 405–407
  process of, 383–388
  psychomotor domain and, 387–388
  psychosocial climate and, 384–385
  purposes, 380
  rating scales, 393–395
  self-evaluation, 410–411
  significance of, 79
  simulations and, 408–410, 417
  summative, 79, 155–156, 381, 410, 416, 421, 427
  types of, 382
  videotape and, 395–396
  written communication methods, 396–404, 417
    case study, 399–400
    nursing care plan, 396–399

nursing notes, 403-405
process recording, 401-402
teaching plan, 400-401
See also Grading
Evaluation of clinical setting, *see* Clinical setting, evaluation
Evaluation of nursing students, *see* Evaluation, clinical
Experiential learning:
affective skills and, 320
basis of, 165
case study, 169
clinical assignment and, 165-167
clinical experience value, 50
experiential diary, 170
games, 174
learning and experience, 27-29
learning log, 170
nursing care plans, 168-169
process recording, 169-171
purpose of, 165, 200
role play, 174
significance of, 48
simulation and, 172-176
teaching plan, 169
written assignments, 167-168
Externship programs, 199

Faculty, *see* Teachers
Fawcett, J., 11, 13, 94
Feedback, 146, 154, 266, 380-381, 384
Field dependent, *see* Cognitive style
Field independent, *see* Cognitive style
Field trips, as teaching tool, 184-185
Fine motor skills, *see* Psychomotor skills
Fleishman, E. A., 257, 260, 269
Formative evaluation, *see* Evaluation, clinical
Fries, J., 473-474
Frisch, N. A., 221, 304
Fry, S., 3, 11, 297

Gadow, S., 297, 328
Games, as teaching tools, 169. *See also* Simulation
Gardner, J. W., 311-312
Gilligan, C., 304, 319
Goodnow, J. J., 98, 209
Gordon, M., 62-63, 65, 69, 70, 75, 94, 223
Grace, H., 465-466

Grading:
clinical performance, 119, 434-436. *See also* Clinical performance grading systems
computation methods, 427-429, 437-446
criterion-referenced, 428
data base variation, 426-427
faculty attitude toward, 423
goal-free learning, 446
meaning of, 421-424, 447
normal curve, 428
norm-referenced, 428
reliability of, 445
self-referenced, 428
standards of, 427
student attitude toward, 423-424
student learning and, 424-425
system types, 431-434
use for, 429-431
Grading systems:
five-dimensional, 431-432
two-dimensional, 431-432, 435
Graduate degree programs, 12
Graves, J., 455-456
Gross, M., 455-456

Hall, E., 39, 50, 57
Handling ambiguity, *see* Ambiguity, management of
Hands-on care, as teaching tool, 328-329
Hanna, D. R., 172, 174
Harrington, C., 112, 465
Health care costs:
community responsibilities and, 472-477
crisis issues, 463-466
future direction of, 464-465, 487-489
group practice models, 475
nursing role, future, 469-472
prospective payment system, 466-468
review cost control program, 468-469
technological advances and, 457-458
Health care maintenance organization (HMO), 475
Hedin, B. A., 144, 384
Hegyvary, S. T., 122, 147
Henderson, V., 59, 65
Hergenhahn, B., 27, 31
Higgs, Z. R., 37, 111-112
History of nursing education, 56-57

Hi-Tech/Hi-Touch care, training in, 274, 459-460, 481
Holistic theory approach, 26-27, 32, 58, 95-100
Home care, future directions of, 112, 479-480, 488
Hospital, as practice field, 481
Human science theory, 24-27
Hursh, B., 8, 220
Hypothesis generation skills, 223, 233

Imitation level, psychomotor skill development, 270-271
Implementation:
  defined, 77
  as phase of nursing process, 77
Incident process, critical, 180-181, 392
Independent study, see Self-directed teaching methods, independent study
Infante, M. S., 151
Information processing model of clinical judgment, see Clinical judgment
Instructional process, 151-155. See also Teaching; Teaching methods
Interactions of teacher and student, see Teacher-student relationships
Interactive video (IAV), as teaching tool, 173, 189-191
Internship programs, 200
Intervention strategies, selection of, 74-76
Intuition:
  process of, 214-215
  study of use of, 33
  See also Problem-solving
Issue conference, 183
  as evaluation tool, 407, 417
Itano, J. K., 222-223, 227

Jacox, A. J., 460, 462
Johnson, C., 409-410

Karns, P., 148, 393-394
Keele, S., 252, 254, 258
Kerr, R., 249, 251
Ketefian, S., 305, 319
Kintgen-Andrews, J., 212, 231
Kleehammer, K., 148, 385
Knowing-in-action, 48
Knowledge, definitions of, 207-208

Knowledge deficit, 71
Knox, J. E., 141, 143, 145
Kohlberg, L., 302-303, 319

Labeling, consequences of, 86, 329-330
Law of Pragnaz, 30
Lawther, J. D., 258-259, 266
Learner:
  assessment of, 153-154, 156
  feedback and, 154-155
  field-dependent, see Cognitive style
  field-independent, see Cognitive style
  knowledge of, 41-42, 163, 345-347
  See also Student, knowledge about
Learning:
  cognitive styles, see Cognitive styles
  concept of, 24-40
  cultural determinants, 39-40, 50
  dynamics of, 47, 50
  environment and, see Learning environment
  experience and, 27-29
  experiences, 149-151, 342
  holistic approach to, 26-27, 32
  human science theory, 24-27
  information processing, 35
  insightful, 31-32
  knowledge and, 34-35
  perception and, 29-32
  process of, 24-29, 46-47, 485
  relationship to teaching, 40-47
  theories of, 6-7, 19
  thinking and, 32-34
  transfer of, 34, 260-261
Learning environment:
  development of, 117
  faculty and, 117-120, 148-149
  significance of, 45-46, 50, 109, 155
  See also Clinical setting
Learning contracts, see Self-directed teaching methods
Learning experiences:
  activities, 353-355
  selection of, 149-151
Learning log, as evaluation tool, 402-403, 417
Learning Resources Laboratory, 262-263
Legal issues, 119-120
Leininger, M., 3, 297, 311
Lens decision model, 224-225

Lessner, M. W., 119-120
Leveling of objectives in nursing curriculum, 345-346
Lowman, J., 139, 144
Lynaugh, J., 463, 469, 471

Mahdi, E., 6, 33, 483
Manipulation level, psychomotor skill development, 270-271
Manual skills, *see* Psychomotor skills
Maraldo, P., 460-461, 463-464, 469, 476
Marriner, A., 55, 72
Mastery, defined, 273
Mastery of learning theory, 43, 50, 273, 282, 427
Matthews, R., 189, 396, 409
Mead, M., 39, 50
Media, *see* Multimedia
Meleis, A. I., 13, 34
Meyers, C., 32-34, 44, 166, 217-218, 231, 239
Miller, M. A., 166, 218, 232
Miller, V. G., 214-215
Milo, N., 474, 476
Milton, O., 43, 422-425, 428-430, 433
Mistakes, acceptance of, 118
Mitchell, C., 71-72
Modeling, as teaching tool, 330-331
Models, simulation, 173-174
Module, *see* Self-directed teaching, self-paced module
Moral reasoning, development of, 302-305, 319
Morality, defined, 305-306
Morrill, L. S., 111, 300, 304-305, 318-319
Multimedia:
  in evaluation, 409
  role as teaching tool, 187-191
Multiplicity, 219
Myrick, F., 197-198

Naisbitt, J., 453-454, 458, 462
National League for Nursing:
  Council of Research in Nursing Education, The, 483
  Nursing Agenda for Health Care Reform, 470
Naturalization level, psychomotor skill development, 270-272, 277-278
Nehring, V., 141-143, 145
Networking, need for, 461-463

Nightingale, Florence, 15-16, 56
Nonprint media, 187
Norris, C., 298-299
North American Nursing Diagnosis Association (NANDA):
  collaborative diagnosis, 71
  diagnostic categories, 64, 66, 69, 71
Northouse, L. L., 121
Nurse-patient process recording, *see* Process recording, as evaluation tool
Nursing:
  defined, 55-56
  goals of, 76
  philosophy of, 343
  roles and responsibilities, 458-463
Nursing & Health Care, 478
Nursing Agenda for Health Care Reform, 470
Nursing care plan:
  computerization of, 398-399
  difficulties of, 398
  effectiveness of, 398, 417
  as evaluation tool, 396-399
  format of, 396-399
  purpose of, 168, 239
  significance of, 101-102
Nursing centers, 111-112, 476
Nursing education:
  future of clinical setting, 477-489
  history of, 56-57
Nursing ethics, theory development, 297-298. *See also* Ethics
Nursing frameworks, *see* Nursing theories
Nursing Information System (NIS):
  documentation and, 403-404
  introduction of, 60
  uses of, 455-456
Nursing models, *see* Nursing theories
Nursing/multidisciplinary conferences, as evaluation tool, 407-408
Nursing notes:
  computers and, 403-404
  evaluation of, 403
  importance of, 403
Nursing practice:
  future directions of, 451-453, 476-477, 484-487
  role/responsibilities changes, 458-463
  theories of, *see* Practice theories

504 INDEX

Nursing process:
 cognitive skill development, *see* Cognitive skills, development of
 comparison with teaching process, 40-41
 defined, 55-56
 development of, 56-60
 example of, 96-97
 holistic theory and, 58
 issues, 58-60
 nature of, 60-61
 nursing theories, 80-93
 phases of, 59, 61, 103. *See also specific phases*
 problem-solving and, 58-60
 skills in, 98
 teaching of, 95-103
Nursing rounds, as teaching tool, 185-186
Nursing theories, 80-93
Nursing Theories Conference Group, intervention forms, 75

Objectives:
 affective domain, 291, 308, 321-325, 331-332
 clinical, 152, 348-353
 cognitive domain, 99, 234, 241
 curriculum, 344-346, 348-349, 353, 356
 evaluation, relation to objectives, 385-388
 psychomotor domain, 250, 273-275
 teaching, relation to teaching, 162
Observation:
 in clinical setting, 184
 components of, 389
 demonstrations, 186-187
 difficulties of, 389-390
 discussion of, 389
 as evaluation tool, 387-390
 field trips, 184-185
 nursing rounds, 185-186
 purpose of, 183-184, 201
Oermann, M., 3, 41, 44, 56, 102, 110, 112, 139, 145, 155, 170, 179, 183, 186-187, 189, 191, 197-199, 217-218, 222, 234, 274, 322, 344, 381, 383, 389, 391-396, 468
Oral communication evaluation methods, 329-330
Orb, A., 94, 343

Organization level, affective domain, 324-325
O'Shea, H. S., 144, 150
Overlearning/repetition, 259

Patient, concerns of:
 Bill of Rights for Patients, 314
 individualized intervention, 48, 75
Peer review:
 benefits of, 102
 conference, 183
Perceptual style of learners, 257
Performance, defined, 250-251
Perry, W. G., Jr., 34, 50, 219-221, 304, 319
Personal causation, development of, 9-10, 19, 486-487
Phenomenology theory:
 and clinical judgment, 225
 perspectives, 25-26
Planning, nursing process:
 ethical issues, 86-87
 evaluation, 77-79
 goal setting, 73
 implementation of, 77
 intervention strategy selection, 74-77
 priority setting, 73-74
Plunkett, E. J., 173, 239
Poulton, E. C., 254, 268
Practical nursing programs, 12
Practice, *see* Clinical practice
Practice theories:
 action theories, 13-15, 19
 espoused theory, 15
 theory in use, 15
Preceptorship, role of, 196-201
Precision level, psychomotor skill development, 270-271, 277
Print media, 187
Priority setting skills, 73-74
Problem-solving:
 decision-making and, 215-217
 development of, 8-9, 211-212, 240
 individualized patient care and, 48
 intuition and, 214-215
 process of, 212-214
 requirements of, 30
 teaching methods:
  critical incident, 180-181
  decision-making situations, 179-180
  problem-solving situations, 177-179

purpose of, 177, 200-201
  strategies for, 229-233
  teaching principles regarding, 233, 237-240
Process of care, evaluation of, 78
Process recording, as evaluation tool, 401-402, 417
Productive thinking, defined, 32-33
Professional autonomy, significance of, 460-461, 485-486
Program objectives, examples of, 344-345
Psychomotor domain:
  cognitive process and, 267-268
  concepts regarding, 248-251
  curriculum selection, 273-275
  evaluation and, 387-388
  intervention strategies and, 76
  knowledge of patient, 264, 268
  learning transfer factors, 260-261
  practice:
    distribution of, 258
    individual response to, 255-256
    length/frequency of, 257-259
    patterns of, 257
    perceptual variation, 256-257
    setting for, *see* Psychomotor domain, setting for
    significance of, 265
    overlearning/repetition and, 259
    performance criteria, 270-273
    performance grid, 277-282, 284
    process of, 269
    reminiscence and, 259-260
    results and, 266-267
    retention and, 259
  setting for:
    clinical, 263-264, 284
    learning resources laboratory, 262-263, 275-276, 284
  skill classification, 250, 275-276
  skills development, 248-251
  studies regarding, 274-275
  taxonomy of, 269-270, 284
  teaching framework for, 261-262
  teaching methods, 283-284
  testing methods, 277
  theoretical models:
    adaptation, 254-255
    behavioral cybernetic, 252
    information processing, 252-253
    whole *vs.* part approach to, 264-266
Putzier, D. J., 99, 222-223

Quantitative allocation for grading, 426-427. *See also* Grading

Rate of learning, 150
Raths, L. E., 300-301, 318, 322
Rating scales:
  benefits of, 395
  development of, 394
  difficulties of, 393-394
  as evaluation tool, 393-395
  limitations of, 394-395
  parts of, 393
  purpose of, 393
  validity/reliability, 394
Receiving level, affective domain, 322
Reflective thinking:
  cognitive field theory and, 50
  defined, 32
Reilly, D., 17, 44, 56, 79, 94, 102, 139, 155, 170, 179, 183, 217, 218, 234, 269, 274-275, 296, 300-301, 310, 318-319, 322, 325, 343-344, 381, 383, 386, 389, 391-396, 480, 483
Relativism, 219-220
Reminiscence, defined, 259-260
Research of future educational programs, need for, 482-484
Responding level, affective domain, 324
Retention, defined, 259-260
Rogers, C., 32-33, 50, 147-148, 193
Role play, as teaching tool, 174

Saba, V. K., 404, 455
Schein, E. H., 5, 7, 308-309
Schon, D., 2-4, 7, 9, 13, 15, 34, 44-45, 50, 114-116, 166, 213-214, 310, 399, 484
Selection and evaluation of clinical setting, *see* Clinical setting, evaluation and selection
Self-directed teaching methods:
  independent study, 193
  learning contract and, 192-195
  purpose of, 192, 201
  self-paced module, 193, 195-196
Self-evaluation, importance of, 410-411
Shinn, R. L., 326, 331

Shulman, L. S., 222-224
Siegel, H., 217-218
Silberman, C. E., 433-434
Simulation:
  computer, 191, 239
  as evaluation tool, 409, 417
  as teaching tool, 172-176, 211
Simulation games, see Games; Simulation
Singer, R., 249-250, 252-255, 257, 259-260, 265-266
Skills, see Affective domain, skills development; Cognitive domain, skills development; Psychomotor domain, skills development
Social Policy Statement of the American Nurses Association, nursing definition, 11-12
Standards of nursing practice, 315-316
Steele, S. M., 300, 318-319
Stelmach, G. E., 253-254, 258
Student, knowledge of:
  program entry factor, 43
  significance of, 41-42
Summative evaluation, see Evaluation, clinical
Sweeney, M. A., 274, 279

Tanner, C., 99, 110, 168, 222-223, 225, 398
Taxonomy:
  affective domain and, 321-325
  cognitive domain and, 233-237
  psychomotor skill development and, 269-270
Taxonomy I Diagnosis Revised, 66
Teacher(s):
  belief system of, 101
  bias of, 327
  characteristics of effective teacher, 140-145, 146
  clinical competence, 141-142, 156
  concept of evaluation, 383
  interaction with learner, 44, 145-149, 156. See also Teacher-student relationships
  knowledge of, 140-141, 156
  personal characteristics, 144
  preparation of, 482
  qualities of, 140-145
  responsibilities of, 44-45, 117-120, 122, 149
  skills of, 142-143, 163
  students, relationships with, see Teacher-student relationships
Teacher-student relationships:
  caring behaviors, 143, 145, 147
  conferences and, 182
  empathetic understanding, 147
  establishment of, 143-149
  interaction, 156
  studies regarding, 147-148
  trust and, 147
Teaching:
  climate for, 45-46, 50, 109. See also Learning environment
  as diagnostic process, 41-42
  dynamics of, 46-47, 50
  intervention and, 43-44
  learning and, 40-41
  process in clinical, 151-155
  teacher(s) and, see Teacher(s)
Teaching-learning process:
  framework for, 23-24, 40-49
  requirements of, 46
Teaching methods:
  clinical, see specific teaching methods
  selection criteria, 162-164, 201
Teaching plan:
  development of, 102
  as evaluation tool, 400-401, 417
Technological advances, impact of:
  computerization, see Computer technology, introduction to
  hospital care and, 456-458
  instrumentation, 454
Technology, 453-463
Testing, sex bias in, 304. See also Grading
Theories:
  action, 4-5, 13-15, 19
  intervention, 15
  nursing action, 4-5, 13-15
  practice, 13-15, 19
  problem solving, 211-217
Thinking like professionals, 8-9, 485-486
Transcultural nursing, 310-312

Values:
  clarification of, 318, 332
  defined, 300-301

inquiry process, 318-319, 332
  sources of, 312-317
  See also Affective domain
Valuing level, affective domain, 324-325
Van Ort, S. R., 126, 343
Videotape:
  as evaluation tool, 395-396
  as teaching tool, 189, 283

Walker, D., 119-120, 478
Warren, J. R., 422, 429-430, 445-446
Waters, V., 111, 200
Watson, J., 3, 297
Werley, H., 66, 456

Wertheimer, M., 30, 32
White, N. E., 238
Whole learning theory, 264-265, 283
Witkin, H. A., 36, 42
Written assignment:
  cognitive skills development and, 239
  for evaluation, 396-405
  as teaching tool, 167-168

Yinger, R. J., 217-218
Yura, H., 55, 57, 72

Ziegler, S., 55, 71
Zwolski, K., 458-459